Digitization in Dentistry: Clinical Applications

Digitization in Dentistry: Clinical Applications

Editor: Shon Kinder

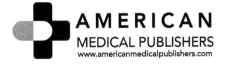

AMERICAN
MEDICAL PUBLISHERS
www.americanmedicalpublishers.com

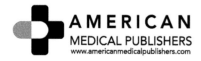

Cataloging-in-Publication Data

Digitization in dentistry : clinical applications / edited by Shon Kinder.
    p. cm.
Includes bibliographical references and index.
ISBN 978-1-63927-660-8
1. Dentistry. 2. Dental informatics. 3. Dentistry--Data processing.
4. Mouth--Diseases--Treatment. I. Kinder, Shon.
RK240 .D54 2023
617.600 285--dc23

American Medical Publishers,
41 Flatbush Avenue,
1st Floor, New York,
NY 11217, USA

ISBN 978-1-63927-660-8 (Hardback)

Contents

Preface..VII

Chapter 1   **3D Printing Approach in Dentistry: The Future for Personalized Oral Soft Tissue Regeneration**...1
Dobrila Nesic, Birgit M. Schaefer, Yue Sun, Nikola Saulacic and Irena Sailer

Chapter 2   **3D Printed Temporary Veneer Restoring Autotransplanted Teeth in Children: Design and Concept Validation Ex Vivo**................................22
Ali Al-Rimawi, Mostafa EzEldeen, Danilo Schneider, Constantinus Politis and Reinhilde Jacobs

Chapter 3   **Dental Restorative Digital Workflow: Digital Smile Design from Aesthetic to Function**...32
Gabriele Cervino, Luca Fiorillo, Alina Vladimirovna Arzukanyan, Gianrico Spagnuolo and Marco Cicciù

Chapter 4   **Accuracy of 3-Dimensionally Printed Full-Arch Dental Models**.........44
Yasaman Etemad-Shahidi, Omel Baneen Qallandar, Jessica Evenden, Frank Alifui-Segbaya and Khaled Elsayed Ahmed

Chapter 5   **Digital Undergraduate Education in Dentistry**...................................62
Nicola U. Zitzmann, Lea Matthisson, Harald Ohla and Tim Joda

Chapter 6   **Impact of Aging on the Accuracy of 3D-Printed Dental Models: An In Vitro Investigation**...85
Tim Joda, Lea Matthisson and Nicola U. Zitzmann

Chapter 7   **Dental Practice Integration into Primary Care: A Microsimulation of Financial Implications for Practices**...92
Sung Eun Choi, Lisa Simon, Jane R. Barrow, Nathan Palmer, Sanjay Basu and Russell S. Phillips

Chapter 8   **Clinical Performance of Partial and Full-Coverage Fixed Dental Restorations Fabricated from Hybrid Polymer and Ceramic CAD/CAM Materials**...105
Nadin Al-Haj Husain, Mutlu Özcan, Pedro Molinero-Mourelle and Tim Joda

Chapter 9   **Recent Trends and Future Direction of Dental Research in the Digital Era**.......131
Tim Joda, Michael M. Bornstein, Ronald E. Jung, Marco Ferrari, Tuomas Waltimo and Nicola U. Zitzmann

Chapter 10   **Efficacy of Plasma-Polymerized Allylamine Coating of Zirconia after Five Years**.......138
Nadja Rohr, Katja Fricke, Claudia Bergemann, J Barbara Nebe and Jens Fischer

Chapter 11   **Big Data and Digitalization in Dentistry: A Systematic Review of the Ethical Issues**..**150**
Maddalena Favaretto, David Shaw, Eva De Clercq, Tim Joda and
Bernice Simone Elger

Chapter 12   **Marginal and Internal Fit of Ceramic Restorations Fabricated Using Digital Scanning and Conventional Impressions**...**165**
Jeong-Hyeon Lee, Keunbada Son and Kyu-Bok Lee

Chapter 13   **Digital Oral Medicine for the Elderly**..**176**
Christian E. Besimo, Nicola U. Zitzmann and Tim Joda

Chapter 14   **Influence of Preparation Design, Marginal Gingiva Location and Tooth Morphology on the Accuracy of Digital Impressions for Full-Crown Restorations: An In Vitro Investigation**...**181**
Selina A. Bernauer, Johannes Müller, Nicola U. Zitzmann and Tim Joda

Chapter 15   **Current Applications, Opportunities and Limitations of AI for 3D Imaging in Dental Research and Practice**...**189**
Kuofeng Hung, Andy Wai Kan Yeung, Ray Tanaka and Michael M. Bornstein

Chapter 16   **Dental Caries Diagnosis and Detection Using Neural Networks**...........................**207**
María Prados-Privado, Javier García Villalón, Carlos Hugo Martínez-Martínez,
Carlos Ivorra and Juan Carlos Prados-Frutos

Permissions

List of Contributors

Index

Preface

This book was inspired by the evolution of our times; to answer the curiosity of inquisitive minds. Many developments have occurred across the globe in the recent past which has transformed the progress in the field.

Digital dentistry denotes utilization of dental devices or technologies, which incorporate computerized or digitally controlled components for carrying out various dental procedures, in place of using electrical or mechanical tools. It is helpful in performing dental procedures in an efficient manner, as compared to mechanical tools, for both diagnostic and restorative purposes. Digital technologies that are used in dentistry involve CAD/CAM, intraoral cameras, 3D printing, digital radiography, dental lasers, digital X-rays, etc. The image acquiring devices such as computer tomography, and intra and extra oral scanners are used to convert patient tissue shapes into 3D data. This data is further edited by making use of CAD software. Limitations of digitalization in the dental industry involve misunderstanding of the novel technologies, lack of motivation to adapt emerging technologies and cost. This book is a valuable compilation of topics, ranging from the basic to the most complex clinical applications of digitization in dentistry. It is appropriate for those seeking detailed information in this area.

This book was developed from a mere concept to drafts to chapters and finally compiled together as a complete text to benefit the readers across all nations. To ensure the quality of the content we instilled two significant steps in our procedure. The first was to appoint an editorial team that would verify the data and statistics provided in the book and also select the most appropriate and valuable contributions from the plentiful contributions we received from authors worldwide. The next step was to appoint an expert of the topic as the Editor-in-Chief, who would head the project and finally make the necessary amendments and modifications to make the text reader-friendly. I was then commissioned to examine all the material to present the topics in the most comprehensible and productive format.

I would like to take this opportunity to thank all the contributing authors who were supportive enough to contribute their time and knowledge to this project. I also wish to convey my regards to my family who have been extremely supportive during the entire project.

Editor

1

3D Printing Approach in Dentistry: The Future for Personalized Oral Soft Tissue Regeneration

Dobrila Nesic [1,*] , **Birgit M. Schaefer** [2] , **Yue Sun** [1] , **Nikola Saulacic** [3] and **Irena Sailer** [1]

1   Division of Fixed Prosthodontics and Biomaterials, University Clinic of Dental Medicine,
    University of Geneva, Rue Michel-Servet 1, CH-1211 Geneva 4, Switzerland; Yue.Sun@unige.ch (Y.S.);
    irena.sailer@unige.ch (I.S.)
2   Geistlich Pharma AG, Bahnhofstrasse 40, CH-6110 Wolhusen, Switzerland; birgit.schaefer@geistlich.ch
3   Department of Cranio-Maxillofacial Surgery, Inselspital, Bern University Hospital, University of Bern,
    Freiburgstrasse 10, CH-3010 Bern, Switzerland; nikola.saulacic@insel.ch
*   Correspondence: dobrila.nesic@unige.ch

Abstract: Three-dimensional (3D) printing technology allows the production of an individualized 3D object based on a material of choice, a specific computer-aided design and precise manufacturing. Developments in digital technology, smart biomaterials and advanced cell culturing, combined with 3D printing, provide promising grounds for patient-tailored treatments. In dentistry, the "digital workflow" comprising intraoral scanning for data acquisition, object design and 3D printing, is already in use for manufacturing of surgical guides, dental models and reconstructions. 3D printing, however, remains un-investigated for oral mucosa/gingiva. This scoping literature review provides an overview of the 3D printing technology and its applications in regenerative medicine to then describe 3D printing in dentistry for the production of surgical guides, educational models and the biological reconstructions of periodontal tissues from laboratory to a clinical case. The biomaterials suitable for oral soft tissues printing are outlined. The current treatments and their limitations for oral soft tissue regeneration are presented, including "off the shelf" products and the blood concentrate (PRF). Finally, tissue engineered gingival equivalents are described as the basis for future 3D-printed oral soft tissue constructs. The existing knowledge exploring different approaches could be applied to produce patient-tailored 3D-printed oral soft tissue graft with an appropriate inner architecture and outer shape, leading to a functional as well as aesthetically satisfying outcome.

Keywords: 3D printing; oral soft tissues; gingiva; biomaterials; tissue engineering; PRF

1. Introduction

Recent years have seen an expansion of the field of three-dimensional (3D) printing, also referred to as additive manufacturing or solid freeform fabrication [1,2]. 3D printing technology allows the production of an individualized 3D object based on a material of choice and a specific computer-aided design. In the medical field, the possibility to include living cells in the procedure has lifted 3D printing to another level and opened a myriad of possibilities for the creation of different tissues. The new opportunities are now paving the way towards patient-tailored treatments. Several factors have contributed to the emerging applications of the 3D printing approaches. The development of a variety of printable biomaterials now offers more precise control of scaffold inner architecture and outer shape. The available analytical digital tools offer quick and precise acquisition and documentation of the patient-specific situation in 3D. An easy transfer of digital data allows the design of anatomically perfectly shaped structures that can be customized for each patient. The expiration of the key 3D printing patents has substantially decreased the cost of printers. The rapid developments of these technologies bring new and exciting approaches in all medical fields, including dentistry. A timeline illustrating the major discoveries of the 3D printing technologies and their applications in medicine is provided in Table 1.

Table 1. A timeline depicting the evolution of the three-dimensional (3D) printing technologies of importance for the medical field.

Year	Key Developments
1984	Invention of stereolithography (SLA) 3D printing (Charles Hull)
1986	Invention of the selective laser sintering (SLS) process (Carl Deckard)
1988	Bioprinting by 2D micro-positioning of cells and the first commercial SLA 3D printer (Charles Hull)
1989	Patenting of a fused deposition modelling (Lisa and Scott Crump)
1999	First 3D-printed organ—a bladder—used for transplantation (Wake Forest Institute for Regenerative Medicine)
2000	EnvisionTEC launched the first commercial extrusion-based bioprinter, the 3D-Bioplotter
2002	First early stage kidney prototype bioprinted via microextrusion (Wake Forest Institute for Regenerative Medicine)
2003	First inkjet bioprinter (modified HP standard inkjet printer)
2005	Founding of RepRap, an open source initiative to build a 3D printer that can print most of its own components
2007	Selective laser sintering printer becomes available, for 3D parts fabrication from fused metal/plastic
2008	First 3D-printed prosthetic leg
2009	First 3D-printed blood vessels (Organovo)
2012	First 3D-printed jaw
2014	First 3D-printed human liver tissue (Organovo), and first desk-top bioprinter (Allevi)
2015	First implanted 3D-printed bioresorbable scaffold for periodontal repair (University of Michigan)
2018	First commercial 3D-printed full human tissue (skin) model Poieskin (Poietis)
2019	First 3D-printed heart that contracts, with blood vessels (University of Tel Aviv) and 3D-printed lung air-sac with surrounding blood vessels (Volumetric)
2020	3D printer for personalized medicine M3DIMAKER (FabRx)

Adapted from GlobalData, "The history of 3D printing", Carlos Gonzales, ASME, and [3].

The 3D printing process begins with a design of a 3D model, created by a computer-aided design (CAD) software. The model is then converted into cross-sectional slices and sent to the 3D printer, which deposits layer after layer of the chosen material to produce an object. Such "additive manufacturing" has several advantages over conventional, subtractive manufacturing: (1) it allows the production of a controlled inner structure, (2) it reduces material waste, (3) the object is produced as a single unit instead of being assembled from individual parts, and (4) the designed files can be transferred electronically, easily shared and indefinitely stored without occupying physical space. Consequently, production time and costs are decreased.

In the last decade, 3D printing technology has been broadly used in different medical fields including regenerative medicine, the production of anatomical models and surgical guides as well as for drug formulations [4–7]. In parallel, the development of 3D printable biomaterials to build tissue models without or with cells enables studying the processes of complex cellular interactions during tissue formation, maturation and disease, as well as toxicology testing and drug screening [4,8–10]. 3D-printed models have been used for presurgical planning in craniomaxillofacial surgery [11], cardiology [12], cerebral aneurysm [13] as well as in orthopaedics [14]. Today, physical models are employed as cutting guides for tumor resection as well as templates for shaping patient's specific implants and prostheses [15–17]. Finally, 3D printing has found use in producing anatomical models for education and training [18,19]. This scoping review provides a brief summary of 3D printing approaches in the medicinal field, with a particular emphasis on the current status of 3D printing in dentistry, and the possibilities it offers for personalized soft tissue volume augmentation.

2. The 3D Printing Technology

In 3D printing, objects are fabricated automatically by adding material(s) layer-after-layer, to form a 3D volumetric structure [20]. As with any new technology, technical standards had to be established for a wide range of materials, products, systems, and services. The American Section of the International Association for Testing Materials (ASTM) International Standard Organization committee F42 on AM technologies has named seven additive manufacturing categories: binder jetting, direct energy deposition, material extrusion, material jetting, powder bed fusion, sheet lamination, and vat photopolymerization [21]. In the biomedical field, the mainly employed printing methods can be broadly divided into acellular techniques comprising stereolithography (SLA), powder-fusion printing (PFP), solid freeform fabrication (SFF) and techniques including cells: inkjet-based, extrusion-based, and laser-assisted bioprinting (LAB) (reviewed in [3]). SLA is based on beaming a laser or a light source onto a photosensitive polymer to harden its surface. The continuous vertical lifting of the container with a polymer results in a gradual hardening of the material and emergence of a 3D object. SLA was used to print biodegradable polymers, ceramic acrylate, or hydroxyapatite for bone reconstruction [22–24]. Lithography-based ceramics manufacturing (LCM) was employed for the high precision fabrication of glass ceramic dental replacements [25]. Another 3D printing technology, the digital light processing (DLP) based on photopolymerization, was employed for the fabrication of zirconia implants [26,27]. In selective laser sintering (SLS), a powder fusion printing (PFP) technique, granules of metal, raisin or plastic are beamed with a laser to fuse in a layer-after-layer fashion [28]. Tricalcium phosphate and hydroxyapatite were used with this technique to produce scaffolds for bone regeneration [29]. The advantage of the PFP techniques is the possibility to print melting metals such as titanium, magnesium or cobalt chromium, employed in medicine and dentistry. Solid form fabrication (SFF) allows deposition of strands by a nozzle via a precise XYZ axes positioning system. Upon extrusion, however, the material must retain its shape. As an example, polycaprolactone (PCL) was combined with alginate to print scaffolds for cartilage repair [30].

The 3D printing technology that includes cells has been named "bioprinting", and the hydrogels, in which cells reside for the printing purpose, have been named "bioinks" [31]. Hydrogels offer modifiable chemical composition, and adjustable mechanical and biodegradation properties [32]. Hydrogels represent attractive materials for bioinks due to their biocompatibility, low cytotoxicity, and high water content [33,34]. A hydrogel suitable for 3D bioprinting must be viscous enough to keep its shape during printing, without squeezing cells, and have cross-linking abilities to allow retention of the 3D structure after printing. In extrusion bioprinting, pneumatic (pressure) or mechanical (plunger) force extrudes filaments. Fast gelation for retention of the desired outer form and inner structure ensues. As examples, alginate is combined with calcium, and fibrinogen with thrombin. The main advantage of extrusion bioprinting is the possibility to use multiple materials and cell types in different combinations [5]. Laser-assisted bioprinting (LAB) is based on a laser pulse that produces local heating of a cell-containing solution causing dropping of cells in an orderly manner on the other side of a platform/substrate [35]. Laser-direct-writing, a type of LAB, was successfully used to deposit different cells types and biomaterials [36]. In inkjet bioprinting, a defined volume of fluid (with or without cells) is jetted onto a platform to obtain a precise pattern [5]. Droplets are deposited using either thermal or piezoelectric energy. The major advantage is the speed achieved in building the complex cell-laden tissue mimicking equivalents, and a multi-head approach for bioprinting different cell types and biomaterials. The main disadvantage is that cells or bioactive molecules must be in a liquid state to allow deposition, and subsequently solidify into the required structure. The commonly used hydrogels in LAB techniques are cross-linked using physical, chemical, pH, or ultraviolet light methods [37]. A comprehensive comparison of both types of 3D printing techniques relevant for tissue constructs has been recently published [3].

3. 3D Printing for Tissue Engineering

3D printing has been very successful in making biomaterial scaffolds with custom-designed geometries and is becoming an important technology for tissue engineering [38]. The tissue engineering approach aims at rebuilding a functional tissue that could either replace or facilitate the regeneration of the missing tissue [39]. The tissue engineering triangle comprises biomimetic scaffolds as the initial structural support, cells as tissue masons and bioactive molecules as the instructors providing the necessary signals [40]. In the past, the production of a tissue relied on scaffold fabrication techniques with limited possibilities to reproduce the tissue complexity. Today, the 3D printing approach has a distinct advantage in that it can produce various geometries to perfectly fit any tissue defect as well as mimic complex inner tissue architecture and heterogeneity via the precise positioning of different materials and/or cell types [1,2]. For hard tissues, 3D printing of bone graft scaffolds comprised approaches using natural and synthetic biomaterials [41,42] assembled in a biomimetic scaffold [43]. For soft tissues, 3D printing mainly relied on various hydrogels combined with cells to produce tissues like cartilage [44–48], vascular as well as cardiovascular tissues [49–51], liver [52], and skin [53–59]. Recently, modular assembly, with separate 3D-printed biological components (cells, cell aggregates or microtissue units) combined with the corresponding biomimicking scaffolds, has been applied for 3D printing of blood vessels, osteochondral grafts or liver constructs [60]. Companies have also exploited 3D printing to biofabricate different types of tissues. exVive3D™ Liver (Organovo, San Diego, CA, USA) is a bioprinted human hepatic tissue successfully used for toxicity assessment to complement in vitro and preclinical testing [61]. TeVido (TeVido Biodevices, Austin, TX, USA) is developing breast reconstructions for cancer patients based on their own cells, and l'Oréal (Paris, France) and Poietis (Pessac, France) work together to tackle hair loss by 3D printing hair follicles [62]. A recent detailed and comprehensive description of different 3D printing methods with their advantages and disadvantages, clinical applications, the necessary biomaterial considerations and bioprinting strategies provides an excellent guidance for the biofabrication of tissue constructs [63].

4. 3D Printing in Dentistry: A Brief Overview

3D printing in the dental field was introduced more than a decade ago and its application continues to increase, with 139 publications and 1800 citations in 2019 (Figure 1). SLA manufacturing of implant-drill-guides for guided surgery procedures and laser–sintered alloys were the first additive fabrication technologies applied in dentistry. The development of digital image acquisition, and the application of the CAD/CAM technology allowed the emergence of a fully digitalized dental treatment [64]. Intraoral-scanning has been replacing plastic imprints to produce computer-aided manufactured (CAM) digital physical models. Hence, the manual handling is being replaced throughout the three processing steps, and this novel approach has been termed "digital workflow" [65]. The first step comprises data acquisition through various scanning technologies. The most common techniques are computerized tomography (CT), cone beam computed tomography (CBCT), magnetic resonance imaging (MRI), and laser digitizing with extraoral or intraoral scanning devices. The second step is the data processing and the model design with a computer-aided design (CAD) software. The resulting STL file is imported into the printer software. The building variables and parameters for segmentation are next specified, together with the support structures, to generate the information needed to run the 3D printer. In the third step, the processed data are used to manufacture structures with the chosen material through the CAM step [65]. 3D-printed objects have been successfully used in prosthodontics, orthodontics, orthognathics, endodontics, craniofacial, and oral and maxillofacial surgical procedures [66]. The benefits include simplification, minimal invasiveness, greater accuracy, a reduction in operating times, and improvement in patient comfort and aesthetics.

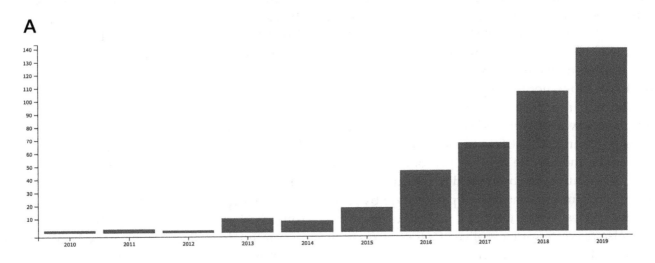

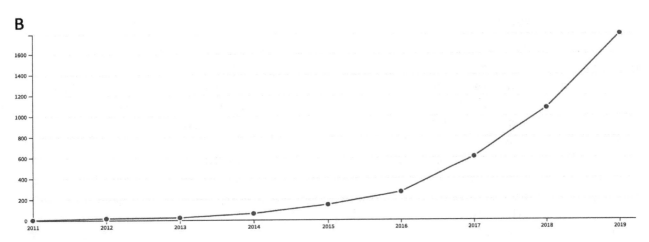

Figure 1. A notable increase in the number of articles (**A**) and citations (**B**) published on 3D printing in the dental field during the last decade. Source: Web of Science.

4.1. Presurgical Virtual Planning and Dental Surgical Guides

Haptics technology exploits the sense of touch and its interaction with the virtual environment. The convergence of haptics and virtual reality technology and integration with 3D imaging data resulted in the emergence of dental haptic simulators. Created virtual oral anatomy and facilitated the simulation of dental procedures offer real-time visual, tactile and auditory planning as well as feedback [67,68]. Combination of haptic instruments with 3D printing contributed towards the development of patient-specific instrumentation, in particular, surgical guide instruments that increase accuracy during surgery while decreasing the risk of infections and operation time/cost.

Customized design of surgical splints and stainless-steel arch-wires through 3D digital treatment simulation allows for precise fabrication as well as the prediction of dental and jaw movements. This approach reduces treatment time, reinforces decompensatory tooth movements, and rapidly improves aesthetics [69]. Several commercial applications have been developed to facilitate 3D virtual treatment planning, although the biomechanical planning of tooth movements requires further development. Surgical planning software including Virtual Surgical Planning (VSP®) Technology (3D Systems; Littleton, CO, USA), ProPlan CMF™ (Materialise, Leuven, Belgium), IPS CaseDesigner® (KLS MÂRTIN Group, Tuttlingen, Germany), and InVivo6® (Anatomage, San Jose, CA, USA) integrate CT/Cone Beam CT (CBCT) data, 3D stereophotogrammetry, and intra-oral occlusal scans to generate a comprehensive 3D model. Dental movements and surgical osteotomies can be simulated interactively between the surgeon, orthodontist, and engineer. The final clinical plan is used to generate an intermediate and a final splint, both of which are fabricated via 3D printing. Virtual orthodontic movements can be similarly planned and applied. Software such as InVivo[6®] (Anatomage, San Jose, CA, USA) and Orchestrate[®] (Orchestrate3D, Rialto, CA, USA) incorporate data either from CBCT or intraoral scans and allow for individual tooth movements to be programmed and sequenced. The orthodontist creates a virtual set-up of the final occlusion, as well as the sequence and the pathway for tooth movements. Sequenced models or aligners can be fabricated with a relatively inexpensive 3D printer in a dental laboratory or in the orthodontist's office. Similar approaches using fixed appliances were developed by SureSmile[®] (OraMetrix; Richardson, TX, USA) and Insignia[®] (Ormco, Orange County, CA, USA) to fabricate custom arch-wires or orthodontic brackets. The possibility to determine the precise sequence of tooth movements results in their perfect alignment.

3D printing has been used to produce surgical guides for pulp canal obliteration based on CBCT scans. To diminish the risk of perforation by producing a correct path of canal and instrumentation access, guides were printed and utilized to target burs to otherwise elusive canal spaces [70]. 3D printing was also used to print a replica of a tooth to be autotransplanted, in order to prepare the implantation site and decrease PDL damage from repeated insertion/removal cycles during fitting [71].

4.2. Educational Models in Dentistry

In academia, in the past, dental students had to rely on extracted teeth, human cadavers, resin blocks or commercially prepared teeth replicas for the simulation of cases during their studies [72,73]. In clinics, printed tooth reproductions were used in preparation for the treatment of complicated cases to simulate optimal access, instrumentation and obturation [74]. Today, 3D-printed objects represent a teaching aid for students to improve their understanding of the complexity of different oral structures, to simulate functions and to train for the optimal intervention. Duplicate 3D-printed models are used for standardized students' skill assessments as well as individual student skill progression.

In dental practice, 3D-printed models could improve communication between the practitioner and the patient. Better understanding of the proposed treatment leads to a compliant attitude and develops mutual understanding and trust [75].

In research, a three-dimensional organ-germ culture method that generated a structurally correct tooth [76,77] was replaced by a 3D-printed bioengineered tooth replica for in vitro and in vivo experiments toward understanding the whole-tooth morphogenesis [78] as well as regeneration [78,79].

4.3. 3D Printing for Reconstruction of Oral Tissues

The periodontal ligament (PDL) is the fibrous connective tissue structure that anchors alveolar bone to tooth cement [80]. By resisting compressive loading, PDL allows tooth movement upon mastication and speech. During the initial inflammatory processes and subsequent periodontium wound healing, the blood supply through the PDL vascular plexus and the neural network play critical roles [79,81]. Hence, the loss of PDL impairs not only teeth physiological movement but also the defense against infection [82]. PDL-derived cells possess mesenchymal stem cell-like properties and have been considered as a source for the reconstruction of periodontal tissues [83,84]. More than two decades ago, PDL-derived cells were used with the "cell sheet technology", i.e., cell detachment without enzymatic treatment [85] for periodontal regeneration. Preclinical and clinical studies demonstrated periodontal regeneration with inserted PDL fibers and newly formed cementum in periodontal defects [86–91]. The major drawback of the cell-sheet approach was the compromised biomechanical stability and the demanding surgical technique. The improvements of the cell sheets' biomechanical properties included layering of several sheets, supporting the sheets with hydrogels, and adding ECM components to the thermo-responsive surface [90,92]. With the development of additive manufacturing, a 3D-printed calcium phosphate (CaP)-coated PCL scaffold was combined with cell sheets from different human cell types resulting in significant periodontal attachment [93]. In another approach, decellularized periodontal ligament cell sheets were transferred onto melt electrospun PCL membranes. The retained intact extracellular matrix and resident growth factors supported repopulation by allogeneic cells [94]. A recent study demonstrated the formation of a periodontal-like structure around a titanium implant. PDL cell sheets were cultured on an acid-etched, blasted titanium surface coated with calcium phosphate to mimic the environment around a natural tooth [95].

The 3D printing approach could prove particularly valuable in answering the need for the complex hierarchical organization of periodontium consisting of gingiva, PDL, cementum, and alveolar bone. The periodontium is a highly organized tissue that supports the teeth and plays an important role in transmitting mechanical forces [80,96]. Reconstruction of periodontal tissue necessitates coordinated spatiotemporal control of the healing process via volume maintenance, wound stabilization and selective cell repopulation [97]. The approach with multiphasic biomaterial constructs could recapitulate the structural integrity of tooth-supporting tissues destroyed as a consequence of trauma, chronic infection or surgical resection. A series of consecutive studies aimed at developing 3D-printed biomimetic composite hybrid polymeric scaffolds to reproduce the dentin–PDL–bone interfaces [98–100]. The studies relied on a differential structural design for the alveolar bone and PDL parts, using 3D printing with PCL for bone and PGA for PDL, genetically modified human cells and human tooth dentin slice [98]. The newly formed tissues consisted of parallel and obliquely oriented fibers that grew within the PCL/PGA constructs forming tooth cementum-like tissue, ligament, and bone structures. In the next study, PCL was combined with human cells for producing PDL and bone structures and evaluated in an in situ rat mandible defect model [99]. The design of perpendicularly oriented micro-channels of the PDL part allowed the formation of oriented anchoring ligaments linking cement and alveolar bone [99,100]. The "guided" fiber PDL architecture permitted control of tissue infiltration and optimal organization of both ligament interfaces. This knowledge was subsequently applied for the treatment of the periodontal reconstruction case following the "digital workflow" approach [101]. After the CBCT scan of the defect area, an STL file was created and used to design the osseous defect together with guided PDL channels. PCL was combined with hydroxyapatite and 3D printed. The construct was additionally submerged in bb-PDGF. The treated site remained intact for one year, after which the construct presented problems and had to be removed. Further research on the refinement of the guided "pillars" for PDL identified combined mesoscale and microscale hierarchical features allowing cell alignment for a more precise PDL formation [102]. An approach from another group consisted of a 3D-printed triphasic PCL/hydroxyapatite scaffold corresponding to cementum, PDL, and alveolar bone, each loaded with the three corresponding cell types and timely delivery of growth factors [103]. In vivo implantation resulted in aligned PDL-like collagen fibers that inserted into bone-like and dentin/cementum tissues. This approach illustrates a strategy for the regeneration of multiphase periodontal tissues by spatiotemporal delivery of several cell types and signaling proteins. Together, these studies demonstrate the potential of 3D printing to generate customized periodontal scaffolds for the regeneration of multi-tissue interfaces required for oral, dental and even craniofacial engineering applications.

5. Biomaterials Used for 3D Printing of Oral Tissues

Scaffolds produced from biomaterials provide an initial mechanical support and allow for cell population, adhesion and differentiation to foster guided tissue regeneration. The majority of the raw materials for additive manufacturing used for dental and medical purposes can be grouped into binder/powder material combinations including polymers (resins and thermoplastics), ceramics, and metals [104]. Biomaterials for tissue fabrication can be broadly divided into inorganic, mainly used for bone regeneration and organic, predominantly used for soft tissue regeneration. Inorganic biomaterials need to be mechanically stable, resorb slowly, and not induce an inflammatory reaction [105]. Hydroxyapatite is stoichiometrically similar to the mineral phase of the natural bone ensuring biocompatibility yet has reduced mechanical resistance and a long resorption time. Calcium phosphate binds chemically to bone, it is easier to manufacture into desired shapes and resorbs faster compared to hydroxyapatite [106]. In contrast to hydroxyapatite and calcium phosphate, the production of bioglass allows for an extremely versatile composition leading to a controlled resorption rate and modulation of cell migration and tissue revascularization [107]. Organic biomaterials are polymers of natural origin such as agarose, alginate, collagen, gelatin, chitosan, fibrin, or synthetic such as polylactide (PLA), poly glycolic acid (PGA), poly-lactic-*co*-glycolic acid (PLGA), and polycaprolactone (PCL) [106]. Hydrogels used for soft tissue regeneration can be either curable polymers, producing mechanically solid scaffolds upon solidification, or soft, injectable hydrogels. Both can be combined with cells; in the first case, cells are seeded after curing to avoid harsh printing/curing conditions; in the second, cells reside within the bioink during printing (bioprinting). A hybrid barrier membrane has been recently produced for guided tissue regeneration by 3D printing by combining gelatin (for cell adhesion), elastin (for membrane long-term stability and elasticity) and sodium hyaluronate (for cell-signaling), and cross-linked by 1-Ethyl-3-(3-dimethylaminopropyl) carbodiimide (EDC) [108]. The membrane has small pores on one side and large pores on the other side to accommodate osteoblasts, fibroblasts, and keratinocytes population on the different sides. The in vitro analysis indicated biocompatibility, mechanical strength, degradation rates, as well as tensile modulus for easy surgical handling.

Hydrogels are capable of absorbing and retaining large quantities of water. They can be classified into naturally-derived hydrogels such as agarose, alginate, fibrin, collagen type I, chitosan, gelatin, hyaluronic acid, Matrigel^{TM}, and synthetically-derived and synthetically-derived such as Pluronic®-127, polyethylene glycol (PEG) or various methacrylated combinations including gelatin (GelMA), hyaluronic acid (HAMA), silk fibroin (SilMA), and pectin (PECMA) [1,106,109,110]. The bioprintability of hydrogels is governed by their rheological properties and the target bioprinting modality, and includes three bioprinting techniques: extrusion-based, droplet-based and laser-based (cell transfer or photopolymerization) [110]. Two printing approaches: extrusion-based bioprinting for cell-encapsulating hydrogels and melt electro-writing for aligned sub-micrometer fibers were converged to produce a mechanically stable construct with viable cells [111]. Bioink gelation can be achieved via physical (temperature, ions), chemical (glutaraldehyde, genipin, irradiation-induced photo-polymerization) or enzymatic (thrombin) crosslinking. Due to hydrogels' high permeability to oxygen, nutrients and other water-soluble compounds, they are considered as attractive materials for the fabrication of tissue constructs. Another important advantage of the 3D printing approach with hydrogels is the easy incorporation of bioactive agents [112]. The presence of such signaling molecules can provide the necessary instructions to residing, host-tissue cells or externally delivered cells for facilitated tissue regeneration. Bioinks were also produced from decellularized matrix components, cellulose or silk [31]. Bioinks derived from decellularized extracellular matrices present major advantages: they contain all tissue components preserved in the correct proportions, and the tissue-specific signaling factors, therefore providing an optimal instructive environment for cell migration, proliferation and differentiation [113]. Such bioinks have been successfully bioprinted into porcine liver, heart, skin, cartilage and skeletal muscle tissues, and human adipose tissue [114,115].

6. Oral Soft Tissue Regeneration: Current Treatments and Limitations

Oral soft tissue plays an important role in the structure and function of the oral cavity. The oral mucosa covers the inside of the oral cavity and consists of: (1) the masticatory mucosa (gingiva and cover of the hard palate), (2) the specialized mucosa (cover of the tongue), and (3) lining mucosa [80]. Gingiva belongs to masticatory mucosa, covering the alveolar bone and surrounding the teeth. Structurally, it consists of the oral epithelium and the underlying connective tissue, lamina propria. The non-attached alveolar mucosa consists of a thin, non-keratinized stratified squamous epithelium and loosely connected collagen fibers. In contrast, the attached mucosa contains the thick, keratinized squamous epithelium and well-organized and dense collagen fibers. The hard palate and attached gingiva are made of the keratinized type of attached mucosa. The attached keratinized mucosa is indispensable for the maintenance of teeth, PDL, as well as dental implants. It forms a protective barrier against harmful environmental agents such as pathogens, chemicals, and constant abrasion [116]. The insufficiency of oral mucosa due to gingival recessions, infections, trauma, and tumors require oral mucosa reconstruction. Soft tissue augmentation is frequently used to regain reduced or lost tissue in edentulous patients, cover an exposed root or implant, increase buccal mucosal soft tissue thickness or coronal soft tissue height [117,118]. The treatment of choice must comply with functional mastication, speech, and aesthetics. Depending on the location and the need, various techniques are used, most relying on the autologous tissue grafts. For the soft tissue volume augmentation, subepithelial connective tissue graft (SCTG) gave a better clinical outcome compared to free gingival grafts (FGG), and it is used at implant sites or in partially edentulous patients [117,119]. However, the use of an autologous tissue graft presents several disadvantages and limitations: the height, length, and thickness of the palate depends on the anatomical position and varies among patients; the harvesting technique is surgically demanding, a limited amount of tissue can be gained per intervention, and patients complain about prolonged postsurgical pain and numbness [120–124]. To reduce the morbidity caused by graft harvesting, soft tissue substitutes have been sought [125,126]. The requirements for an ideal non-autologous graft for soft tissue augmentation comprise biocompatibility, volume and mechanical stability, concomitant biodegradability and tissue integration, easy handling, and low cost without compromised efficacy [126]. Freeze-dried skin allografts were among the first products introduced in mucogingival surgery. They were initially used as a replacement for FGG in combination with an apically positioned flap for the augmentation of keratinized tissue [127]. Later in the 1980s, allogenic dermal substitutes such as the acellular dermal matrix graft, Alloderm®, (Life Cell Corporation, The Woodlands, TX, USA), originally developed for covering full-thickness burn wounds [128], were introduced to increase keratinized tissue, cover exposed roots, deepen the vestibular fornix, and augment localized alveolar defects [129–132]. Unfortunately, the outcomes were associated with difficult clinical handling and high shrinkage rates of the grafted areas. Moreover, histology analysis indicated a significant difference in comparison to the natural tissue [133]. To reduce scar retraction and enhance the healing process, a novel collagen matrix, Geistlich Mucograft® (Geistlich Pharma AG, Wolhusen, Switzerland), was designed and evaluated as a replacement for autogenous tissue to increase the width of keratinized tissue and cover gingival recessions [134–138]. Clinical data indicated strong enhancement of the keratinized tissue width with similar outcomes in comparison to the FGG [139–142]. Another matrix, Mucoderm® (Botiss Dental, Berlin, Germany), a porcine dermis-derived acellular matrix, was used for the treatment of oral dehiscence, ridge preservation, root coverage and vertical augmentation [143]. Finally, a highly porous yet volume stable 3D matrix consisting of slightly cross-linked reconstituted collagen fibers has been introduced (Geistlich Fibro-Gide®, Geistlich Pharma AG, Wolhusen, Switzerland) and shown to increase soft tissue volume similarly to SCTG [144–146]. These promising biological scaffolds reduce morbidity, decrease surgical time as well as costs. However, they must be tailored for each individual defect, do not reproduce the inner architecture of a particular oral site, and remain surgically demanding.

7. Platelet Rich Fibrin (PRF) for Oral Soft Tissue Regeneration

The first steps during the wound healing process, including oral soft tissue, are haemostasis and formation of granulation tissue, both orchestrated by the signaling molecules released by various cell types. To accelerate the healing process at a surgery site, blood concentrates rich in platelets and autologous growth factors have been developed [147,148]. The first blood concentrate, platelet rich plasma (PRP), was obtained after platelets separation from red blood cells during a centrifugation process [147,149]. This preparation required an anticoagulant and relied on thrombin for subsequent clotting. The alternative concentrate, platelet rich fibrin (PRF), was obtained without anti-coagulants, with clotting taking place gradually and naturally [150]. While fast coagulation (PRP) results in a quick release of growth factors and dense fibers formation, slow coagulation (PRF) leads to long-term growth factors release from a more compact matrix rich in fibers [151,152]. Both blood preparations, PRP and PRF, have been extensively studied for a plethora of clinical problems [153]. Over the years, PRF has gained more interest, as it is less time consuming, does not require an anti-coagulant or thrombin, and due to the preserved fibrin matrix ultimately favors neovascularization. Several improvements have been made to the initial PRF preparation to increase cells and matrix longevity. The centrifugation speed was decreased resulting in an increase in the number of platelets and leukocytes, and a more balanced distribution of cells within the matrix [154]. An additional decrease in the centrifugation time further improved cell survival and growth factor release [155]. This low-speed centrifugation concept was also applied for the liquid injectable PRF, with similar results: selective enrichment of platelets, growth factors and leukocytes [156,157].

For soft tissue augmentation in dentistry, PRF was mainly employed for the treatment of extraction sockets, gingival recessions, and palatal wound closure [158]. Although beneficial effects were seen, conclusions were difficult to draw due to the lack of proper controls in study designs. A recent review analyzed studies that used PRF for different dental treatments, namely in endodontics, implantology, sinus lift, socket preservation, bone regeneration, and socket preservation, orthodontics and periodontology [159]. In periodontology, PRF was often combined with biomaterials and demonstrated beneficial outcome. The authors hypothesize that PRF made the acellular matrix more cell-friendly, fostering better adhesion, cell–cell communication, and tissue integration. A similar role for PRF can be envisioned for the 3D-printed, individualized acellular scaffolds. However, the main limitation remains the lack of standardized protocol of PRF preparations among clinicians.

8. Monitoring Soft Tissue Augmentation

For an accurate and standardized assessment of the soft tissue augmentation requirements and the subsequent different treatment outcomes, measurement of the surface and thickness, i.e., volume of the soft tissue, is crucial. A recent review addressed technological developments from 2D to 3D methods outlining advantages and drawbacks [160]. Traditional, 2D methods for measurement of soft tissue comprise a periodontal probe, oral photography and ultrasonic devices. Their main advantages are their relative non-invasiveness and accuracy of 0.1–0.5 mm. The significant limitation for all three methods is the need for a connection to a 3D design software in order to obtain 3D information of the defect areas. 3D methods comprise CBCT, Moiré method and laser CAD/CAM devices. CBCT is limited due to linear measurements, scattering effect, limited accuracy and radiation exposure, but it is painless. The Moiré method is time-consuming, requires casting with risks of displacement and dimensional changes during impression, but provides more accuracy compared to CBCT. Lasers were proven as the most accurate and offer a choice between scanning of an imprinted cast and a direct oral digital scanning. Digital optical scanning and assessment methods have been introduced to measure and longitudinally quantify soft tissue volume loss or gain [161,162]. Therefore, the "digital workflow" can also be employed for the initial assessment (diagnostic), virtual planning and evaluation of the efficacy of treatment options and future 3D printing of soft tissues required for gingival soft tissue augmentation.

9. Tissue Engineering for Oral Soft Tissue Regeneration

Tissue engineering approaches have already been developed with the aim to establish 3D organotypic cultures resembling the natural gingiva for clinical as well as research purposes. An ideal full-thickness tissue engineered gingiva should consist of: (1) a supporting connective tissue, i.e., lamina propria containing fibroblasts within a vascularized ECM; (2) a continuous basement membrane which separates lamina propria from the epithelium, and (3) a stratified squamous epithelium containing densely packed keratinocytes that undergo differentiation as they move towards the surface. Initially, keratinocytes were cultured in cell sheets with a cell feeder layer [163], resulting in a fragile, difficult to handle and retractable tissue. Subsequently, incorporation of fibroblasts and collagen provided the support of a lamina propria substitute and led to the fabrication of the first gingiva equivalent tested in clinics [164]. Scaffolds that were developed and used in gingiva tissue engineering in the past decades can be classified into: (1) naturally derived (acellular human dermis), (2) collagen-based, (3) fibrin-based,

(4) gelatin-based, (5) synthetic (PCL) or hybrid [165]. For clinical applications, the primary cell source was cells isolated from autologous biopsies in contrast to the in vitro studies which often favored immortalized cell lines for the sake of availability, reproducibility, and standardization. However, cancer-derived cell lines regularly present compromised physiological responses. Keratinocytes and fibroblasts were therefore "physiologically" immortalized by the expression of Telomerase Reverse Transcriptase [166]. These cells allowed the formation of a full-thickness gingival equivalent that closely reproduced the native gingival tissue architecture [167]. Such organotypic models provide invaluable tools to study oral mucosa biology and could also replace animal studies for drug targeting, vaccination development, and testing of new therapeutics. In laboratories, they are used to understand the physiological role of human oral mucosa barrier properties as well as different pathologies, including oral cancer, bacterial and fungal infections. Additionally, oral mucosa models are used for cytotoxicity and biocompatibility testing of oral health care products [168]. In clinics, tissue engineered gingiva was used to augment keratinized tissue around teeth [169] and has recently been up-scaled for large (over 15 cm^2) soft tissue defects [170]. Gingival grafts cultured on a biodegradable collagen scaffold were also employed in periodontal plastic surgery to treat patients with insufficiency of the attached gingiva [171,172].

Several companies have ventured into developing gingival tissue models. SkinEthic Laboratories (Nice, France) offers an epithelial gingival model based on the air–liquid interface culture of normal gingival keratinocytes. This keratinized, stratified, squamous epithelium can be used as a screening tool for corrosion, irritation, permeability and metabolism testing of new compounds as well as for investigating the effects of anti-inflammatory or antibiotic formulations [173]. MatTek Corporation developed EpiOral™, a model of human oral (buccal) stratified non-keratinized epithelium, and EpiGingival™, a model of gingival stratified keratinized epithelium for screening newly developed oral care products as well as for studying innate immunity, drug delivery, and pathology of the oral mucosa.

10. The Future: 3D Printing for Oral Soft Tissue Regeneration

3D printing could prove an ideal approach to produce scaffolds for soft tissue augmentation by addressing the variability in the soft tissue shape, inner architecture, thickness, volume, mechanics, and function associated with the position in the oral cavity. Importantly, 3D printing would allow application of the "digital workflow", resulting in the production of the patient-tailored grafts. Several decisions would need to be made to establish the 3D printing approach of oral mucosa [6]: the most appropriate imaging acquisition, the choice of biomaterial to best correspond to gingiva in its chemical, biological and mechanical properties, inclusion or not of cells (and the source), and finally the choice of the printing technique. Digital imaging of bone, soft tissue, and blood vessels during pre-operative virtual planning for face reconstruction has been accomplished with Haptics system [67]. With the intraoral scan digital acquisition, the level and the anatomy of tissue insufficiency, as well as the vascular network, can be determined. The desired characteristics of 3D printable biomaterials comprise biocompatibility, high porosity to promote cell population, tissue in-growth and vessel formation, biodegradability according to the rate of new matrix deposition (tissue generation), and mechanical stability. The appropriate macro-architecture characteristics would ensure timely neovascularization, as recently demonstrated for the regeneration of dental pulp [174]. A smart biomaterial containing all instruction cues could circumvent the need for growth factors or cells. However, in certain pathological cases such as inflammation, infection or necrosis, different anti-inflammatory, and immunomodulatory drugs or antibiotics could be incorporated and released in a timely and concentration-controlled manner. The inclusion of approved autologous blood concentrate preparations, such as PRF or PRP, could facilitate the healing process via the release of natural growth factors. From the dentist's point of view, the "digital workflow" would have to be easy to plan and execute, with the final soft tissue graft that is effortless to handle and suture and provides satisfactory functional as well as esthetical results. A schematic illustration of the potential future "digital workflow" is depicted in Figure 2.

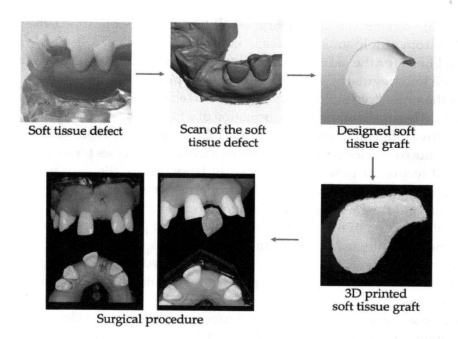

Figure 2. "Digital workflow" for soft tissue augmentation. The soft tissue defect is scanned (intraorally or from the imprint-derived cast); the ideal graft is designed and converted into an STL file. Upon 3D printing of a defect-tailored graft for optimal volume augmentation, the graft is surgically placed to fit the defect, and sutured.

In summary, 3D printing is a versatile manufacturing technology offering vast patterning possibilities, precise manufacturing, and abundant choices of biomaterials for a cost-effective patient-tailored end construct. This interdisciplinary approach pursues the integration of technologies from the fields of engineering, digital imaging, materials science, biology, chemistry, and medicine. 3D printing technology has already been largely employed in numerous biomedical applications to make tissues, organs, and medical devices, as well as to provide surgical planning aids and educational models. Continuous expansion and adaptation of 3D printers' abilities, combined with reduced costs, increased speed, and use of a broader range of printable materials will bring this technology to the forefront of biomedical applications. New challenges, needs, and achievements can be envisioned in the field of bioprinting as more researchers with different backgrounds and research questions employ 3D printers. In dentistry, particularly for soft tissue regeneration, application of the "digital workflow" to achieve a perfect-fit patient-tailored graft according to the defect, with an adjusted inner architecture and outer shape to maximize tissue mimicry, will result in functional as well as aesthetically pleasing tissue restoration.

Author Contributions: D.N. conceptualization, writing and editing; I.S. conceptualization and critical reviewing; D.N., B.M.S., Y.S., and N.S. critical reviewing and editing the manuscript. All authors have read and agreed to the published version of the manuscript.

Acknowledgments: The authors would like to thank Hyeonjong Lee Department of Prosthodontics, School of Dentistry, Pusan National University for his assistance in generating and printing the soft tissue graft depicted in Figure 2.

References

1.   Matai, I.I.; Kaur, G.G.; Seyedsalehi, A.A.; McClinton, A.A.; Laurencin, C.T.C. Progress in 3D bioprinting technology for tissue/organ regenerative engineering. *Biomaterials* **2020**, *226*, 119536. [CrossRef] [PubMed]

2.   Sun, W.W.; Starly, B.B.; Daly, A.C.A.; Burdick, J.A.J.; Groll, J.J.R.; Skeldon, G.G.; Shu, W.W.; Sakai, Y.Y.; Shinohara, M.M.; Nishikawa, M.M.; et al. The bioprinting roadmap. *Biofabrication* **2020**, *12*, 022002. [CrossRef] [PubMed]

3. Sears, N.A.; Seshadri, D.R.; Dhavalikar, P.S.; Cosgriff-Hernandez, E. A Review of Three-Dimensional Printing in Tissue Engineering. *Tissue Eng. Part B Rev.* **2016**, *22*, 298–310. [CrossRef]

4. Goole, J.; Amighi, K. 3D printing in pharmaceutics: A new tool for designing customized drug delivery systems. *Int. J. Pharm.* **2016**, *499*, 376–394. [CrossRef] [PubMed]

5. Kang, H.W.; Lee, S.J.; Ko, I.K.; Kengla, C.; Yoo, J.J.; Atala, A. A 3D bioprinting system to produce human-scale tissue constructs with structural integrity. *Nat. Biotechnol.* **2016**, *34*, 312–319. [CrossRef] [PubMed]

6. Murphy, S.V.; Atala, A. 3D bioprinting of tissues and organs. *Nat. Biotechnol.* **2014**, *32*, 773–785. [CrossRef] [PubMed]

7. Ventola, C.L. Medical Applications for 3D Printing: Current and Projected Uses. *Pharm. Ther.* **2014**, *39*, 704–711.

8. Shafiee, A.; Atala, A. Printing Technologies for Medical Applications. *Trends Mol. Med.* **2016**, *22*, 254–265. [CrossRef]

9. Vanderburgh, J.; Sterling, J.A.; Guelcher, S.A. 3D Printing of Tissue Engineered Constructs for In Vitro Modeling of Disease Progression and Drug Screening. *Ann. Biomed. Eng.* **2017**, *45*, 164–179. [CrossRef]

10. Zadpoor, A.A.; Malda, J. Additive Manufacturing of Biomaterials, Tissues, and Organs. *Ann. Biomed. Eng.* **2017**, *45*, 1–11. [CrossRef]

11. Hsieh, T.Y.; Vong, S.; Strong, E.B. Orbital reconstruction. *Curr. Opin. Otolaryngol. Head Neck Surg.* **2015**, *23*, 388–392. [CrossRef]

12. Jacobs, S.; Grunert, R.; Mohr, F.W.; Falk, V. 3D-Imaging of cardiac structures using 3D heart models for planning in heart surgery: A preliminary study. *Interact. Cardiovasc. Thorac. Surg.* **2008**, *7*, 6–9. [CrossRef] [PubMed]

13. Kono, K.; Shintani, A.; Okada, H.; Terada, T. Preoperative simulations of endovascular treatment for a cerebral aneurysm using a patient-specific vascular silicone model. *Neurol. Med. Chir.* **2013**, *53*, 347–351. [CrossRef] [PubMed]

14. Eltorai, A.E.; Nguyen, E.; Daniels, A.H. Three-Dimensional Printing in Orthopedic Surgery. *Orthopedics* **2015**, *38*, 684–687. [CrossRef] [PubMed]

15. Bellanova, L.; Paul, L.; Docquier, P.L. Surgical guides (patient-specific instruments) for pediatric tibial bone sarcoma resection and allograft reconstruction. *Sarcoma* **2013**, *2013*, 787653. [CrossRef]

16. D'Urso, P.S.; Earwaker, W.J.; Barker, T.M.; Redmond, M.J.; Thompson, R.G.; Effeney, D.J.; Tomlinson, F.H. Custom cranioplasty using stereolithography and acrylic. *Br. J. Plast. Surg.* **2000**, *53*, 200–204. [CrossRef]

17. Zopf, D.A.; Hollister, S.J.; Nelson, M.E.; Ohye, R.G.; Green, G.E. Bioresorbable airway splint created with a three-dimensional printer. *N. Engl. J. Med.* **2013**, *368*, 2043–2045. [CrossRef]

18. Kiarashi, N.; Nolte, A.C.; Sturgeon, G.M.; Segars, W.P.; Ghate, S.V.; Nolte, L.W.; Samei, E.; Lo, J.Y. Development of realistic physical breast phantoms matched to virtual breast phantoms based on human subject data. *Med. Phys.* **2015**, *42*, 4116–4126. [CrossRef]

19. Suzuki, R.; Taniguchi, N.; Uchida, F.; Ishizawa, A.; Kanatsu, Y.; Zhou, M.; Funakoshi, K.; Akashi, H.; Abe, H. Transparent model of temporal bone and vestibulocochlear organ made by 3D printing. *Anat. Sci. Int.* **2018**, *93*, 154–159. [CrossRef]

20. Derby, B. Printing and prototyping of tissues and scaffolds. *Science* **2012**, *338*, 921–926. [CrossRef]

21. ASTM. ISO/ASTM52900-15. *Standard Terminology for Additive Manufacturing—General Principles—Terminology*; ASTM International: West Conshohocken, PA, USA, 2015. [CrossRef]

22. Chu, T.M.; Hollister, S.J.; Halloran, J.W.; Feinberg, S.E.; Orton, D.G. Manufacturing and characterization of 3-d hydroxyapatite bone tissue engineering scaffolds. *Ann. N. Y. Acad. Sci.* **2002**, *961*, 114–117. [CrossRef] [PubMed]

23. Langton, C.M.; Whitehead, M.A.; Langton, D.K.; Langley, G. Development of a cancellous bone structural model by stereolithography for ultrasound characterisation of the calcaneus. *Med. Eng. Phys.* **1997**, *19*, 599–604. [CrossRef]

24. Leukers, B.; Gulkan, H.; Irsen, S.H.; Milz, S.; Tille, C.; Schieker, M.; Seitz, H. Hydroxyapatite scaffolds for bone tissue engineering made by 3D printing. *J. Mater. Sci. Mater. Med.* **2005**, *16*, 1121–1124. [CrossRef] [PubMed]

25. Schönherr, J.A.; Baumgartner, S.; Hartmann, M.; Stampfl, J. Stereolithographic Additive Manufacturing of High Precision Glass Ceramic Parts. *Materials* **2020**, *13*, 1492. [CrossRef]

26. Anssari Moin, D.; Hassan, B.; Wismeijer, D. A novel approach for custom three-dimensional printing of a zirconia root analogue implant by digital light processing. *Clin. Oral Implant. Res.* **2017**, *28*, 668–670. [CrossRef]

27. Osman, R.B.; van der Veen, A.J.; Huiberts, D.; Wismeijer, D.; Alharbi, N. 3D-printing zirconia implants; a dream or a reality? An in-vitro study evaluating the dimensional accuracy, surface topography and mechanical properties of printed zirconia implant and discs. *J. Mech. Behav. Biomed. Mater.* **2017**, *75*, 521–528. [CrossRef]

28. Yang, S.; Leong, K.F.; Du, Z.; Chua, C.K. The design of scaffolds for use in tissue engineering. Part I. Traditional factors. *Tissue Eng.* **2002**, *8*, 1–11. [CrossRef]

29. Shuai, C.; Mao, Z.; Lu, H.; Nie, Y.; Hu, H.; Peng, S. Fabrication of porous polyvinyl alcohol scaffold for bone tissue engineering via selective laser sintering. *Biofabrication* **2013**, *5*, 015014. [CrossRef]

30. Kundu, J.; Shim, J.H.; Jang, J.; Kim, S.W.; Cho, D.W. An additive manufacturing-based PCL-alginate-chondrocyte bioprinted scaffold for cartilage tissue engineering. *J. Tissue Eng. Regen. Med.* **2015**, *9*, 1286–1297. [CrossRef]

31. Gopinathan, J.; Noh, I. Recent trends in bioinks for 3D printing. *Biomater. Res.* **2018**, *22*, 11. [CrossRef]

32. Chimene, D.; Kaunas, R.; Gaharwar, A.K. Hydrogel Bioink Reinforcement for Additive Manufacturing: A Focused Review of Emerging Strategies. *Adv. Mater.* **2020**, *32*, e1902026. [CrossRef] [PubMed]

33. Guillotin, B.; Guillemot, F. Cell patterning technologies for organotypic tissue fabrication. *Trends Biotechnol.* **2011**, *29*, 183–190. [CrossRef] [PubMed]

34. Morgan, F.L.; Moroni, L.; Baker, M.B. Dynamic Bioinks to Advance Bioprinting. *Adv. Healthc. Mater.* **2020**, e1901798. [CrossRef] [PubMed]

35. Odde, D.J.; Renn, M.J. Laser-guided direct writing for applications in biotechnology. *Trends Biotechnol.* **1999**, *17*, 385–389. [CrossRef]

36. Guillemot, F.; Souquet, A.; Catros, S.; Guillotin, B.; Lopez, J.; Faucon, M.; Pippenger, B.; Bareille, R.; Remy, M.; Bellance, S.; et al. High-Throughput Laser Print. *Cells Biomater. Tissue Engineering. Acta Biomater.* **2010**, *6*, 2494–2500. [CrossRef]

37. Murphy, S.V.; Skardal, A.; Atala, A. Evaluation of hydrogels for bio-printing applications. *J. Biomed. Mater. Res. Part A* **2013**, *101*, 272–284. [CrossRef] [PubMed]

38. Hollister, S.J. Porous scaffold design for tissue engineering. *Nat. Mater.* **2005**, *4*, 518–524. [CrossRef]

39. Vacanti, J.P.; Langer, R. Tissue engineering: The design and fabrication of living replacement devices for surgical reconstruction and transplantation. *Lancet* **1999**, *354*, SI32–SI34. [CrossRef]

40. Langer, R.; Vacanti, J.P. Tissue engineering. *Science* **1993**, *260*, 920–926. [CrossRef]

41. Roseti, L.; Parisi, V.; Petretta, M.; Cavallo, C.; Desando, G.; Bartolotti, I.; Grigolo, B. Scaffolds for Bone Tissue Engineering: State of the art and new perspectives. *Mater. Sci. Eng. C Mater. Biol. Appl.* **2017**, *78*, 1246–1262. [CrossRef] [PubMed]

42. Wen, Y.; Xun, S.; Haoye, M.; Baichuan, S.; Peng, C.; Xuejian, L.; Kaihong, Z.; Xuan, Y.; Jiang, P.; Shibi, L. 3D printed porous ceramic scaffolds for bone tissue engineering: A review. *Biomater. Sci.* **2017**, *5*, 1690–1698. [CrossRef] [PubMed]

43. Kim, H.D.; Amirthalingam, S.; Kim, S.L.; Lee, S.S.; Rangasamy, J.; Hwang, N.S. Biomimetic Materials and Fabrication Approaches for Bone Tissue Engineering. *Adv. Healthc. Mater.* **2017**, *6*, 1700612. [CrossRef] [PubMed]

44. Abbadessa, A.; Mouser, V.H.; Blokzijl, M.M.; Gawlitta, D.; Dhert, W.J.; Hennink, W.E.; Malda, J.; Vermonden, T. A Synthetic Thermosensitive Hydrogel for Cartilage Bioprinting and Its Biofunctionalization with Polysaccharides. *Biomacromolecules* **2016**, *17*, 2137–2147. [CrossRef]

45. Apelgren, P.; Amoroso, M.; Lindahl, A.; Brantsing, C.; Rotter, N.; Gatenholm, P.; Kolby, L. Chondrocytes and stem cells in 3D-bioprinted structures create human cartilage in vivo. *PLoS ONE* **2017**, *12*, e0189428. [CrossRef] [PubMed]

46. Nyberg, E.L.; Farris, A.L.; Hung, B.P.; Dias, M.; Garcia, J.R.; Dorafshar, A.H.; Grayson, W.L. 3D-Printing Technologies for Craniofacial Rehabilitation, Reconstruction, and Regeneration. *Ann. Biomed. Eng.* **2017**, *45*, 45–57. [CrossRef] [PubMed]

47. You, F.; Eames, B.F.; Chen, X. Application of Extrusion-Based hydrogel Bioprinting for Cartilage Tissue Engineering. *Int. J. Mol. Sci.* **2017**, *18*, 1597. [CrossRef] [PubMed]

48. Abbadessa, A.; Blokzijl, M.M.; Mouser, V.H.; Marica, P.; Malda, J.; Hennink, W.E.; Vermonden, T. A thermo-responsive and photo-polymerizable chondroitin sulfate-based hydrogel for 3D printing applications. *Carbohydr. Polym.* **2016**, *149*, 163–174. [CrossRef] [PubMed]

49. Borovjagin, A.V.; Ogle, B.M.; Berry, J.L.; Zhang, J. From Microscale Devices to 3D Printing: Advances in Fabrication of 3D Cardiovascular Tissues. *Circ. Res.* **2017**, *120*, 150–165. [CrossRef] [PubMed]

50. Duan, B. State-of-the-Art Review of 3D Bioprinting for Cardiovascular Tissue Engineering. *Ann. Biomed. Eng.* **2017**, *45*, 195–209. [CrossRef]

51. Richards, D.; Jia, J.; Yost, M.; Markwald, R.; Mei, Y. 3D Bioprinting for Vascularized Tissue Fabrication. *Ann. Biomed. Eng.* **2017**, *45*, 132–147. [CrossRef] [PubMed]

52. Ikegami, T.; Maehara, Y. Transplantation: 3D printing of the liver in living donor liver transplantation. *Nat. Rev. Gastroenterol. Hepatol.* **2013**, *10*, 697–698. [CrossRef] [PubMed]

53. Albanna, M.; Binder, K.W.; Murphy, S.V.; Kim, J.; Qasem, S.A.; Zhao, W.; Tan, J.; El Amin, I.B.; Dice, D.; Marco, J.; et al. Situ Bioprinting Autologous Ski. Cells Accel. Wound Heal. Extensive Excisional Full-Thick. *Wounds. Sci. Rep.* **2019**, *9*, 1856. [CrossRef]

54. Baltazar, T.T.n.; Merola, J.J.; Catarino, C.C.; Xie, C.B.C.; Kirkiles Smith, N.C.N.; Lee, V.V.; Hotta, S.S.; Dai, G.G.; Xu, X.X.; Ferreira, F.C.F.; et al. Three Dimensional Bioprinting of a Vascularized and Perfusable Skin Graft Using Human Keratinocytes, Fibroblasts, Pericytes, and Endothelial Cells. *Tissue Eng. Part A* **2020**, *26*, 227–238. [CrossRef] [PubMed]

55. Cubo, N.; Garcia, M.; Del Canizo, J.F.; Velasco, D.; Jorcano, J.L. 3D bioprinting of functional human skin: Production and in vivo analysis. *Biofabrication* **2016**, *9*, 015006. [CrossRef] [PubMed]

56. Derr, K.K.; Zou, J.J.; Luo, K.K.; Song, M.J.M.; Sittampalam, G.S.M.; Zhou, C.C.; Michael, S.S.; Ferrer, M.M.; Derr, P.P. Fully Three-Dimensional Bioprinted Skin Equivalent Constructs with Validated Morphology and Barrier Function. *Tissue Eng. Part C Methods* **2019**, *25*, 334–343. [CrossRef] [PubMed]

57. Kim, B.S.; Kwon, Y.W.; Kong, J.S.; Park, G.T.; Gao, G.; Han, W.; Kim, M.B.; Lee, H.; Kim, J.H.; Cho, D.W. 3D cell printing of in vitro stabilized skin model and in vivo pre-vascularized skin patch using tissue-specific extracellular matrix bioink: A step towards advanced skin tissue engineering. *Biomaterials* **2018**, *168*, 38–53. [CrossRef]

58. Pourchet, L.J.; Thepot, A.; Albouy, M.; Courtial, E.J.; Boher, A.; Blum, L.J.; Marquette, C.A. Human Skin 3D Bioprinting Using Scaffold-Free Approach. *Adv. Healthc. Mater.* **2017**, *6*, 1601101. [CrossRef]

59. Rimann, M.; Bono, E.; Annaheim, H.; Bleisch, M.; Graf-Hausner, U. Standardized 3D Bioprinting of Soft Tissue Models with Human Primary Cells. *J. Lab. Autom.* **2016**, *21*, 496–509. [CrossRef]

60. Schon, B.S.; Hooper, G.J.; Woodfield, T.B. Modular Tissue Assembly Strategies for Biofabrication of Engineered Cartilage. *Ann. Biomed. Eng.* **2017**, *45*, 100–114. [CrossRef]

61. Visk, D. Will Advances in preclinical In Vitro modeels Lower the Costs of Drug Development? *Appl. In Vitro Toxicol.* **2015**, *1*, 79–82. [CrossRef]

62. Liaw, C.Y.; Guvendiren, M. Current and emerging applications of 3D printing in medicine. *Biofabrication* **2017**, *9*, 024102. [CrossRef] [PubMed]

63. Pedde, R.D.; Mirani, B.; Navaei, A.; Styan, T.; Wong, S.; Mehrali, M.; Thakur, A.; Mohtaram, N.K.; Bayati, A.; Dolatshahi-Pirouz, A.; et al. Emerging Biofabrication Strategies for Engineering Complex Tissue Constructs. *Adv. Mater.* **2017**, *29*, 1606061. [CrossRef] [PubMed]

64. Dawood, A.; Marti Marti, B.; Sauret-Jackson, V.; Darwood, A. 3D printing in dentistry. *Br. Dent. J.* **2015**, *219*, 521–529. [CrossRef]

65. Van Noort, R. The future of dental devices is digital. *Dent. Mater.* **2012**, *28*, 3–12. [CrossRef] [PubMed]

66. Shah, P.; Chong, B.S. 3D imaging, 3D printing and 3D virtual planning in endodontics. *Clin. Oral Investig.* **2018**, *22*, 641–654. [CrossRef] [PubMed]

67. Patzelt, A.; Patzelt, S. *The Virtual Patient*, 1st ed.; Wiley-Blackwell: Oxford, UK, 2015.

68. Rhienmora, P.; Haddawy, P.; Dailey, M.N.; Khanal, P.; Suebnukarn, S. Development of a dental skills training simulator using virtual reality and Haptic device. *Nectec. Tech. J.* **2008**, *8*, 140–147.

69. Jheon, A.H.; Oberoi, S.; Solem, R.C.; Kapila, S. Moving towards precision orthodontics: An evolving paradigm shift in the planning and delivery of customized orthodontic therapy. *Orthod. Craniofacial Res.* **2017**, *20*, 106–113. [CrossRef]

70. Anderson, J.; Wealleans, J.; Ray, J. Endodontic applications of 3D printing. *Int. Endod. J.* **2018**. [CrossRef]

71. Verweij, J.P.; Jongkees, F.A.; Anssari Moin, D.; Wismeijer, D.; van Merkesteyn, J.P.R. Autotransplantation of teeth using computer-aided rapid prototyping of a three-dimensional replica of the donor tooth: A systematic literature review. *Int. J. Oral Maxillofac. Surg.* **2017**, *46*, 1466–1474. [CrossRef]

72. Nassri, M.R.; Carlik, J.; da Silva, C.R.; Okagawa, R.E.; Lin, S. Critical analysis of artificial teeth for endodontic teaching. *J. Appl. Oral Sci.* **2008**, *16*, 43–49. [CrossRef]

73. Spenst, A.; Kahn, H. The use of a plastic block for teaching root canal instrumentation and obturation. *J. Endod.* **1979**, *5*, 282–284. [CrossRef]

74. Kfir, A.; Telishevsky-Strauss, Y.; Leitner, A.; Metzger, Z. The diagnosis and conservative treatment of a complex type 3 dens invaginatus using cone beam computed tomography (CBCT) and 3D plastic models. *Int. Endod. J.* **2013**, *46*, 275–288. [CrossRef] [PubMed]

75. Rengier, F.; Mehndiratta, A.; von Tengg-Kobligk, H.; Zechmann, C.M.; Unterhinninghofen, R.; Kauczor, H.U.; Giesel, F.L. 3D printing based on imaging data: Review of medical applications. *Int. J. Comput. Assist. Radiol. Surg.* **2010**, *5*, 335–341. [CrossRef]

76. Ishida, K.; Murofushi, M.; Nakao, K.; Morita, R.; Ogawa, M.; Tsuji, T. The regulation of tooth morphogenesis is associated with epithelial cell proliferation and the expression of Sonic hedgehog through epithelial-mesenchymal interactions. *Biochem. Biophys. Res. Commun.* **2011**, *405*, 455–461. [CrossRef] [PubMed]

77. Nakao, K.; Morita, R.; Saji, Y.; Ishida, K.; Tomita, Y.; Ogawa, M.; Saitoh, M.; Tomooka, Y.; Tsuji, T. The development of a bioengineered organ germ method. *Nat. Methods* **2007**, *4*, 227–230. [CrossRef] [PubMed]

78. Ikeda, E.; Morita, R.; Nakao, K.; Ishida, K.; Nakamura, T.; Takano-Yamamoto, T.; Ogawa, M.; Mizuno, M.; Kasugai, S.; Tsuji, T. Fully functional bioengineered tooth replacement as an organ replacement therapy. *Proc. Natl. Acad. Sci. USA* **2009**, *106*, 13475–13480. [CrossRef]

79. Zhang, W.; Ahluwalia, I.P.; Yelick, P.C. Three dimensional dental epithelial-mesenchymal constructs of predetermined size and shape for tooth regeneration. *Biomaterials* **2010**, *31*, 7995–8003. [CrossRef]

80. Lindhe, J.; Karring, T.; Araujo, M. Anatomy of Periodontal Tissue. In *Clinical Periodontology and Implant Dentistry*; Lang, P.N., Lindhe, J., Eds.; John Wiley & Sons: Oxford, UK, 2015; pp. 1–46.

81. Oshima, M.; Mizuno, M.; Imamura, A.; Ogawa, M.; Yasukawa, M.; Yamazaki, H.; Morita, R.; Ikeda, E.; Nakao, K.; Takano-Yamamoto, T.; et al. Functional tooth regeneration using a bioengineered tooth unit as a mature organ replacement regenerative therapy. *PLoS ONE* **2011**, *6*, e21531. [CrossRef]

82. Ericsson, I. Biology and Pathology of Peri-Implant Soft Tissues. In *Optimal Implant Positioning & Soft Tissue Management for the Branemark System*; Palacci, P., Ericsson, I., Engstrand, P., Rongert, B., Eds.; Quintessence Pub Co: Chicago, IL, USA, 1995.

83. Nagatomo, K.; Komaki, M.; Sekiya, I.; Sakaguchi, Y.; Noguchi, K.; Oda, S.; Muneta, T.; Ishikawa, I. Stem cell properties of human periodontal ligament cells. *J. Periodontal Res.* **2006**, *41*, 303–310. [CrossRef]

84. Seo, B.M.; Miura, M.; Gronthos, S.; Bartold, P.M.; Batouli, S.; Brahim, J.; Young, M.; Robey, P.G.; Wang, C.Y.; Shi, S. Investigation of multipotent postnatal stem cells from human periodontal ligament. *Lancet* **2004**, *364*, 149–155. [CrossRef]

85. Okano, T.; Yamada, N.; Sakai, H.; Sakurai, Y. A novel recovery system for cultured cells using plasma-treated polystyrene dishes grafted with poly (N-isopropylacrylamide). *J. Biomed. Mater. Res.* **1993**, *27*, 1243–1251. [CrossRef] [PubMed]

86. Akizuki, T.; Oda, S.; Komaki, M.; Tsuchioka, H.; Kawakatsu, N.; Kikuchi, A.; Yamato, M.; Okano, T.; Ishikawa, I. Application of periodontal ligament cell sheet for periodontal regeneration: A pilot study in beagle dogs. *J. Periodontal Res.* **2005**, *40*, 245–251. [CrossRef] [PubMed]

87. Flores, M.G.; Yashiro, R.; Washio, K.; Yamato, M.; Okano, T.; Ishikawa, I. Periodontal ligament cell sheet promotes periodontal regeneration in athymic rats. *J. Clin. Periodontol.* **2008**, *35*, 1066–1072. [CrossRef] [PubMed]

88. Hasegawa, M.; Yamato, M.; Kikuchi, A.; Okano, T.; Ishikawa, I. Human periodontal ligament cell sheets can regenerate periodontal ligament tissue in an athymic rat model. *Tissue Eng.* **2005**, *11*, 469–478. [CrossRef] [PubMed]

89. Iwata, T.; Washio, K.; Yoshida, T.; Ishikawa, I.; Ando, T.; Yamato, M.; Okano, T. Cell sheet engineering and its application for periodontal regeneration. *J. Tissue Eng. Regen. Med.* **2015**, *9*, 343–356. [CrossRef] [PubMed]

90. Iwata, T.; Yamato, M.; Tsuchioka, H.; Takagi, R.; Mukobata, S.; Washio, K.; Okano, T.; Ishikawa, I. Periodontal regeneration with multi-layered periodontal ligament-derived cell sheets in a canine model. *Biomaterials* **2009**, *30*, 2716–2723. [CrossRef]

91. Tsumanuma, Y.; Iwata, T.; Washio, K.; Yoshida, T.; Yamada, A.; Takagi, R.; Ohno, T.; Lin, K.; Yamato, M.; Ishikawa, I.; et al. Comparison of different tissue-derived stem cell sheets for periodontal regeneration in a canine 1-wall defect model. *Biomaterials* **2011**, *32*, 5819–5825. [CrossRef]

92. Fujita, H.; Shimizu, K.; Nagamori, E. Application of a cell sheet-polymer film complex with temperature sensitivity for increased mechanical strength and cell alignment capability. *Biotechnol. Bioeng.* **2009**, *103*, 370–377. [CrossRef]

93. Dan, H.; Vaquette, C.; Fisher, A.G.; Hamlet, S.M.; Xiao, Y.; Hutmacher, D.W.; Ivanovski, S. The influence of cellular source on periodontal regeneration using calcium phosphate coated polycaprolactone scaffold supported cell sheets. *Biomaterials* **2014**, *35*, 113–122. [CrossRef]

94. Farag, A.; Vaquette, C.; Theodoropoulos, C.; Hamlet, S.M.; Hutmacher, D.W.; Ivanovski, S. Decellularized periodontal ligament cell sheets with recellularization potential. *J. Dent. Res.* **2014**, *93*, 1313–1319. [CrossRef]

95. Washio, K.; Tsutsumi, Y.; Tsumanuma, Y.; Yano, K.; Srithanyarat, S.S.; Takagi, R.; Ichinose, S.; Meinzer, W.; Yamato, M.; Okano, T.; et al. In Vivo Periodontium Formation Around Titanium Implants Using Periodontal Ligament Cell Sheet. *Tissue Eng. Part A* **2018**. [CrossRef] [PubMed]

96. Schroeder, H.E.; Listgarten, M.A. The gingival tissues: The architecture of periodontal protection. *Periodontology 2000* **1997**, *13*, 91–120. [CrossRef]

97. Vaquette, C.; Pilipchuk, S.P.; Bartold, P.M.; Hutmacher, D.W.; Giannobile, W.V.; Ivanovski, S. Tissue Engineered Constructs for Periodontal Regeneration: Current Status and Future Perspectives. *Adv. Healthc. Mater.* **2018**, *7*, e1800457. [CrossRef] [PubMed]

98. Park, C.H.; Rios, H.F.; Jin, Q.; Bland, M.E.; Flanagan, C.L.; Hollister, S.J.; Giannobile, W.V. Biomimetic hybrid scaffolds for engineering human tooth-ligament interfaces. *Biomaterials* **2010**, *31*, 5945–5952. [CrossRef]

99. Park, C.H.; Rios, H.F.; Jin, Q.; Sugai, J.V.; Padial-Molina, M.; Taut, A.D.; Flanagan, C.L.; Hollister, S.J.; Giannobile, W.V. Tissue engineering bone-ligament complexes using fiber-guiding scaffolds. *Biomaterials* **2012**, *33*, 137–145. [CrossRef] [PubMed]

100. Park, C.H.; Rios, H.F.; Taut, A.D.; Padial-Molina, M.; Flanagan, C.L.; Pilipchuk, S.P.; Hollister, S.J.; Giannobile, W.V. Image-based, fiber guiding scaffolds: A platform for regenerating tissue interfaces. *Tissue Eng. Part C Methods* **2014**, *20*, 533–542. [CrossRef]

101. Rasperini, G.; Pilipchuk, S.P.; Flanagan, C.L.; Park, C.H.; Pagni, G.; Hollister, S.J.; Giannobile, W.V. 3D-printed Bioresorbable Scaffold for Periodontal Repair. *J. Dent. Res.* **2015**, *94*, 153S–157S. [CrossRef] [PubMed]

102. Pilipchuk, S.P.; Monje, A.; Jiao, Y.; Hao, J.; Kruger, L.; Flanagan, C.L.; Hollister, S.J.; Giannobile, W.V. Integration of 3D Printed and Micropatterned Polycaprolactone Scaffolds for Guidance of Oriented Collagenous Tissue Formation In Vivo. *Adv. Healthc. Mater.* **2016**, *5*, 676–687. [CrossRef]

103. Lee, C.H.; Hajibandeh, J.; Suzuki, T.; Fan, A.; Shang, P.; Mao, J.J. Three-dimensional printed multiphase scaffolds for regeneration of periodontium complex. *Tissue Eng. Part A* **2014**, *20*, 1342–1351. [CrossRef]

104. Guvendiren, M.; Molde, J.; Soares, R.M.; Kohn, J. Designing Biomaterials for 3D Printing. *ACS Biomater. Sci. Eng.* **2016**, *2*, 1679–1693. [CrossRef]

105. Polo-Corrales, L.; Latorre-Esteves, M.; Ramirez-Vick, J.E. Scaffold design for bone regeneration. *J. Nanosci. Nanotechnol.* **2014**, *14*, 15–56. [CrossRef]

106. Fahmy, M.D.; Jazayeri, H.E.; Razavi, M.; Masri, R.; Tayebi, L. Three-Dimensional Bioprinting Materials with Potential Application in Preprosthetic Surgery. *J. Prosthodont. Off. J. Am. Coll. Prosthodont.* **2016**, *25*, 310–318. [CrossRef] [PubMed]

107. Ceccarelli, G.; Presta, R.; Benedetti, L.; Cusella De Angelis, M.G.; Lupi, S.M.; Rodriguez, Y.B.R. Emerging Perspectives in Scaffold for Tissue Engineering in Oral Surgery. *Stem Cells Int.* **2017**, *2017*, 4585401. [CrossRef] [PubMed]

108. Tayebi, L.; Rasoulianboroujeni, M.; Moharamzadeh, K.; Almela, T.K.D.; Cui, Z.; Ye, H. 3D-printed membrane for guided tissue regeneration. *Mater. Sci. Eng. C Mater. Biol. Appl.* **2018**, *84*, 148–158. [CrossRef]

109. Choi, G.; Cha, H.J. Recent advances in the development of nature-derived photocrosslinkable biomaterials for 3D printing in tissue engineering. *Biomater. Res.* **2019**, *23*, 18. [CrossRef]

110. Hospodiuk, M.; Dey, M.; Sosnoski, D.; Ozbolat, I.T. The bioink: A comprehensive review on bioprintable materials. *Biotechnol. Adv.* **2017**, *35*, 217–239. [CrossRef] [PubMed]

111. De Ruijter, M.; Ribeiro, A.; Dokter, I.; Castilho, M.; Malda, J. Simultaneous Micropatterning of Fibrous Meshes and Bioinks for the Fabrication of Living Tissue Constructs. *Adv. Healthc. Mater.* **2018**, *8*, e1800418. [CrossRef] [PubMed]

112. Wang, P.; Berry, D.; Moran, A.; He, F.; Tam, T.; Chen, L.; Chen, S. Controlled Growth Factor Release in 3D-Printed Hydrogels. *Adv. Healthc. Mater.* **2019**, e1900977. [CrossRef]

113. Han, W.; Singh, N.K.; Kim, J.J.; Kim, H.; Kim, B.S.; Park, J.Y.; Jang, J.; Cho, D.W. Directed differential behaviors of multipotent adult stem cells from decellularized tissue/organ extracellular matrix bioinks. *Biomaterials* **2019**, *224*, 119496. [CrossRef]

114. Dzobo, K.; Motaung, K.S.; Adesida, A. Recent Trends in Decellularized Extracellular Matrix Bioinks for 3D Printing: An Updated Review. *Int. J. Mol. Sci.* **2019**, *18*, 4628. [CrossRef]

115. Kim, B.S.; Kim, H.; Gao, G.; Jang, J.; Cho, D.W. Decellularized extracellular matrix: A step towards the next generation source for bioink manufacturing. *Biofabrication* **2017**, *9*, 034104. [CrossRef]

116. Presland, R.B.; Boggess, D.; Lewis, S.P.; Hull, C.; Fleckman, P.; Sundberg, J.P. Loss of normal profilaggrin and filaggrin in flaky tail (ft/ft) mice: An animal model for the filaggrin-deficient skin disease ichthyosis vulgaris. *J. Investig. Dermatol.* **2000**, *115*, 1072–1081. [CrossRef] [PubMed]

117. Thoma, D.S.; Benic, G.I.; Zwahlen, M.; Hammerle, C.H.; Jung, R.E. A systematic review assessing soft tissue augmentation techniques. *Clin. Oral Implant. Res.* **2009**, *20*, 146–165. [CrossRef] [PubMed]

118. Thoma, D.S.; Naenni, N.; Figuero, E.; Hammerle, C.H.; Schwarz, F.; Jung, R.E.; Sanz Sanchez, I. Effects of soft tissue augmentation procedures on peri-implant health or disease: A systematic review and meta-analysis. *Clin. Oral Implant. Res.* **2018**, *29*, 32–49. [CrossRef]

119. Thoma, D.S.; Buranawat, B.; Hammerle, C.H.; Held, U.; Jung, R.E. Efficacy of soft tissue augmentation around dental implants and in partially edentulous areas: A systematic review. *J. Clin. Periodontol.* **2014**, *41* (Suppl. 15), S77–S91. [CrossRef]

120. Benninger, B.; Andrews, K.; Carter, W. Clinical measurements of hard palate and implications for subepithelial connective tissue grafts with suggestions for palatal nomenclature. *J. Oral Maxillofac. Surg.* **2012**, *70*, 149–153. [CrossRef] [PubMed]

121. Del Pizzo, M.; Modica, F.; Bethaz, N.; Priotto, P.; Romagnoli, R. The connective tissue graft: A comparative clinical evaluation of wound healing at the palatal donor site: A preliminary study. *J. Clin. Periodontol.* **2002**, *29*, 848–854. [CrossRef] [PubMed]

122. Griffin, T.J.; Cheung, W.S.; Zavras, A.I.; Damoulis, P.D. Postoperative complications following gingival augmentation procedures. *J. Periodontol.* **2006**, *77*, 2070–2079. [CrossRef]

123. Soileau, K.M.; Brannon, R.B. A histologic evaluation of various stages of palatal healing following subepithelial connective tissue grafting procedures: A comparison of eight cases. *J. Periodontol.* **2006**, *77*, 1267–1273. [CrossRef]

124. Zucchelli, G.; Mele, M.; Stefanini, M.; Mazzotti, C.; Marzadori, M.; Montebugnoli, L.; de Sanctis, M. Patient morbidity and root coverage outcome after subepithelial connective tissue and de-epithelialized grafts: A comparative randomized-controlled clinical trial. *J. Clin. Periodontol.* **2010**, *37*, 728–738. [CrossRef]

125. Vignoletti, F.; Nunez, J.; Sanz, M. Soft tissue wound healing at teeth, dental implants and the edentulous ridge when using barrier membranes, growth and differentiation factors and soft tissue substitutes. *J. Clin. Periodontol.* **2014**, *41*, S23–S35. [CrossRef] [PubMed]

126. Zuhr, O.; Baumer, D.; Hurzeler, M. The addition of soft tissue replacement grafts in plastic periodontal and implant surgery: Critical elements in design and execution. *J. Clin. Periodontol.* **2014**, *41*, S123–S142. [CrossRef]

127. Yukna, R.A.; Sullivan, W.M. Evaluation of resultant tissue type following the intraoral transplantation of various lyophilized soft tissues. *J. Periodontal Res.* **1978**, *13*, 177–184. [CrossRef]

128. Wainwright, D.J. Use of an acellular allograft dermal matrix (AlloDerm) in the management of full-thickness burns. *Burns* **1995**, *21*, 243–248. [CrossRef]

129. Aichelmann-Reidy, M.E.; Yukna, R.A.; Evans, G.H.; Nasr, H.F.; Mayer, E.T. Clinical evaluation of acellular allograft dermis for the treatment of human gingival recession. *J. Periodontol.* **2001**, *72*, 998–1005. [CrossRef]

130. Batista, E.L., Jr.; Batista, F.C.; Novaes, A.B., Jr. Management of soft tissue ridge deformities with acellular dermal matrix. Clinical approach and outcome after 6 months of treatment. *J. Periodontol.* **2001**, *72*, 265–273. [CrossRef] [PubMed]

131. Harris, R.J. Root coverage in molar recession: Report of 50 consecutive cases treated with subepithelial connective tissue grafts. *J. Periodontol.* **2003**, *74*, 703–708. [CrossRef] [PubMed]

132. Wei, P.C.; Laurell, L.; Geivelis, M.; Lingen, M.W.; Maddalozzo, D. Acellular dermal matrix allografts to achieve increased attached gingiva. Part 1: A clinical study. *J. Periodontol.* **2000**, *71*, 1297–1305. [CrossRef] [PubMed]

133. Wei, P.C.; Laurell, L.; Lingen, M.W.; Geivelis, M. Acellular dermal matrix allografts to achieve increased attached gingiva. Part 2: A histological comparative study. *J. Periodontol.* **2002**, *73*, 257–265. [CrossRef]

134. Lee, K.H.; Kim, B.O.; Jang, H.S. Clinical evaluation of a collagen matrix to enhance the width of keratinized gingiva around dental implants. *J. Periodontal Implant Sci.* **2010**, *40*, 96–101. [CrossRef]

135. Maiorana, C.; Beretta, M.; Pivetti, L.; Stoffella, E.; Grossi, G.B.; Herford, A.S. Use of a Collagen Matrix as a Substitute for Free Mucosal Grafts in Pre-Prosthetic Surgery: 1 Year Results From a Clinical Prospective Study on 15 Patients. *Open Dent. J.* **2016**, *10*, 395–410. [CrossRef] [PubMed]

136. McGuire, M.K.; Scheyer, E.T. Xenogeneic collagen matrix with coronally advanced flap compared to connective tissue with coronally advanced flap for the treatment of dehiscence-type recession defects. *J. Periodontol.* **2010**, *81*, 1108–1117. [CrossRef] [PubMed]

137. Nevins, M.; Nevins, M.L.; Kim, S.W.; Schupbach, P.; Kim, D.M. The use of mucograft collagen matrix to augment the zone of keratinized tissue around teeth: A pilot study. *Int. J. Periodontics Restor. Dent.* **2011**, *31*, 367–373.

138. Vignoletti, F.; Nunez, J.; Discepoli, N.; De Sanctis, F.; Caffesse, R.; Munoz, F.; Lopez, M.; Sanz, M. Clinical and histological healing of a new collagen matrix in combination with the coronally advanced flap for the treatment of Miller class-I recession defects: An experimental study in the minipig. *J. Clin. Periodontol.* **2011**, *38*, 847–855. [CrossRef] [PubMed]

139. Froum, S.J.; Khouly, I.; Tarnow, D.P.; Froum, S.; Rosenberg, E.; Corby, P.; Kye, W.; Elian, N.; Schoor, R.; Cho, S.C. The use of a xenogeneic collagen matrix at the time of implant placement to increase the volume of buccal soft tissue. *Int. J. Periodontics Restor. Dent.* **2015**, *35*, 179–189. [CrossRef]

140. Lorenzo, R.; Garcia, V.; Orsini, M.; Martin, C.; Sanz, M. Clinical efficacy of a xenogeneic collagen matrix in augmenting keratinized mucosa around implants: A randomized controlled prospective clinical trial. *Clin. Oral Implant. Res.* **2012**, *23*, 316–324. [CrossRef]

141. Sanz, M.; Lorenzo, R.; Aranda, J.J.; Martin, C.; Orsini, M. Clinical evaluation of a new collagen matrix (Mucograft prototype) to enhance the width of keratinized tissue in patients with fixed prosthetic restorations: A randomized prospective clinical trial. *J. Clin. Periodontol.* **2009**, *36*, 868–876. [CrossRef]

142. Schmitt, C.M.; Moest, T.; Lutz, R.; Wehrhan, F.; Neukam, F.W.; Schlegel, K.A. Long-term outcomes after vestibuloplasty with a porcine collagen matrix (Mucograft®) versus the free gingival graft: A comparative prospective clinical trial. *Clin. Oral Implant. Res.* **2016**, *27*, e125–e133. [CrossRef]

143. Nocini, P.F.; Castellani, R.; Zanotti, G.; Gelpi, F.; Covani, U.; Marconcini, S.; de Santis, D. Extensive keratinized tissue augmentation during implant rehabilitation after Le Fort I osteotomy: Using a new porcine collagen membrane (Mucoderm). *J. Craniofacial Surg.* **2014**, *25*, 799–803. [CrossRef]

144. Chappuis, V.; Shahim, K.; Buser, R.; Koller, E.; Joda, T.; Reyes, M.; Buser, D. Novel Collagen Matrix to Increase Tissue Thickness Simultaneous with Guided Bone Regeneration and Implant Placement in Esthetic Implant Sites: A Feasibility Study. *Int. J. Periodontics Restor. Dent.* **2018**, *38*, 575–582. [CrossRef]

145. Thoma, D.S.; Zeltner, M.; Hilbe, M.; Hammerle, C.H.; Husler, J.; Jung, R.E. Randomized controlled clinical study evaluating effectiveness and safety of a volume-stable collagen matrix compared to autogenous connective tissue grafts for soft tissue augmentation at implant sites. *J. Clin. Periodontol.* **2016**, *43*, 874–885. [CrossRef] [PubMed]

146. Thoma, D.S.; Gasser, T.J.; Jung, R.E.; Hammerle, C.H. Randomized controlled clinical trial comparing implant sites augmented with a volume-stable collagen matrix or an autogenous connective tissue graft: 3-year data after insertion of reconstructions. *J. Clin. Periodontol.* **2020**, *47*, 630–639. [CrossRef] [PubMed]

147. Marx, R.E.; Carlson, E.R.; Eichstaedt, R.M.; Schimmele, S.R.; Strauss, J.E.; Georgeff, K.R. Platelet-rich plasma: Growth factor enhancement for bone grafts. *Oral Surg. Oral Med. Oral Pathol. Oral Radiol. Endod.* **1998**, *85*, 638–646. [CrossRef]

148. Whitman, D.H.; Berry, R.L.; Green, D.M. Platelet gel: An autologous alternative to fibrin glue with applications in oral and maxillofacial surgery. *J. Oral Maxillofac. Surg.* **1997**, *55*, 1294–1299. [CrossRef]

149. Knighton, D.R.; Ciresi, K.F.; Fiegel, V.D.; Austin, L.L.; Butler, E.L. Classification and treatment of chronic nonhealing wounds. Successful treatment with autologous platelet-derived wound healing factors. *Ann. Surg.* **1986**, *204*, 322–330. [CrossRef] [PubMed]

150. Dohan, D.M.; Choukroun, J.; Diss, A.; Dohan, S.L.; Dohan, A.J.; Mouhyi, J.; Gogly, B. Platelet-rich fibrin (PRF): A second-generation platelet concentrate. Part I: Technological concepts and evolution. *Oral Surg. Oral Med. Oral Pathol. Oral Radiol. Endod.* **2006**, *101*, e37–e44. [CrossRef]

151. Kobayashi, E.; Fluckiger, L.; Fujioka-Kobayashi, M.; Sawada, K.; Sculean, A.; Schaller, B.; Miron, R.J. Comparative release of growth factors from PRP, PRF, and advanced-PRF. *Clin. Oral Investig.* **2016**, *20*, 2353–2360. [CrossRef]

152. Schaer, M.O.; Diaz-Romero, J.; Kohl, S.; Zumstein, M.A.; Nesic, D. Platelet-rich concentrates differentially release growth factors and induce cell migration in vitro. *Clin. Orthop. Relat. Res.* **2015**, *473*, 1635–1643. [CrossRef]

153. Miron, R.J.; Fujioka-Kobayashi, M.; Bishara, M.; Zhang, Y.; Hernandez, M.; Choukroun, J. Platelet-Rich Fibrin and Soft Tissue Wound Healing: A Systematic Review. *Tissue Eng. Part B Rev.* **2017**, *23*, 83–99. [CrossRef]

154. Ghanaati, S.; Booms, P.; Orlowska, A.; Kubesch, A.; Lorenz, J.; Rutkowski, J.; Landes, C.; Sader, R.; Kirkpatrick, C.; Choukroun, J. Advanced platelet-rich fibrin: A new concept for cell-based tissue engineering by means of inflammatory cells. *J. Oral Implantol.* **2014**, *40*, 679–689. [CrossRef]

155. Fujioka-Kobayashi, M.; Miron, R.J.; Hernandez, M.; Kandalam, U.; Zhang, Y.; Choukroun, J. Optimized Platelet-Rich Fibrin with the Low-Speed Concept: Growth Factor Release, Biocompatibility, and Cellular Response. *J. Periodontol.* **2017**, *88*, 112–121. [CrossRef] [PubMed]

156. Choukroun, J.; Ghanaati, S. Reduction of relative centrifugation force within injectable platelet-rich-fibrin (PRF) concentrates advances patients' own inflammatory cells, platelets and growth factors: The first introduction to the low speed centrifugation concept. *Eur. J. Trauma Emerg. Surg.* **2018**, *44*, 87–95. [CrossRef] [PubMed]

157. Wend, S.; Kubesch, A.; Orlowska, A.; Al-Maawi, S.; Zender, N.; Dias, A.; Miron, R.J.; Sader, R.; Booms, P.; Kirkpatrick, C.J.; et al. Reduction of the relative centrifugal force influences cell number and growth factor release within injectable PRF-based matrices. *J. Mater. Sci. Mater. Med.* **2017**, *28*, 188. [CrossRef]

158. Miron, R.J.; Zucchelli, G.; Pikos, M.A.; Salama, M.; Lee, S.; Guillemette, V.; Fujioka-Kobayashi, M.; Bishara, M.; Zhang, Y.; Wang, H.-L.; et al. Use of platelet-rich fibrin in regenerative dentistry: A systematic review. *Clin. Oral Investig.* **2017**, *21*, 1913–1927. [CrossRef] [PubMed]

159. Ghanaati, S.; Herrera-Vizcaino, C.; Al-Maawi, S.; Lorenz, J.; Miron, R.J.; Nelson, K.; Schwarz, F.; Choukroun, J.; Sader, R. Fifteen years of platelet rich fibrin (PRF) in dentistry and oromaxillofacial surgery: How high is the level of scientific evidence? *J. Oral Implantol.* **2018**. [CrossRef]

160. Marzadori, M.S.M.; Mazzotti, C.; Ganz, S.; Sharma, P.; Zucchelli, G. Soft-tissue augmentation procedures in edentulous esthetic areas. *Periodontology 2000* **2018**, *77*, 111–122. [CrossRef]

161. Sanz-Martin, I.; Sailer, I.; Hammerle, C.H.; Thoma, D.S. Soft tissue stability and volumetric changes after 5 years in pontic sites with or without soft tissue grafting: A retrospective cohort study. *Clin. Oral Implant. Res.* **2016**, *27*, 969–974. [CrossRef]

162. Thoma, D.S.; Jung, R.E.; Schneider, D.; Cochran, D.L.; Ender, A.; Jones, A.A.; Gorlach, C.; Uebersax, L.; Graf-Hausner, U.; Hammerle, C.H. Soft tissue volume augmentation by the use of collagen-based matrices: A volumetric analysis. *J. Clin. Periodontol.* **2010**, *37*, 659–666. [CrossRef]

163. Rheinwald, J.G.; Green, H. Serial cultivation of strains of human epidermal keratinocytes: The formation of keratinizing colonies from single cells. *Cell* **1975**, *6*, 331–343. [CrossRef]

164. Ueda, M.; Ebata, K.; Kaneda, T. In vitro fabrication of bioartificial mucosa for reconstruction of oral mucosa: Basic research and clinical application. *Ann. Plast. Surg.* **1991**, *27*, 540–549. [CrossRef]

165. Moharamzadeh, K.; Brook, I.M.; Van Noort, R.; Scutt, A.M.; Thornhill, M.H. Tissue-engineered oral mucosa: A review of the scientific literature. *J. Dent. Res.* **2007**, *86*, 115–124. [CrossRef] [PubMed]

166. Smits, J.P.H.; Niehues, H.; Rikken, G.; van Vlijmen-Willems, I.; van de Zande, G.; Zeeuwen, P.; Schalkwijk, J.; van den Bogaard, E.H. Immortalized N/TERT keratinocytes as an alternative cell source in 3D human epidermal models. *Sci. Rep.* **2017**, *7*, 11838. [CrossRef] [PubMed]

167. Buskermolen, J.K.; Reijnders, C.M.; Spiekstra, S.W.; Steinberg, T.; Kleverlaan, C.J.; Feilzer, A.J.; Bakker, A.D.; Gibbs, S. Development of a Full-Thickness Human Gingiva Equivalent Constructed from Immortalized Keratinocytes and Fibroblasts. *Tissue Eng. Part C Methods* **2016**, *22*, 781–791. [CrossRef] [PubMed]

168. Moharamzadeh, K.; Colley, H.; Murdoch, C.; Hearnden, V.; Chai, W.L.; Brook, I.M.; Thornhill, M.H.; Macneil, S. Tissue-engineered oral mucosa. *J. Dent. Res.* **2012**, *91*, 642–650. [CrossRef]

169. Izumi, K.; Feinberg, S.E.; Iida, A.; Yoshizawa, M. Intraoral grafting of an ex vivo produced oral mucosa equivalent: A preliminary report. *Int. J. Oral Maxillofac. Surg.* **2003**, *32*, 188–197. [CrossRef]

170. Kato, H.; Marcelo, C.L.; Washington, J.B.; Bingham, E.L.; Feinberg, S.E. Fabrication of Large Size Ex Vivo-Produced Oral Mucosal Equivalents for Clinical Application. *Tissue Eng. Part C Methods* **2015**, *21*, 872–880. [CrossRef]

171. Mohammadi, M.; Mofid, R.; Shokrgozar, M.A. Peri-implant soft tissue management through use of cultured gingival graft: A case report. *Acta Med. Iran.* **2011**, *49*, 319–324.

172. Mohammadi, M.; Shokrgozar, M.A.; Mofid, R. Culture of human gingival fibroblasts on a biodegradable scaffold and evaluation of its effect on attached gingiva: A randomized, controlled pilot study. *J. Periodontol.* **2007**, *78*, 1897–1903. [CrossRef] [PubMed]

173. De Brugerolle, A. SkinEthic Laboratories, a company devoted to develop and produce in vitro alternative methods to animal use. *Altex* **2007**, *24*, 167–171. [CrossRef]

174. Athirasala, A.; Lins, F.; Tahayeri, A.; Hinds, M.; Smith, A.J.; Sedgley, C.; Ferracane, J.; Bertassoni, L.E. A Novel Strategy to Engineer Pre-Vascularized Full-Length Dental Pulp-like Tissue Constructs. *Sci. Rep.* **2017**, *7*, 3323. [CrossRef]

2

3D Printed Temporary Veneer Restoring Autotransplanted Teeth in Children: Design and Concept Validation Ex Vivo

Ali Al-Rimawi [1,2,†], Mostafa EzEldeen [1,3,*,†] , Danilo Schneider [1], Constantinus Politis [1] and Reinhilde Jacobs [1,4]

1   OMFS IMPATH Research Group, Faculty of Medicine, Department of Imaging and Pathology, KU Leuven and Oral and Maxillofacial Surgery, University Hospitals Leuven, 3000 Leuven, Belgium; dr.alirimawi@gmail.com (A.A.-R.); drdaniloschneider@gmail.com (D.S.); constantinus.politis@uzleuven.be (C.P.); reinhilde.jacobs@uzleuven.be (R.J.)
2   Department of Dentistry, Royal Medical Services, Jordanian Armed Forces, 00962 Amman, Jordan
3   Department of Oral Health Sciences, KU Leuven and Paediatric Dentistry and Special Dental Care, University Hospitals Leuven, 3000 Leuven, Belgium
4   Department of Dental Medicine, Karolinska Institute, SE-171 77 Stockholm, Sweden
*   Correspondence: mostafa.ezeldeen@kuleuven.be
†   These authors contributed equally to this work.

Abstract: (1) Background: Three-dimensional printing is progressing rapidly and is applied in many fields of dentistry. Tooth autotransplantation offers a viable biological approach to tooth replacement in children and adolescents. Restoring or reshaping the transplanted tooth to the anterior maxilla should be done as soon as possible for psychological and aesthetic reasons. However, to avoid interfering with the natural healing process, reshaping of transplanted teeth is usually delayed three to four months after transplantation. This delay creates a need for simple indirect temporary aesthetic restoration for autotransplanted teeth. The aim of this study was to develop and validate a digital solution for temporary restoration of autotransplanted teeth using 3D printing. (2) Methods: Four dry human skulls and four dry human mandibles were scanned using cone beam computed tomography to create 3D models for 15 premolars. Digital impression of the maxillary arch of one of the skulls was captured by intra oral scanner. The digital work flow for the design and fabrication of temporary veneers is presented. The seating and adaptation of the 3D printed veneers were evaluated using stereomicroscopy and micro-computed tomography. (3) Results: Evaluation of the veneer seating using stereomicroscopy showed that the mean marginal gap at all of the sides was below the cut-off value of 200 μm. The overall mean marginal gap was 99.9 ± 50.7 μm (median: 87.8 (IQR 64.2–133 μm)). The internal adaptation evaluation using micro-computed tomography showed an average median gap thickness of 152.5 ± 47.7 (IQR 129–149.3 μm). (4) Conclusions: The present concept of using temporary veneers that are designed and fabricated with CAD/CAM (computer-aided design/computer-aided manufacturing) technology using a DLP (digital light processing) printer may present a viable treatment option for restoration of autotransplanted teeth.

Keywords: CBCT; CAD/CAM; 3D printing; DLP; tooth autotransplantation

1. Introduction

Computer-aided design/computer-aided manufacturing (CAD/CAM) use in dentistry started in the early nineties with subtractive manufacturing [1,2]. Recently, additive manufacturing technology, three dimensional (3D) printing, has been progressing rapidly and is applied in many fields of dentistry [3] such as: fabrication of surgical guides for placement of dental implants [4–7], guides for endodontic access and apical surgeries [8,9], fabrication of surgical guides and tooth replicas for tooth autotransplantation (TAT) [10–12], construction of physical models for orthodontics [13], manufacturing of dental implants [14], and study models, splints, and guides in orthognathic surgeries [15–17].

The process of 3D printing in dentistry goes through three stages, starting with data acquisition using low dose cone beam computed tomography (CBCT) [18,19] and/or intraoral scanner (IOS) [20,21], followed by processing and designing using dedicated software tools, and, finally, printing [12,22–24].

Different 3D printing technologies are being used in dentistry, which can be technically classified into: fused deposition modelling (FDM), stereolithography (SLA), PolyJet printing, MultiJet printing, ColorJet printing, selective laser sintering, and digital light processing (DLP) [3,24].

As aforementioned, CAD/CAM and 3D printing technology are already being applied in tooth autotransplantation (TAT) procedures [10,12]. TAT offers a viable biological approach to tooth replacement in children and adolescents after traumatic dental injuries (TDIs), agenesis, developmental anomalies, or specific orthodontic problems [25–29]. The treatment options available, for example implant placement, are limited by the ongoing dentoalveolar development [30], while orthodontic tooth alignment is challenging unless skeletal anchorage is applied [31,32]. TAT allows for periodontal healing and enables preservation of the alveolar ridge, maintaining the possibility of function and growth [25,33–35]. Restoring or reshaping the transplanted tooth to the anterior maxilla should be done as soon as possible for psychological and aesthetic reasons [36]. However, to avoid interfering with the natural healing process [33,37], reshaping of transplanted teeth is usually delayed three to four months after transplantation [38]. This delay creates a need for a simple indirect temporary aesthetic restoration for TAT, which so far has not yet been reported.

The aim of this study was to develop and validate a digital solution for temporary restoration of autotransplanted teeth using 3D printing technology.

2. Materials and Methods

2.1. Image Acquisition

Four dry human skulls and four dry human mandibles were scanned using a CBCT machine NewTom VGI EVO (QR Verona, Verona, Italy) Ethical Review Board of the University Hospitals Leuven (S55619 ML9535, University Hospitals Leuven). Scanning parameters were set for a standard mode, 360° rotation, 200 μm voxel size, and a field of view of 80 mm × 80 mm at 110 kV (x-ray tube voltage) and automatic tube current modulation. All data sets were exported using the Digital Imaging and Communications in Medicine (DICOM) file format with an isotropic voxel size of 200 μm and a slice interval and thickness of 200 μm.

2.2. Segmentation Protocol

CBCT scans were imported into MeVisLab (MeVis Medical Solutions AG, Bremen, Germany). Regions of interest including the single rooted first or second premolar were selected. All regions of interest images were normalized using an intensity windowing filter and then a median filter to suppress any noise and decrease confounding variables between the images.

All single rooted premolars were then segmented using a dedicated tool that was developed in MeVisLab and validated for accurate tooth/root canal space segmentation as described [39] (Figure 1A). The tool applies interactive livewire boundary extraction to create a set of orthogonal contours around the tooth of interest. Livewire allows for a semi-interactive segmentation of structures with prominent edge image features [40]. Internally, the module generates a graph representation of the image to work on; the graph's nodes represent image pixels and edges connect neighbouring pixels. The edges are weighted based on the cost function (image gradient magnitude). If starting and ending points are defined on such a graph, the shortest path (minimal cost path) is computed using dynamic programming (F * algorithm) [41]. This was followed by a variational interpolation algorithm that reconstructs the surface of an object with energy-minimizing, smooth, and implicit functions in order to create a 3D mask of the tooth surface (Figure 1A) [42].

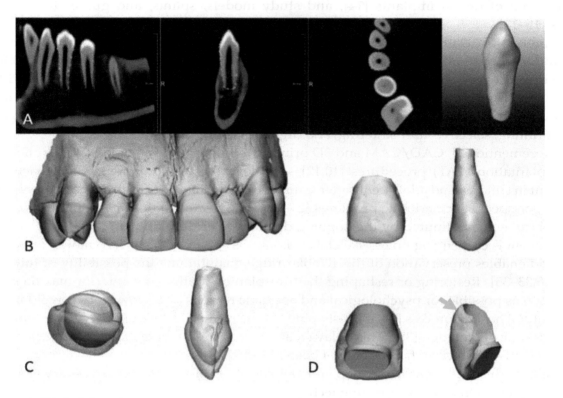

Figure 1. Digital flow for temporary veneer preparation. (**A**) Premolar segmentation; (**B**) designing temporary veneer based on the shape of the contralateral incisor (to mimic the clinical situation where one maxillary central incisor will be lost, a mirror image of the contralateral maxillary incisor was used to design the temporary veneer that will fit the transplanted premolar); (**C**) checking veneer thickness to ensure optimal printing; (**D**) final veneer design: removing undercuts, beveling the edges (green arrow), and inspecting the surface thickness is done to avoid print failure spots.

After segmentation, the 3D triangle-based surfaces of the 15 premolars (four skulls: seven premolars, four mandibles: eight premolars) were reconstructed and saved as Standard Triangle Language (STL) files.

The digital impression of the maxillary arch of one of the skulls was captured by Trios IOS (Trios® 3 Cart wired, 3Shape, Copenhagen, Denmark).

2.3. Designing of Temporary Veneers

The steps of veneer designing are illustrated in Figure 1. The digital 3D model of the maxillary central incisors was acquired using the Trios intra-oral scanner and the 3D models of the segmented premolars were imported to 3-matic version 12.0 (Materialise; Leuven, Belgium) (Figure 1B,C).

To mimic the clinical situation where one maxillary central incisor will be lost, a mirror image of the contralateral maxillary incisor was used to design the temporary veneer that will fit the transplanted premolar (Figure 1B). The crown of the central incisor was isolated from the 3D model which was created by the intra-oral scanner (Figure 1C) and was then moved to overlap the crown of the premolar. The transparency of the central incisor was then changed into medium transparency in order to control the thickness of the desired veneer during the design process (Figure 1C).

Subsequently, the 3D model of the premolar was subtracted from the 3D model of the maxillary central incisor (Figure 1D). The generated subtraction object represented the temporary veneer design; the design was further optimized and was then exported as an STL file, ready for printing (Figure 1D).

This process was repeated for the 15 3D models of the segmented premolars using the same maxillary central incisor. As a result, 15 digital models of temporary veneers were generated.

2.4. Three-Dimensional Printing of Temporary Veneers

The 3D models of the veneers and assigned premolars were exported to the Raydent studio software and were printed in a Raydent (RAM500, RayMedical, Seoul, South-Korea) DLP 3D printer. The printer utilizes liquid crystal planar solidification technology and was loaded with its specific resin material (crown and bridge resin).

The printed veneers were cleaned in an ultrasonic bath using IPA 90% (Isopropyl alcohol) to remove residual resin and were then post cured with Curing Unit (RPC500). Figure 2A presents an example for the 3D printed temporary veneer.

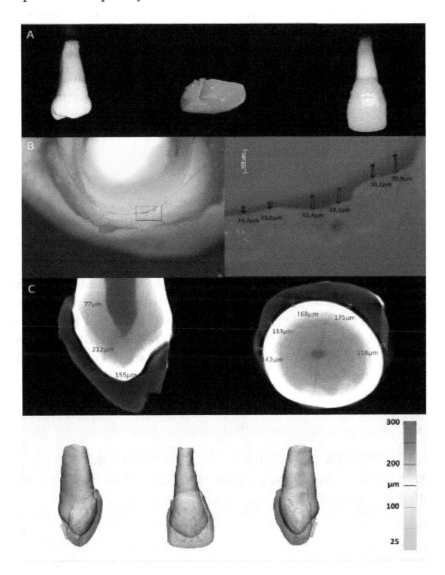

Figure 2. 3D printed veneer and evaluation methods. (**A**) 3D printed veneer and fitting to premolar; (**B**) evaluation of veneer seating using stereomicroscopy; (**C**) internal gap evaluation using micro-computed tomography, D: quantitative analysis of gap thickness.

2.5. Evaluation of Veneer Seating and Marginal Adaptation

All premolars were removed from the skulls and mandibles. Then, each veneer was seated onto its corresponding tooth. To ensure the correct seating of each veneer, corresponding to the designed position, a special holder was designed using in 3-matic version 12.0 (Materialise; Leuven, Belgium) and was 3D printed using the Connex printer (Object 360, Stratasys, MN, USA).

The cervical, mesial, and distal veneer margins were examined under a stereomicroscope (Olympus, Singapore) (Figure 2B). For each side, digital images for detected gaps were captured at 50 x magnification. Six measurements were made at each image resulting in 18 readings for each veneer.

2.6. Evaluation of Internal Adaptation Using Micro-Computed Tomographic Imaging

Image Acquisition

To check internal adaptation, the fitted veneers were scanned with the SkyScan 1172 micro-computed tomographic (μCT) system (Bruker, Antwerp, Belgium) (Figure 2C). The μCT parameters were 12.8 μm voxel size, 40 kVp, 250 mA, 0.5 mm aluminum filter, angular rotation step of 0.7°, 360° scanning, and exposure time of 0.295 s with a total scan duration of 22.5 min.

The x-ray projections were reconstructed using volumetric reconstruction software (SkyScan, Nrecon), beam hardening correction of 2%, and ring artefact correction were used for the reconstruction. Reconstructed slices were exported as DICOM files.

2.7. Segmentation Protocol, 3D Reconstruction, and Quantitative Analysis of Gap Thickness

To assess the internal adaptation, the gap between the veneer and the tooth was segmented using an indirect protocol applying logical operations. DICOM files of reconstructed images were imported into a dedicated tool which was developed in MeVisLab (MeVis Medical Solutions AG, Bremen, Germany).

The gap and enamel were segmented together as a single entity and were then saved as a binary image and as an intensity image. The intensity image was loaded, then the enamel was thresholded and saved as a separate binary image. The segmented binary images of the gap and enamel and the enamel separately were used to reconstruct two 3D models. The enamel 3D model was then subtracted from the 3D model of the gap and enamel, resulting in the 3D model of the gap (3matic, Materialise; Leuven, Belgium). The thickness of the resulting gap 3D model was then analyzed and expressed as a color-coded map (Figure 2D).

3. Statistical Analysis

Statistical analysis and graph plotting were performed using the statistical software package GraphPad Prism 7.00 (GraphPad Software, La Jolla, CA, USA). One-way way ANOVA was used to test for statistical differences at $p < 0.05$.

4. Results

The resulting 3D printed temporary veneer is presented in Figure 2A. Evaluation of veneer seating using stereomicroscopy showed that the mean marginal gap at all sides was below the cut-off value of 200 μm (Figure 3A). The overall mean marginal gap was 99.9 ± 50.7 μm [median: 87.8 (IQR 64.2–133 μm)]. Cervically, the mean marginal gap was 92.4 ± 48.1 μm [median: 87.8 (IQR 50.2–133 μm)]. On the mesial side, the mean marginal gap was 111 ± 59.2 μm [median: 89.1 (IQR 81.8–155 μm)] and on the distal side, the mean marginal gap was 96 ± 44.9 μm [median: 89.8 (IQR 63.4–140 μm) (Figure 3A). Differences between the gap thickness measured at different positions did not show any statistically significant differences ($p > 0.05$).

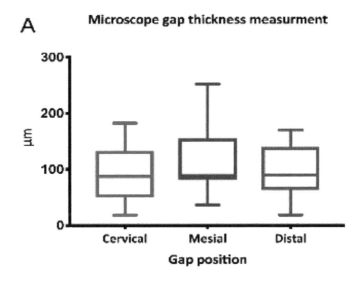

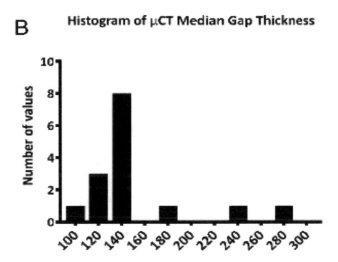

Figure 3. (**A**) stereomicroscopy gap measurements; (**B**) distribution of the gap thickness between the veneer and the tooth.

Internal adaptation evaluation using μCT showed an average median gap thickness of 152.5 ± 47.7 (IQR 129–149.3 μm). Figure 2D presents a color-coded map for 3D gap thickness analysis demonstrating the homogenous thickness below the cut-off value of 200 μm. Moreover, the overall distribution of the gap thickness between the veneer and the tooth was below the cut-off value of 200 μm in the majority of the samples.

5. Discussion

Tooth autotransplantation TAT offers a viable biological approach to tooth replacement in children and adolescents after traumatic dental injuries (TDIs), agenesis, developmental anomalies, or specific orthodontic problems [25–29]. In a recent systematic review, Akhlef et al. [28] reported an overall survival rate for conventional TAT ranging between 93% and 100% (weighted mean: 96.7%, median: 100%) after 9 months to 22 years of observation (median: 8.75 years). The survival rates for conventional TAT of teeth with incomplete root formation was reported to be 97.4, 97.8, and 96.3% after 1, 5, and 10 years, respectively [29]. Studies reporting on the aesthetic results after TAT are limited [28]. Czochrowska et al. [38] reported a clinical assessment of a reshaped autotransplanted tooth using composite build-ups compared to a natural contralateral tooth according to objective parameters.

The authors reported a 59% match, 27% deviation, and 14% mismatch with the natural contralateral tooth [38].

While restoring or reshaping transplanted teeth to the anterior maxilla is essential for psychological and aesthetic reasons [36], reshaping of transplanted teeth is usually delayed three to four months after transplantation to avoid interfering with the natural healing process [28,29,38,43]. This interval could be bridged using a simple indirect temporary aesthetic restoration for autotransplanted teeth.

The current report proposes a digital technique for designing and fabricating temporary veneers for autotransplanted teeth via chair side 3D printing technology, namely DLP. Simultaneously, the accuracy of this printing technology was validated by examining the marginal and internal adaptation of these temporary veneers.

A precise fit is an essential requirement for any dental restoration or prostheses. Ill-fitting prostheses will result in damage for the periodontium, tooth structure, and the prosthesis itself [23,44,45]. This study applied two methods for evaluating the adaptation of the veneers: direct view with microscope to measure the marginal fit, and μCT to evaluate the internal adaptation. Although there is no consensus about the best method to examine the marginal adaptation of fixed dental prosthesis, a direct view method is the most used method and with the most reproducible results. In the present study, marginal gaps were measured by stereomicroscopy (direct viewing method), resulting in a mean of a marginal gap of 100 μm, which is below the clinically acceptable value of marginal gaps of 120 μm [46,47].

To assess internal adaptation, μCT scans of the maxillary central incisor shaped veneers fitted on premolars, simulating the clinical situation, were used. The majority of the studies where μCT was used to assess internal adaptation performed two dimensional measurements of the internal gaps on cross sectional slides [48,49], while in this study, three-dimensional evaluation of the internal gap was applied. The average median thickness of the internal gaps in the present study was 152 μm, which is within the accepted values [50–52].

In a 2-year follow-up study on the use of 3D printed veneers, values of internal adaptation of porcelain laminate veneers ranged from 195 to 202 μm, which is higher than our values, while clinical performance was rated 100% satisfactory over the 2-year period [52].

One of the potential limitations of the suggested protocol is the use of one specific 3D printing technology and one specific printing material. Future studies are needed to study different 3D printing technologies other than DLP, while using other printing materials.

With the development of 3D printing technology and new resin materials developed specifically for dental restorations, it is expected that the use of this technique could be expanded for applications other than in autotransplanted teeth, especially in clinical situations where treatment should be done in a short amount of time, for example dental treatment under general anesthesia, trauma, and uncooperative children.

6. Conclusions

The present concept of using temporary veneers designed and fabricated with CAD/CAM technology using a DLP printer may present a viable treatment option for restoration of autotransplanted teeth. For the current design, values of marginal and internal adaptation were found to be within the clinically acceptable ranges.

Author Contributions: Conceptualization, M.E. and R.J.; methodology, A.A.-R., M.E. and R.J.; software, A.A.-R., M.E. and C.P.; validation, A.A.-R., M.E., and D.S.; formal analysis, A.A.-R., and M.E.; investigation, A.A.-R., M.E., D.S., C.P., and R.J.; resources, C.P and R.J.; data curation, A.A.-R., M.E., and D.S; writing—original draft preparation, A.A.-R., and M.E; writing—review and editing, A.A.-R., M.E., D.S., C.P. and R.J.; visualization, A.A.-R., M.E., and D.S.; supervision, M.E., C.P. and R.J.; project administration, M.E., C.P. and R.J.; funding acquisition, C.P. and R.J.

References

1. Duret, F.; Preston, J.D. CAD/CAM imaging in dentistry. *Curr. Opin. Dent.* **1991**, *1*, 150–154. [PubMed]
2. Miyazaki, T.; Hotta, Y.; Kunii, J.; Kuriyama, S.; Tamaki, Y. A review of dental CAD/CAM: Current status and future perspectives from 20 years of experience. *Dent. Mater. J.* **2009**, *28*, 44–56. [CrossRef] [PubMed]
3. Torabi, K.; Farjood, E.; Hamedani, S. Rapid prototyping technologies and their applications in prosthodontics, a Review of Literature. *J. Dent. (Shiraz)* **2015**, *16*, 1–9.
4. Van Assche, N.; Vercruyssen, M.; Coucke, W.; Teughels, W.; Jacobs, R.; Quirynen, M. Accuracy of computer-aided implant placement. *Clin. Oral. Implants. Res.* **2012**, *23*, 112–123. [CrossRef] [PubMed]
5. Vercruyssen, M.; Coucke, W.; Naert, I.; Jacobs, R.; Teughels, W.; Quirynen, M. Depth and lateral deviations in guided implant surgery: An RCT comparing guided surgery with mental navigation or the use of a pilot-drill template. *Clin. Oral. Implants Res.* **2015**, *26*, 1315–1320. [CrossRef] [PubMed]
6. Vercruyssen, M.; van de Wiele, G.; Teughels, W.; Naert, I.; Jacobs, R.; Quirynen, M. Implant- and patient-centred outcomes of guided surgery, a 1-year follow-up: An RCT comparing guided surgery with conventional implant placement. *J. Clin. Periodontol.* **2014**, *41*, 1154–1160. [CrossRef] [PubMed]
7. Colombo, M.; Mangano, C.; Mijiritsky, E.; Krebs, M.; Hauschild, U.; Fortin, T. Clinical applications and effectiveness of guided implant surgery: A critical review based on randomized controlled trials. *BMC Oral Health* **2017**, *17*, 150. [CrossRef] [PubMed]
8. Krastl, G.; Zehnder, M.S.; Connert, T.; Weiger, R.; Kuhl, S. Guided Endodontics: A novel treatment approach for teeth with pulp canal calcification and apical pathology. *Dent. Traumatol.* **2016**, *32*, 240–246. [CrossRef] [PubMed]
9. Torres, A.; Shaheen, E.; Lambrechts, P.; Politis, C.; Jacobs, R. Microguided Endodontics: A case report of a maxillary lateral incisor with pulp canal obliteration and apical periodontitis. *Int. Endod. J.* **2018**. [CrossRef] [PubMed]
10. Lee, S.J.; Jung, I.Y.; Lee, C.Y.; Choi, S.Y.; Kum, K.Y. Clinical application of computer-aided rapid prototyping for tooth transplantation. *Dent. Traumatol.* **2001**, *17*, 114–119. [CrossRef]
11. Shahbazian, M.; Jacobs, R.; Wyatt, J.; Denys, D.; Lambrichts, I.; Vinckier, F.; Willems, G. Validation of the cone beam computed tomography-based stereolithographic surgical guide aiding autotransplantation of teeth: Clinical case-control study. *Oral Surg. Oral Med. Oral Pathol. Oral Radiol.* **2013**, *115*, 667–675. [CrossRef] [PubMed]
12. Shahbazian, M.; Jacobs, R.; Wyatt, J.; Willems, G.; Pattijn, V.; Dhoore, E.; Van Lierde, C.; Vinckier, F. Accuracy and surgical feasibility of a CBCT-based stereolithographic surgical guide aiding autotransplantation of teeth: In vitro validation. *J. Oral Rehabil.* **2010**, *37*, 854–859. [CrossRef] [PubMed]
13. Kim, S.Y.; Shin, Y.S.; Jung, H.D.; Hwang, C.J.; Baik, H.S.; Cha, J.Y. Precision and trueness of dental models manufactured with different 3-dimensional printing techniques. *Am. J. Orthod. Dentofacial Orthop.* **2018**, *153*, 144–153. [CrossRef] [PubMed]
14. Dawood, A.; Marti Marti, B.; Sauret-Jackson, V.; Darwood, A. 3D printing in dentistry. *Br. Dent. J.* **2015**, *219*, 521–529. [CrossRef] [PubMed]
15. Shaheen, E.; Alhelwani, A.; Van De Casteele, E.; Politis, C.; Jacobs, R. Evaluation of dimensional changes of 3D printed models after sterilization: A pilot study. *Open Dent. J.* **2018**, *12*, 72–79. [CrossRef] [PubMed]
16. Shaheen, E.; Coopman, R.; Jacobs, R.; Politis, C. Optimized 3D virtually planned intermediate splints for bimaxillary orthognathic surgery: A clinical validation study in 20 patients. *J. Craniomaxillofac. Surg.* **2018**, *46*, 1441–1447. [CrossRef] [PubMed]
17. Shaheen, E.; Sun, Y.; Jacobs, R.; Politis, C. Three-dimensional printed final occlusal splint for orthognathic surgery: Design and validation. *Int. J. Oral Maxillofac. Surg.* **2017**, *46*, 67–71. [CrossRef] [PubMed]
18. EzEldeen, M.; Stratis, A.; Coucke, W.; Codari, M.; Politis, C.; Jacobs, R. As low dose as sufficient quality: Optimization of cone-beam computed tomographic scanning protocol for tooth autotransplantation planning and follow-up in children. *J. Endod.* **2017**, *43*, 210–217. [CrossRef] [PubMed]
19. Loubele, M.; Bogaerts, R.; Van Dijck, E.; Pauwels, R.; Vanheusden, S.; Suetens, P.; Marchal, G.; Sanderink, G.; Jacobs, R. Comparison between effective radiation dose of CBCT and MSCT scanners for dentomaxillofacial applications. *Eur. J. Radiol.* **2009**, *71*, 461–468. [CrossRef]
20. Albdour, E.A.; Shaheen, E.; Vranckx, M.; Mangano, F.G.; Politis, C.; Jacobs, R. A novel in vivo method to evaluate trueness of digital impressions. *BMC Oral Health* **2018**, *18*, 117. [CrossRef]

21. Mangano, F.; Gandolfi, A.; Luongo, G.; Logozzo, S. Intraoral scanners in dentistry: A review of the current literature. *BMC Oral Health* **2017**, *17*, 149. [CrossRef] [PubMed]

22. Stanley, M.; Paz, A.G.; Miguel, I.; Coachman, C. Fully digital workflow, integrating dental scan, smile design and CAD-CAM: Case report. *BMC Oral Health* **2018**, *18*, 134. [CrossRef] [PubMed]

23. Joda, T.; Zarone, F.; Ferrari, M. The complete digital workflow in fixed prosthodontics: A systematic review. *BMC Oral Health* **2017**, *17*, 124. [CrossRef] [PubMed]

24. Kim, G.B.; Lee, S.; Kim, H.; Yang, D.H.; Kim, Y.H.; Kyung, Y.S.; Kim, C.S.; Choi, S.H.; Kim, B.J.; Ha, H.; et al. Three-dimensional printing: Basic principles and applications in medicine and radiology. *Korean J. Radiol.* **2016**, *17*, 182–197. [CrossRef] [PubMed]

25. Czochrowska, E.M.; Stenvik, A.; Album, B.; Zachrisson, B.U. Autotransplantation of premolars to replace maxillary incisors: A comparison with natural incisors. *Am. J. Orthod. Dentofacial Orthop.* **2000**, *118*, 592–600. [CrossRef] [PubMed]

26. Day, P.; Duggal, M. Autotransplantation for failing and missing anterior teeth. *Pediatr. Dent.* **2008**, *30*, 286–287. [PubMed]

27. Paulsen, H.U.; Andreasen, J.O.; Schwartz, O. Tooth loss treatment in the anterior region: Autotransplantation of premolars and cryopreservation. *World J. Orthod.* **2006**, *7*, 27–34. [CrossRef] [PubMed]

28. Akhlef, Y.; Schwartz, O.; Andreasen, J.O.; Jensen, S.S. Autotransplantation of teeth to the anterior maxilla: A systematic review of survival and success, aesthetic presentation and patient-reported outcome. *Dent. Traumatol.* **2018**, *34*, 20–27. [CrossRef] [PubMed]

29. Rohof, E.C.M.; Kerdijk, W.; Jansma, J.; Livas, C.; Ren, Y. Autotransplantation of teeth with incomplete root formation: A systematic review and meta-analysis. *Clin. Oral Investig.* **2018**, *22*, 1613–1624. [CrossRef]

30. Sharma, A.B.; Vargervik, K. Using implants for the growing child. *J. Calif. Dent. Assoc.* **2006**, *34*, 719–724.

31. Kanavakis, G.; Ludwig, B.; Rosa, M.; Zachrisson, B.; Hourfar, J. Clinical outcomes of cases with missing lateral incisors treated with the 'T'-Mesialslider. *J. Orthod.* **2014**, *41*, S33–S38. [CrossRef] [PubMed]

32. Becker, K.; Wilmes, B.; Grandjean, C.; Vasudavan, S.; Drescher, D. Skeletally anchored mesialization of molars using digitized casts and two surface-matching approaches: Analysis of treatment effects. *J. Orofac. Orthop.* **2018**, *79*, 11–18. [CrossRef] [PubMed]

33. Andreasen, J.O.; Paulsen, H.U.; Yu, Z.; Schwartz, O. A long-term study of 370 autotransplanted premolars. Part III. Periodontal healing subsequent to transplantation. *Eur. J. Orthod.* **1990**, *12*, 25–37. [CrossRef] [PubMed]

34. Kallu, R.; Vinckier, F.; Politis, C.; Mwalili, S.; Willems, G. Tooth transplantations: A descriptive retrospective study. *Int. J. Oral Maxillofac. Surg.* **2005**, *34*, 745–755. [CrossRef] [PubMed]

35. Denys, D.; Shahbazian, M.; Jacobs, R.; Laenen, A.; Wyatt, J.; Vinckier, F.; Willems, G. Importance of root development in autotransplantations: A retrospective study of 137 teeth with a follow-up period varying from 1 week to 14 years. *Eur. J. Orthod.* **2013**, *35*, 680–688. [CrossRef] [PubMed]

36. Day, P.F.; Kindelan, S.A.; Spencer, J.R.; Kindelan, J.D.; Duggal, M.S. Dental trauma: Part 2. Managing poor prognosis anterior teeth-treatment options for the subsequent space in a growing patient. *J. Orthod.* **2008**, *35*, 143–155. [CrossRef] [PubMed]

37. Andreasen, J.O.; Paulsen, H.U.; Yu, Z.; Bayer, T.; Schwartz, O. A long-term study of 370 autotransplanted premolars. Part II. Tooth survival and pulp healing subsequent to transplantation. *Eur. J. Orthod.* **1990**, *12*, 14–24. [CrossRef]

38. Czochrowska, E.M.; Stenvik, A.; Zachrisson, B.U. The esthetic outcome of autotransplanted premolars replacing maxillary incisors. *Dent. Traumatol.* **2002**, *18*, 237–245. [CrossRef]

39. EzEldeen, M.; Van Gorp, G.; Van Dessel, J.; Vandermeulen, D.; Jacobs, R. 3-dimensional analysis of regenerative endodontic treatment outcome. *J. Endod.* **2015**, *41*, 317–324. [CrossRef]

40. Barrett, W.A.; Mortensen, E.N. Interactive live-wire boundary extraction. *Med. Image Anal.* **1997**, *1*, 331–341. [CrossRef]

41. Suetens, P. *Fundamentals of Medical Imaging*, 2nd ed.; Cambridge University Press: New York, NY, USA, 2009; p. 264.

42. Heckel, F.; Konrad, O.; Hahn, H.K.; Peitgen, H.-O. Interactive 3D medical image segmentation with energy-minimizing implicit functions. *Comput. Gr.* **2011**, *35*, 275–287.

43. Zachrisson, B.U.; Stenvik, A.; Haanæs, H.R. Management of missing maxillary anterior teeth with emphasis on autotransplantation. *Am. J. Orthod. Dentofacial Orthop.* **2004**, *126*, 284–288. [CrossRef]

44.   Bader, J.D.; Rozier, R.G.; McFall, W.T.; Ramsey, D.L. Effect of crown margins on periodontal conditions in regularly attending patients. *J. Prosthet. Dent.* **1991**, *65*, 75–79. [CrossRef]

45.   Bergenholtz, G.; Cox, C.F.; Loesche, W.J.; Syed, S.A. Bacterial leakage around dental restorations: Its effect on the dental pulp. *J. Oral Pathol.* **1982**, *11*, 439–450. [CrossRef] [PubMed]

46.   Fransson, B.; Oilo, G.; Gjeitanger, R. The fit of metal-ceramic crowns, a clinical study. *Dent. Mater.* **1985**, *1*, 197–199. [CrossRef]

47.   McLean, J.W.; von Fraunhofer, J.A. The estimation of cement film thickness by an in vivo technique. *Br. Dent. J.* **1971**, *131*, 107–111. [CrossRef] [PubMed]

48.   Borba, M.; Cesar, P.F.; Griggs, J.A.; Della Bona, Á. Adaptation of all-ceramic fixed partial dentures. *Dent. Mater.* **2011**, *27*, 1119–1126. [CrossRef]

49.   Pelekanos, S.; Koumanou, M.; Koutayas, S.O.; Zinelis, S.; Eliades, G. Micro-CT evaluation of the marginal fit of different In-Ceram alumina copings. *Eur. J. Esthet. Dent.* **2009**, *4*, 278–292.

50.   Harasani, M.H.; Isidor, F.; Kaaber, S. Marginal fit of porcelain and indirect composite laminate veneers under in vitro conditions. *Scand. J. Dent. Res.* **1991**, *99*, 262–268. [CrossRef]

51.   Tetsuya, A.; Ryunosuke, K.; Takashi, O.; Masayoshi, F. Adaptation of laminate veneer restorations fabricated with the CEREC 3 system. *J. Adhes. Dent.* **2006**, *24*, 179–184.

52.   Yuce, M.; Ulusoy, M.; Turk, A.G. Comparison of marginal and internal adaptation of heat-pressed and CAD/CAM porcelain laminate veneers and a 2-Year follow-up. *J. Prosthodont* **2017**. [CrossRef] [PubMed]

Dental Restorative Digital Workflow: Digital Smile Design from Aesthetic to Function

Gabriele Cervino [1][iD], Luca Fiorillo [1][iD], Alina Vladimirovna Arzukanyan [2],
Gianrico Spagnuolo [2,3][iD] and Marco Cicciù [1,*][iD]

[1] Department of Biomedical and Dental Sciences and Morphological and Functional Imaging,
     Messina University, 98100 Messina, Italy; gcervino@unime.it (G.C.); lucafiorillo@live.it (L.F.)
[2] Institute of Dentistry, I. M. Sechenov First Moscow State Medical University, Moscow 119146, Russia;
     aav0218@mail.ru (A.V.A.); gianrico.spagnuolo@gmail.com (G.S.)
[3] Department of Neurosciences, Reproductive and Odontostomatological Sciences, University of Naples
     "Federico II", 80131 Napoli, Italy
[*] Correspondence: mcicciu@unime.it

Abstract: Breakthroughs in technology have not been possible without influencing the medical sciences. Dentistry and dental materials have been fully involved in the technological and information technology evolution, so much so that they have revolutionized dental techniques. In this study, we want to create the first collection of articles on the use of digital techniques and software, such as Digital Smile Design. The aim is to collect all of the results regarding the use of this software, and to highlight the fields of use. Twenty-four articles have been included in the review, and the latter describes the use of Digital Smile Design and, in particular, the field of use. The study intends to be present which dental fields use "digitization". Progress in this field is constant, and will be of increasing interest to dentistry by proposing a speed of treatment planning and a reliability of results. The digital workflow allows for rehabilitations that are reliable both from an aesthetic and functional point of view, as demonstrated in the review. From this study, the current field of use of Digital Smile Design techniques in the various branches of medicine and dentistry have emerged, as well as information about its reliability.

Keywords: Digital Smile Design; restorative dentistry; dentistry software; dentistry design

1. Introduction

In recent years, prosthetic and implant-prosthetic rehabilitation in the dental field have undergone a strong development in aesthetics and cosmetics, benefiting from both the improvement of some laboratory techniques and the definition of some anatomical criteria useful to the aesthetics of the smile. One of the most noteworthy innovations in the field of prosthetics is undoubtedly represented by the advent of computer-aided design and computer-aided manufacturing (CAD/CAM) technology, which allows professionals to guarantee repeatable and remarkable results from an anatomical–functional point of view. The accessible costs, the small size of the machines, and the relative ease of use make this method passable, even in small-scale outpatient facilities. New processing software, for example, aims to make the entire rehabilitative work-flow digital, simplifying the professional's work and also facilitating communication with the patient. A quick search on the main informatics engine indicates all of the software available on the market—among them, an important role is undoubtedly played by the Digital Smile Design method. In this work, we will take into consideration all of the articles in the literature regarding the use of this method. This software allows for excellent communication with our patients on the one hand, but on the other, offers the clinician a tool to make the correct therapeutic choice through algorithms. Rehabilitation follows a digital pathway, and the patient can see the result even before starting. These methods allow for accurate planning and guarantee aesthetic, functional, and predictable results [1–3]. The software in the medical field, 3D technology, and the bioengineering field have been working in synergy in recent years in order to produce excellent therapeutic tools. The possibility of testing three-dimensional structures virtually, before being able to build or test them on patients, is already a huge step forward; this is possible with finite element analyses, for example, with which you can test useful materials for different dental fields, from fixtures to prosthetics, to the simulation of dental movements [4,5]. Digital Smile Design allows for a thorough workflow simulating the rehabilitation of a patient, simply starting with appropriately calibrated photos. The facial study is usually done using the reference lines, from which the standardized parameters have been developed for the frontal and profile views of the face. The horizontal reference lines used in the frontal view include the interpupillary and intercommissural lines, which provide an overall sense of harmony and horizontal perspective, present in an aesthetically pleasing face. However, the main limitation of this kind of therapeutic method is related to the several anatomical features involved in the rehabilitation. The treatment for giving an "aesthetic smile" to patients is related to the different anatomical areas involved in the treatments, like the teeth, gingiva, mucosa, lip, skin, and so on, which rely on symmetry, shape, and golden proportions. The purpose of this study is to evaluate the effective use of Digital Smile Design techniques in dentistry and other medical fields. These techniques are used in different medical fields, and we have analyzed and categorized all of these fields, and have evaluated the reliability and predictability of these digital techniques.

2. Material and Methods

2.1. Protocol and Registration

This review is registered at PROSPERO with ID number 122744. PROSPERO is an international database of prospectively registered systematic reviews in health and social care, welfare, public health, education, crime, justice, and international development, where there is a health-related outcome.

2.2. Focus Question

The following focus questions were developed according to the population, intervention, comparison, and outcome (PICO) study design [6]:

- What are the fields of use of the Digital Smile Design software?
- Is Digital Smile Design bringing improvements in the comfort of patients and in their treatments?

2.3. Information Sources

The search strategy incorporated examinations of electronic databases, supplemented by hand searches. We searched PubMed, Dentistry, and Oral Sciences Source for relevant studies published in English. A hand search of the reference lists in the articles retrieved was carried out in order to source additional relevant publications and to improve on the sensitivity of the search.

2.4. Search

The keywords used in the search of the selected electronic databases included the following:
- "Digital Smile Design"

The choice of keywords was intended to collect and to record as much relevant data as possible, without relying on electronic means alone to refine the search results.

2.5. Selection of Studies

Two independent reviewers singularly analyzed the obtaining papers in order to select the inclusion and exclusion criteria as follows. For the stage of reviewing full-text articles, a complete independent dual revision was performed.

2.6. Types of Selected Manuscripts

The review included studies on humans and animal published in English. Letters, editorials, and PhD theses were excluded.

2.7. Types of Studies

The review included all human prospective and retrospective follow-up studies and clinical trials, cohort studies, case-control studies, case series studies, animal studies, and literature reviews published on using Digital Smile Design for rehabilitation and restorative dentistry.

2.8. Inclusion and Exclusion Criteria

The full texts of all of the studies of possible relevance were obtained for assessment against the following inclusion criteria:

- Digital Smile Design use for restorative dentistry
- Advantages of Digital Smile Design.

The applied exclusion criteria for the studies were as follows:

- Studies involving patients with other specific diseases, immunologic disorders, or other oral risk-related systemic conditions
- Not enough information regarding the selected topic
- No access to the title and the abstract in English.

2.9. Digital Dentistryn

Digital Smile Design

Digital Smile Design is a method that allows us to digitally design the smile of our patients, by obtaining a simulation and pre-visualization of the therapeutic result. Patients are often found by the dentist and are immediately subjected to dental services or therapies, without the dentist himself having planned well or having shared the therapeutic project of a tailor-made smile for the patient with them. On the one hand, Digital Smile Design allows the patient to have awareness from the beginning of the therapeutic plan and for them be the first interpreter in the aesthetic and functional rehabilitation of their mouth, and on the other hand, it allows the specialist to tune in better to the expectations and needs of the patient, in order to pursue their shared goals. These protocols therefore allow for a previsualization of the clinical case and of the therapeutic result, and for presenting the patient, in a clear way, the usefulness of being able to program the rehabilitation and interface clearly with the help of other professional figures. Being able to provide all of the data to the dental technician, or even being able to evaluate the prosthetic–implant–orthodontic rehabilitation is made simpler, by being able to communicate information about the case in a simple and digital way to colleagues [1].

2.10. Sequential Search Strategy

After the first literature analysis, all of the article titles were screened so as to exclude irrelevant publications, case reports, and non-English publications. Then, researches were not selected based on the data obtained from screening the abstracts. The final stage of screening involved reading the full texts in order to confirm each study's eligibility, based on the inclusion and exclusion criteria.

2.11. Data Extraction

The data were independently extracted from the studies in the form of variables, according to the aims and themes of the present review, as listed onwards.

2.12. Data Collections

The data were collected from the included articles, and were arranged in the following fields (Table 1):

"Author (Year)"—revealed the author and year of publication

"Dental Field"—the dental field of Digital Smile Design was used

2.13. Risk of Bias Assessment

Two authors undertook the assessment of risk of bias during the data extraction process. For the included studies, this was conducted using the Cochrane Collaboration's two-part tool for assessing the risk of bias [7,8]. An overall risk of bias was then assigned to each trial, according to Higgins et al. [8]. The levels of bias were classified as follows: low risk, if all of the criteria were met; moderate risk, when only one criterion was missing; high risk, if two or more criteria were missing; and unclear risk, if there were too few details to make a judgement about the certain risk assessment.

3. Results

The results were collected from all of the articles that were taken into consideration. The articles that talk about Digital Smile Design and its use in the field of rehabilitative and restorative dentistry were used. In the article, we have not only taken into consideration the "communicative" utility of the software towards the patients, but also that of therapeutic planning and of aesthetic and functional rehabilitation. The articles included in our review already provide important information regarding the field of use of the current digital techniques. Surely, in the first place, the most common field of use is prosthetic and dental restoration. In second place are the positions that mention digital techniques for periodontal purposes instead. Later, we will review these works more closely. Although these techniques are modern and relatively new, the purpose of this work is not to indicate whether these techniques are reliable or not, because the available data available are still few. The aim is to highlight the use-trend in different dental fields.

3.1. Study Selection

The article review and data extraction were performed according to the Preferred Reporting Items for Systematic Reviews and Metanalyses PRISMA flow diagram (Figure 1). The initial electronic and hand searches retrieved 26 articles. After the titles and abstracts were reviewed, only 24 articles were included.

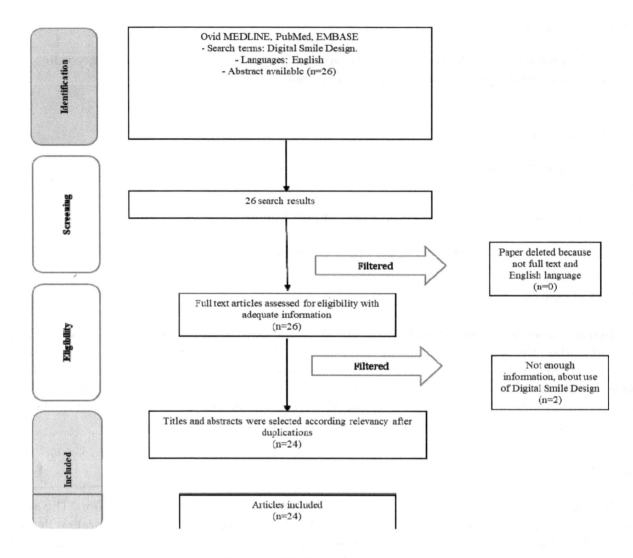

Figure 1. PRISMA flow diagram.

3.2. Study Characteristics

During the selection of the studies, their individual characteristics were evaluated. The characteristics assessed mainly concerned the field of use of Digital Smile Design (Table 1), as follows:

- Restorative dentistry
- Periodontal surgery
- Implantology
- Guided bone regeneration
- Orthodontics
- Maxillofacial surgery

Table 1. Digital Smile Design use.

Author	Year of Publications	Field of Digital Smile Design Use					
		Restorative and Prosthodontics	Periodontal Surgery	Implantology	Guided Bone Regeneration	Orthodontics	Maxillofacial Surgery
Santos et al. [9]	2017	✔	✔				
Meereis et al. [10]	2016	✔					
Cattoni et al. [11]	2016	✔					
Omar et al. [12]	2018		✔				
Arias et al. [13]	2015						
Perez-Davidi [14]	2015	✔					
Tak On et al. [15]	2016						
Daher et al. [16]	2018						
Trushkowsky et al. [17]	2016	✔					
Garcia et al. [18]	2018	✔		✔			
Coachman et al. [19]	2017	✔					
McLaren et al. [20]	2018	✔		✔	✔		
Stanley et al. [21]	2018	✔					
Rojas-Vizcaya et al. [22]	2017	✔				✔	
Pinzan-Vercelino et al. [23]	2017	✔	✔			✔	
Marsango et al. [24]	2014	✔	✔			✔	
Frizzera et al. [25]	2017	✔	✔		✔		
Veneziani [26]	2017	✔					
Pimentel et al. [27]	2015	✔					
Paredes-Gallardo et al. [28]	2017						✔
Halley [29]	2015						
Coachman et al. [30]	2016	✔					
Miranda et al. [31]	2016	✔					

✔: Selected papers after the inclusion criteria.

3.3. Risk of Bias within Studies

Summarizing the risk of bias for each study, most of the studies were classified as unclear risk. More studies were considered as having a low risk of bias.

3.4. Risk of Bias across Studies

There were several limitations present in the current review. The current review includes studies written in English only, which could introduce a publication bias. There were various degrees of heterogeneity in each study design, case selection, and treatment provided among the studies.

4. Discussion

Today, dental care tends to be more conservative than in the past, above all thanks to the advances in medicine. In this section, we want to examine more closely the results obtained by the individual articles evaluated. According to Santos et al., the use of dental planning software can also be used for periodontal surgery. In their article, they considered a case of periodontal plastic surgery appropriately programmed through the Digital Smile Design. Digital Smile Design (DSD) allows for a complete planning of the treatment; the programmed results and those obtained after the surgery are comparable. The increase in the clinical crown is an intervention that must always be appropriately planned. Patients accept better oral surgical techniques if techniques such as DSD are used [9]. In another study, Meereis et al. considered Digital Smile Design for aesthetic rehabilitation, and the usefulness of this tool is again confirmed. In this work, it is considered with the combined approach of gingival plastic surgery and restorative dentistry. In this case, the patient's rehabilitation is performed with lithium disilicate glass ceramic veneers [10]. In the work of Cattoni et al., prosthetic planning is carried out with a digital workflow. The limit of these technologies, according to the authors, is represented by a two-dimensional (2D) workflow—the technique faced by the authors in this case provides a totally digital CAD/CAM process to minimize errors. The three-dimensional (3D) planning is sent to the dental laboratory for the fabrication of the prosthetic products. The technique of combining the Digital Smile Design digital workflow with the .stl files from the digital optical impression allows for the realization of these artefacts in the laboratory [11]. A study by Omar and Duarte published in the Saudi Dentistry journal in 2018 reviewed various programs used for Digital Smile Design, and therefore for treatment planning. In this study, different programs were evaluated (Photoshop CS6, Keynote, Planmeca Romexis Smile Design, CEREC SW 4.2, Aesthetic Digital Smile Design, Smile Designer Pro, DSD App, and VisagiSMile). The authors evaluated the reliability of the latter, although some of the programs were not designed for the dental field. The authors in fact focus on this. The possibility of having functions concerning oral structures, such as teeth or gums, makes the work much quicker and more predictable [12]. In 2015, Arias et al. carried out a further study on the approach using Digital Smile, to perform and plan a periodontal surgery in order to solve a gummy smile [13]. Perez-Davidi carried out a study on prosthetic rehabilitations in monolithic material, with CEREC CAD/CAM systems. There is the possibility, therefore, to perform an immediate mock up and then combine the data from Digital Smile Design and CEREC SW4 for manufacturing [14]. The approach to improve patient aesthetics through Digital Smile Design techniques is further confirmed by other works, such as that by Tak On et al. [15]. The authors confirm the possibility of planning the prosthetic treatment in a preventive manner. Some authors, such as Daher et al., have evaluated the possibility of using cheaper strategies to perform an analysis of Digital Smile Design, such as obtaining images with mobile phones [16]. Trushkowsky et al. [17] confirm the possibility of carrying out aesthetic evaluations for oral rehabilitations. According to Garcia et al., the use of new digital tools offers important perspectives for the daily clinic; in his study, a prosthetic rehabilitation of the anterior maxillary area is evaluated, all planned through Digital Smile Design. According to the authors, in addition to offering a powerful tool to propose treatment plans to patients, by showing them, it is also useful for planning [18]. Coachman et al. also evaluated the use of this software for the planning of total rehabilitations. In this study, the software was used to plan a computer-guided surgery, and a computer-aided design and computer-aided manufacturing (CAD/CAM) of the final prosthetic devices. In this case, therefore, Digital Smile Design was useful for the implant-prosthetic rehabilitation [19]. According to a study by McLaren et al., cosmetic and aesthetic dentistry have undergone a new push from these digital tools. The authors also show how software like Adobe Photoshop can highlight alterations to the smile and can be useful in the analysis of the patient [20]. In 2008, Stanley et al. published an article about digital workflow. The patient of his work, suffering from a Temporo-Mandibular Joint TMJ disorder, underwent a prosthetic rehabilitation with veneers and crowns, with a minimally invasive approach, in order to rehabilitate the loss of vertical dimension and to resolve his joint pains. The protocol was completely digital, using Digital Smile Design for planning and the CAD/CAM techniques for production [21]. An article in the Journal of Prosthetic Dentistry speaks about the possibility of performing a total rehabilitation supported by implants and a guided bone rehabilitation based on Digital Smile Design. The patient suffering from a serious bone deficiency, after a digital planning, therefore, is subjected to a vertical and horizontal bone augmentation. For this reason, surgical templates have been built, and then the fixtures are positioned in order to allow for implant-prosthetic rehabilitation. The final rehabilitation involves a total prosthesis screwed on the implants [22]. Pinzan-Vercelino et al. in their article talk about a multidisciplinary approach using Digital Smile Design for aesthetic rehabilitations in patients with medial diastema of the maxilla [23]. Marsango et al., in Oral and Implantology, talk about the digital workflow. The aesthetic planning and simulation of the dental treatment were carried out on two arches, and subsequently, the scans were sent to a laboratory for production using CAD/CAM techniques. In this case, a prosthetic implant prosthetic rehabilitation was evaluated [24]. A further work taken into consideration sees the use of Digital Smile Design for different dental fields. These techniques, according to the authors, can be used for periodontology, implantology, and prosthetics. Thanks to this software, it is also possible to program pre-prosthetic surgery in detail [25]. Veneziani M. proposed a study on this approach using Digital Smile Design for the treatment of complex cases. In this article, he evaluated the possibility of rehabilitation with veneers, including different branches of dentistry such as periodontal therapy, mucogingival, restorative dentistry, orthodontics, and prosthetics. Therefore, a multidisciplinary approach for the patient thanks to this digital protocol using still porcelain veneers was found [26,27]. Another interesting article talks about the possibility of rehabilitating a second-class brachyphosis patient with a mandibular asymmetry. This complex case involves planning with Digital Smile Design. The multidisciplinary approach in this case includes periodontal, oral, orthodontic, prosthetic, and maxillofacial surgery. The surgical treatment consisted of an osteotomy of the bilateral mandible and a genoplasty; after the surgery, the plates were screwed, and finally removed. Orthodontic treatment followed the surgery and the prosthetic rehabilitation was scheduled [28]. Elaine Halley spoke about the future of dentistry and 3D planning in changing the facial appearance of patients [29]. The latest article to be taken into consideration in this review, in addition to evaluating the use of Digital Smile Design in aesthetic dentistry, sees a case of rehabilitation of the anterior jaw, in this case using metal-free ceramic crowns, passing first for the provisional function of conditioning the gingival tissues [30,31]. In this work, we therefore broadly considered the use of a digital workflow in order to allow for an oral rehabilitation in the different fields of dentistry. Certainly, this technique, already mentioned by some authors [22], is also useful for correcting important bone defects after invasive surgeries in the case of new cancers. Digital techniques can program correct alveolar preservation after extractions with the different techniques present [32]. Soft tissue management and proper planning allow for gingival health to be maintained in our patients [33,34]. In addition, minimally invasive rehabilitations that can be designed allow for the maintenance of dental tissues, while ensuring a correct interface between the dental and prosthetic surfaces, so that there may be correct adhesion [35]. Surely, these types of techniques will progressively tend to replace all of the analog techniques, such as impression techniques, which have different disadvantages [36]. Indeed, with the possibility of being able to provide rehabilitation, it will be possible to make this more predictable. The ideal situation would be to have the advantages from the digital evolution in all of the fields of dentistry—imagine the possibility of knowing precisely the margins of a prosthesis, or even the root canal anatomy, for prosthetic rehabilitation, all the way through to the pins. In this way, it would be possible to predict the angulation and orientation of these beforehand, so as to program the prosthesis, or, for example, by knowing the canal anatomy [37], to know how our instruments will behave during the different therapies [38]. The possibility, in fact, to be able to predict the behavior of the tools that are used by the clinician, would be a very useful target, especially in the aforementioned therapies, where the tools can affect a result if they go against fracture, or experience breakage or wear during treatment. Some materials also suffer, as a result of mechanical fatigue, or even physical or chemical treatments [39]. The latter can also occur within the oral cavity itself [40]. With the improvements in the software over the next few years, it will be possible to program the rehabilitation of a patient by combining the files coming from a CT scan or a Cone Beam, along with the .stl files of an oral impression or a facial scan and a photo. All of this guarantees the rehabilitation desired by the patients as well as guaranteeing their satisfaction [41]. Combining all of this with the predictable wear and tear of different materials, would definitely make rehabilitation more reliable. At this stage, this is the main limitation. Several treatment opportunities, in the field of oral surgery and prosthodontics, as well as dental materials, are available today. Future perspective studies should be directed to managing those different anatomical areas related to the different disciplines. However, the results of the present study still underline how, even if there is significant progress in the field of computer-assisted medicine and dentistry, the clinical evaluation of the patients during the first visit, and therefore the close cooperation between the oral surgeons, radiologists, and prosthodontics, cannot be replaced without compromising the final long term aesthetic and functional results of the patients involved in the treatment. Further clinical studies will help to improve on the management of difficult cases.

Surely, this analysis of the individual articles included in the review has brought to light other evidence regarding the use of digital techniques for dental or medical planning. The fields of use have been clarified, how these techniques are used and what reliability they possess have also been clarified, although it is not possible to obtain statistical results as a result of a lack of data.

Limitations

This work takes into consideration the fields of use of Digital Smile Design, so it does not compare the statistical data from the individual studies.

The low number of studies in the literature for this topic unfortunately represent a disadvantage. This is a very current topic and is still not widely dealt with in the scientific field, and our study clearly explains what the fields of use are in dentistry for using this digital instrument, so it is anticipated to have good scientific confirmation. Having a large number of scientific articles available on this topic that contain detailed information on the reliability, accuracy, and predictability of these methods, would certainly be a good starting point for further review.

5. Conclusions

In could be concluded from all of the articles present in the literature regarding Digital Smile Design, that this tool provides important information to the clinician and patient. Patients can view their rehabilitations even before they start, and this can have important medico-legal functions. In recent years, these digital techniques have undergone a great positive evolution. It is also possible to remember that other techniques, such as engineering finite element analysis, have provided great support to the biomedical field, allowing for the simulation of structures even before being tested on patients, improving the quality of the rehabilitations and the predictability of the latter. With regard to planning, digital instruments appropriately interfaced with other digital files concerning radiographs and dental laboratory machines thus allow for rehabilitations that are more predictable. Indeed, technology has been evolving in this field in recent years, and will continue to include big updates on Digital Smile Design. However, facial scans would be able to make predictions of bone growth in children, to plan orthodontic–orthopedic rehabilitations, and then drive the proper growth of the jaws.

Author Contributions: L.F. was the author responsible for writing the paper. G.C. was the chief reviewer for the collection of data, responsible for the language proofing and revision. G.S. and L.F. were responsible for collecting the data and tables. G.C. and L.F. were responsible for the funding acquisition data. M.C. and L.F. were responsible for the editing, original data, and text preparation. A.V.A. and M.C. was responsible for supervision, and was a corresponding author.

References

1. Consumer Guide to Dentistry. Available online: https://www.yourdentistryguide.com/digital-dentistry/ (accessed on 10 January 2019).

2. Ahrberg, D.; Lauer, H.C.; Ahrberg, M.; Weigl, P. Evaluation of fit and efficiency of CAD/CAM fabricated all-ceramic restorations based on direct and indirect digitalization: A double-blinded, randomized clinical trial. *Clin. Oral Investig.* **2016**, *20*, 291–300. [CrossRef] [PubMed]

3. Moss, B.W.; Russell, M.D.; Jarad, F.D. The use of digital imaging for colour matching and communication in restorative dentistry. *Br. Dent. J.* **2005**, *199*, 43–49. [CrossRef]

4. Cervino, G.; Romeo, U.; Lauritano, F.; Bramanti, E.; Fiorillo, L.; D'Amico, C.; Milone, D.; Laino, L.; Campolongo, F.; Rapisarda, S.; et al. Fem and von mises analysis of OSSTEM® dental implant structural components: Evaluation of different direction dynamic loads. *Open Dent. J.* **2018**, *12*, 219–229. [CrossRef]

5. Lauritano, F.; Runci, M.; Cervino, G.; Fiorillo, L.; Bramanti, E.; Cicciù, M. Three-dimensional evaluation of different prosthesis retention systems using finite element analysis and the Von Mises stress test. *Minerva Stomatologica* **2016**, *65*, 353–367. [PubMed]

6. University Library. Available online: https://researchguides.uic.edu/c.php?g=252338&p=3954402 (accessed on 10 January 2019).

7. Higgins, J.P.T.; Altman, D.G. *Assessing Risk of Bias in Included Studies*; Higgins, J.P.T., Green, S., Eds.; Wiley Blackwellm: Hoboken, NJ, USA, 2008.

8. Higgins, J.P.T.; Altman, D.G.; Gøtzsche, P.C.; Jüni, P.; Moher, D.; Oxman, A.D.; Savović, J.; Schulz, K.F.; Weeks, L.; Sterne, J.A. The Cochrane Collaboration's tool for assessing risk of bias in randomised trials. *BMJ* **2011**, *343*, d5928. [CrossRef]

9. Santos, F.R.; Kamarowski, S.F.; Lopez, C.A.V.; Storrer, C.L.M.; Neto, A.T.; Deliberador, T.M. The use of the digital smile design concept as an auxiliary tool in periodontal plastic surgery. *Dent. Res. J. (Isfahan)* **2017**, *14*, 158–161.

10. Meereis, C.T.; de Souza, G.B.; Albino, L.G.; Ogliari, F.A.; Piva, E.; Lima, G.S. Digital Smile Design for Computer-assisted Esthetic Rehabilitation: Two-year Follow-up. *Oper. Dent.* **2016**, *41*, E13–E22. [CrossRef]

11. Cattoni, F.; Mastrangelo, F.; Gherlone, E.F.; Gastaldi, G. A New Total Digital Smile Planning Technique (3D-DSP) to Fabricate CAD-CAM Mockups for Esthetic Crowns and Veneers. *Int. J. Dent.* **2016**, *2016*, 6282587. [CrossRef]

12. Omar, D.; Duarte, C. The application of parameters for comprehensive smile esthetics by digital smile design programs: A review of literature. *Saudi Dent. J.* **2018**, *30*, 7–12. [CrossRef] [PubMed]

13. Arias, D.M.; Trushkowsky, R.D.; Brea, L.M.; David, S.B. Treatment of the Patient with Gummy Smile in Conjunction with Digital Smile Approach. *Dent. Clin. N. Am.* **2015**, *59*, 703–716. [CrossRef]

14. Perez-Davidi, M. Digital smile design and anterior monolithic restorations chair side fabrication with Cerec Cad/Cam system. *Refuat Hapeh Vehashinayim (1993)* **2015**, *32*, 15–19, 25.

15. Tak On, T.; Kois, J.C. Digital Smile Design Meets the Dento-Facial Analyzer: Optimizing Esthetics While Preserving Tooth Structure. *Compend. Contin. Educ. Dent.* **2016**, *37*, 46–50.

16. Daher, R.; Ardu, S.; Vjero, O.; Krejci, I. 3D Digital Smile Design With a Mobile Phone and Intraoral Optical Scanner. *Compend. Contin. Educ. Dent.* **2018**, *39*, e5–e8. [PubMed]

17. Trushkowsky, R.; Arias, D.M.; David, S. Digital Smile Design concept delineates the final potential result of crown lengthening and porcelain veneers to correct a gummy smile. *Int. J. Esthet. Dent. Autumn* **2016**, *11*, 338–354.

18. Garcia, P.P.; da Costa, R.G.; Calgaro, M.; Ritter, A.V.; Correr, G.M.; da Cunha, L.F.; Gonzaga, C.C. Digital smile design and mock-up technique for esthetic treatment planning with porcelain laminate veneers. *J. Conserv. Dent.* **2018**, *21*, 455–458. [CrossRef] [PubMed]

19. Coachman, C.; Calamita, M.A.; Coachman, F.G.; Coachman, R.G.; Sesma, N. Facially generated and cephalometric guided 3D digital design for complete mouth implant rehabilitation: A clinical report. *J. Prosthet. Dent.* **2017**, *117*, 577–586. [CrossRef] [PubMed]

20. McLaren, E.A.; Goldstein, R.E. The Photoshop Smile Design Technique. *Compend. Contin. Educ. Dent.* **2018**, *39*, e17–e20. [PubMed]

21. Stanley, M.; Paz, A.G.; Miguel, I.; Coachman, C. Fully digital workflow, integrating dental scan, smile design and CAD-CAM: Case report. *BMC Oral Health* **2018**, *18*, 134. [CrossRef] [PubMed]

22. Rojas-Vizcaya, F. Prosthetically guided bone sculpturing for a maxillary complete-arch implant-supported monolithic zirconia fixed prosthesis based on a digital smile design: A clinical report. *J. Prosthet. Dent.* **2017**, *118*, 575–580. [CrossRef]

23. Pinzan-Vercelino, C.R.M.; Pereira, C.C.; Lima, L.R.; Gurgel, J.A.; Bramante, F.S.; Pereira, A.L.P.; Lima, D.M.; Bandeca, M.C. Two-Year Follow-up of Multidisciplinary Treatment Using Digital Smile Design as a Planning Tool for Esthetic Restorations on Maxillary Midline Diastema. *Int. J. Orthod. Milwaukee* **2017**, *28*, 67–70.

24. Marsango, V.; Bollero, R.; D'Ovidio, N.; Miranda, M.; Bollero, P.; Barlattani, A., Jr. Digital work-flow. *Oral Implantol. (Rome)* **2014**, *7*, 20–24. [CrossRef]

25. Frizzera, F.; Tonetto, M.; Cabral, G.; Shibli, J.A.; Marcantonio, E., Jr. Periodontics, Implantology, and Prosthodontics Integrated: The Zenith-Driven Rehabilitation. *Case Rep. Dent.* **2017**, *2017*, 1070292. [CrossRef] [PubMed]

26. Veneziani, M. Ceramic laminate veneers: Clinical procedures with a multidisciplinary approach. *Int. J. Esthet. Dent.* **2017**, *12*, 426–448.

27. Pimentel, W.; Teixeira, M.L.; Costa, P.P.; Jorge, M.Z.; Tiossi, R. Predictable Outcomes with Porcelain Laminate Veneers: A Clinical Report. *J. Prosthodont.* **2016**, *25*, 335–340. [CrossRef]

28. Paredes-Gallardo, V.; García-Sanz, V.; Bellot-Arcís, C. Miniscrew-assisted multidisciplinary orthodontic treatment with surgical mandibular advancement and genioplasty in a brachyfacial Class II patient with mandibular asymmetry. *Am. J. Orthod. Dentofac. Orthop.* **2017**, *152*, 679–692. [CrossRef]

29. Halley, E. The future—3D planning but with the face in motion. *Br. Dent. J.* **2015**, *218*, 326–327. [CrossRef]

30. Coachman, C.; Paravina, R.D. Digitally Enhanced Esthetic Dentistry—From Treatment Planning to Quality Control. *J. Esthet. Restor. Dent.* **2016**, *28* (Suppl. 1), S3–S4. [CrossRef] [PubMed]

31. Miranda, M.E.; Olivieri, K.A.; Rigolin, F.J.; de Vasconcellos, A.A. Esthetic Challenges in Rehabilitating the Anterior Maxilla: A Case Report. *Oper Dent.* **2016**, *41*, 2–7. [CrossRef]

32. Lombardi, T.; Bernardello, F.; Berton, F.; Porrelli, D.; Rapani, A.; Piloni, A.C.; Fiorillo, L.; Di Lenarda, R.; Stacchi, C.; Tozum, T. Efficacy of Alveolar Ridge Preservation after Maxillary Molar Extraction in Reducing Crestal Bone Resorption and Sinus Pneumatization: A Multicenter Prospective Case-Control Study. *BioMed Res. Int.* **2018**, *2018*, 9352130. [CrossRef] [PubMed]

33. Fiorillo, L.; Cervino, G.; Herford, A.S.; Lauritano, F.; D'Amico, C.; Lo Giudice, R.; Laino, L.; Troiano, G.; Crimi, S.; Cicciù, M. Interferon crevicular fluid profile and correlation with periodontal disease and wound healing: A systemic review of recent data. *Int. J. Mol. Sci.* **2018**, *19*, 1908. [CrossRef]

34. Matarese, G.; Ramaglia, L.; Fiorillo, L.; Cervino, G.; Lauritano, F.; Isola, G. Implantology and Periodontal Disease: The Panacea to Problem Solving? *Open Dent. J.* **2017**, *11*, 460–465. [CrossRef] [PubMed]

35. Cervino, G.; Fiorillo, L.; Spagnuolo, G.; Bramanti, E.; Laino, L.; Lauritano, F.; Cicciù, M. Interface between MTA and dental bonding agents: Scanning electron microscope evaluation. *J. Int. Soc. Prev. Community Dent.* **2017**, *7*, 64–68. [PubMed]

36. Cervino, G.; Fiorillo, L.; Herford, A.S.; Laino, L.; Troiano, G.; Amoroso, G.; Crimi, S.; Matarese, M.; D'Amico, C.; Siniscalchi, E.N.; et al. Alginate materials and dental impression technique: A current state of the art and application to dental practice. *Mar. Drugs* **2019**, *19*, 18. [CrossRef] [PubMed]

37. Spagnuolo, G.; Ametrano, G.; D'Antò, V.; Formisano, A.; Simeone, M.; Riccitiello, F.; Amato, M.; Rengo, S. Microcomputed tomography analysis of mesiobuccal orifices and major apical foramen in first maxillary molars. *Open Dent. J.* **2012**, *6*, 118–125. [CrossRef]

38.   Pedullà, E.; Lizio, A.; Scibilia, M.; Grande, N.M.; Plotino, G.; Boninelli, S.; Rapisarda, E.; Lo Giudice, G. Cyclic fatigue resistance of two nickel–titanium rotary instruments in interrupted rotation. *Int. Endod. J.* **2017**, *50*, 194–201. [CrossRef] [PubMed]

39.   Spagnuolo, G.; Ametrano, G.; D'Antò, V.; Rengo, C.; Simeone, M.; Riccitiello, F.; Amato, M. Effect of autoclaving on the surfaces of TiN-coated and conventional nickel-titanium rotary instruments. *Int. Endod. J.* **2012**, *45*, 1148–1155. [CrossRef] [PubMed]

40.   Rongo, R.; Ametrano, G.; Gloria, A.; Spagnuolo, G.; Galeotti, A.; Paduano, S.; Valletta, R.; D'Antò, V. Effects of intraoral aging on surface properties of coated nickel-titanium archwires. *Angle Orthod.* **2014**, *84*, 665–672. [CrossRef] [PubMed]

41.   De Jongh, A.; Cheung, S.; Khoe, L.H.; Asmi, N.E. Cosmetic dental treatment. Its impact on happiness and quality of life. *Ned. Tijdschr. Tandheelkd.* **2011**, *118*, 152–155. [CrossRef] [PubMed]

4

Accuracy of 3-Dimensionally Printed Full-Arch Dental Models

Yasaman Etemad-Shahidi, Omel Baneen Qallandar, Jessica Evenden, Frank Alifui-Segbaya◉ and Khaled Elsayed Ahmed *◉

School of Dentistry and Oral Health, Griffith University, Griffith Health Centre (G40), Office: 7.59, Brisbane, QLD 4215, Australia; yasaman.etemadshahidi@griffithuni.edu.au (Y.E.-S.); omelbaneen.qallandar@griffithuni.edu.au (O.B.Q.); jessica.evenden@griffithuni.edu.au (J.E.); f.alifui-segbaya@griffith.edu.au (F.A.-S.)
* Correspondence: khaled.ahmed@griffith.edu.au

Abstract: The use of additive manufacturing in dentistry has exponentially increased with dental model construction being the most common use of the technology. Henceforth, identifying the accuracy of additively manufactured dental models is critical. The objective of this study was to systematically review the literature and evaluate the accuracy of full-arch dental models manufactured using different 3D printing technologies. Seven databases were searched, and 2209 articles initially identified of which twenty-eight studies fulfilling the inclusion criteria were analysed. A meta-analysis was not possible due to unclear reporting and heterogeneity of studies. Stereolithography (SLA) was the most investigated technology, followed by digital light processing (DLP). Accuracy of 3D printed models varied widely between <100 to >500 μm with the majority of models deemed of clinically acceptable accuracy. The smallest (3.3 μm) and largest (579 μm) mean errors were produced by SLA printers. For DLP, majority of investigated printers ($n = 6/8$) produced models with <100 μm accuracy. Manufacturing parameters, including layer thickness, base design, postprocessing and storage, significantly influenced the model's accuracy. Majority of studies supported the use of 3D printed dental models. Nonetheless, models deemed clinically acceptable for orthodontic purposes may not necessarily be acceptable for the prosthodontic workflow or applications requiring high accuracy.

Keywords: 3-dimensional printing; additive manufacturing; dental models; accuracy; systematic review; full-arch

1. Introduction

Three-dimensional (3D) printing is an additive manufacturing (AM) process that allows conversion of digital models into physical ones through a layer-by-layer deposition printing process. 3D printing has been adopted in dentistry at an increasing rate and construction of dental models is one of the main applications of this promising technology in prosthodontics, orthodontics, implantology and oral and maxillofacial surgery, amongst others [1]. An essential prerequisite of dental models is creating an accurate replication of teeth and the surrounding tissues to serve their intended purposes as diagnostic and restorative aids for assessment, treatment planning and fabrication of various dental appliances and prostheses. Currently, gypsum casts poured from conventional impressions (e.g., alginates silicones, poly-sulphurs, ethers) are considered the gold standard for constructing dental models [2]. However, these cast models suffer a number of limitations, including a need for expedited processing of impressions, depending on the impression material; storage space for resultant casts; the cost of human and laboratory resources involved in fabrication; poor structural durability; and a propensity to dimensional changes over time [3]. In contrast, 3D printed models could offer a more efficient workflow that can be manufactured on demand and are more resilient, less-labour intensive and potentially time-saving [4]. Nonetheless, 3D printed models also present a unique set of limitations. The accuracy of the resultant models depends on several factors that can introduce errors. This includes the data acquisition and image processing of the oral hard and soft tissues, and the myriad of parameters involved in the manufacturing and postprocessing processes [5]. Moreover, models acquired through vat polymerisation and material jetting are prone to shrinkage during the polymerisation stage as well as having stair-step surfaces due to the layering technique used in construction [6]. In addition, a recent study demonstrated that models exhibit dimensional changes postprocessing as they age with their dimensions reported to be significantly different after three-weeks of manufacturing [7].

At present, there is an array of printing technologies available utilising various techniques, with varying outputs and performances, and consequently confounding the issue of a standardised expectation of accuracy. The most commonly used techniques are stereolithography (SLA), digital light processing (DLP), material jetting (MJ) and fused filament fabrication (FFF). Other processes such as continuous liquid interface production (CLIP) and binder jetting (BJ) have also been utilised but are not as common [8]. The earliest and most widely adopted 3D printing technique is SLA, which utilises ultraviolet (UV) scanning laser to sequentially cure liquid photopolymer resin layers. Each layer is solidified in the x-y direction, and the build platform incrementally drops in the z-direction to be recoated by resin and cured [9]. The photopolymerisation of each new layer connects it to the prior layer resulting in models with good strength. DLP uses a conventional light source to polymerise photosensitive liquid resins. However, unlike SLA, each x-y layer is exposed to the light all at once using a selectively masked light source, resulting in shorter production time [10]. Both SLA and DLP are versatile techniques as they can be used with a wide variety of resin systems [11]. CLIP is an advanced form of DLP technology with the advantage of faster printing time. Additionally, this technique utilises a membrane, which allows oxygen permeation to inhibit radical polymerisation. MJ, similar to vat polymerisation techniques (SLA, DLP and CLIP) employs photopolymerisation. This technique allows for deposition of liquid photosensitive resin through multiple jet heads on a platform, which is then cured by UV light [12]. As opposed to SLA and DLP, this technique requires no post-curing. Unlike Vat polymerisation and MJ, which use photopolymer material, FFF relies on the melting of thermoplastic materials, extruded through a fine nozzle, to create objects through layering filaments [11]. BJ technology, on the other hand, utilises selectively deposited liquid bonding agents to fuse powdered material.

The International Organization for Standardization (ISO 5725-1:1994) identifies accuracy as a qualitative concept, with trueness and precision being its quantitative counterparts. Trueness is defined as the 'closeness of agreement between the arithmetic mean of a large number of test results and the true or accepted value'. Precision is defined as the 'closeness of agreement between test results' [13]. There is currently no systematic review of data published on accuracy of dental models manufactured using 3D printing technologies; henceforth, this review aims to investigate the existing literature and evaluate the accuracy of 3D printed dental models using different 3D printing technologies and identify the printing parameters influencing their accuracy.

2. Materials and Methods

2.1. Review Question

The review search question was formulated using the PICO principle (Population, Intervention, Control, Outcome) [14], with dental models as the population cohort, 3D printing as the intervention and accuracy as the outcome. No control was defined. Hence, the formulated question was, "What is the accuracy of dental models manufactured using 3D printing technologies?" The protocol was registered on PROSPERO (registration number: CRD42020164099). The PRISMA guidelines were followed, where applicable [15].

2.2. Eligibility and Search Strategy

An electronic databases search was performed for PubMed, Cochrane Database, Web of Science, Scopus, EMBASE, LILACS, Scientific Electronic Library Online (SciELO) and the first ten pages of Google Scholar, using keywords and MeSH terms (Table 1). The Peer Review of Electronic Search Strategies (PRESS) guidelines were followed with an independent peer-reviewing the suitability of the search strategy [16]. Additionally, hand searching and cross-referencing was performed to identify additional studies. All study designs were included, whether prospective, retrospective, experimental in-vivo or in-vitro. The studies were limited to those published in English in the past 15 years (from 1 January 2005 to 13 March 2020). Abstracts from conferences, letters to the editor and studies that did not assess the accuracy of human dentate dental arches were excluded.

Table 1. Search strategy.

1. Search (print * OR "rapid prototyping" OR "additive manufacturing" OR fabrication OR stereolithography OR "stereo-lithography" OR "stereo lithography" OR photopolymer * OR photopolymer * OR "fused deposition Ωmodelling" OR "fused filament fabrication" OR "material extrusion" OR "material jetting" OR photojet OR polyjet OR "photopolymer jetting" OR "multijet printing" OR "binder jetting" OR "digital light processing" OR "selective laser sintering" OR "continuous liquid interface production" OR photopolymer * OR RP OR AM OR SLA OR SL OR FDM OR FFF OR PPJ OR PJ OR MJP OR MJ OR DLP OR CLIP OR SLS)
2. Search ("dental cast *" OR "dental model *" OR edentulous * OR edentate * OR dentate OR "full arch" OR "replica cast *") AND (3 D OR 3D OR 3 dimensional OR three dimensional)
3. Search (accuracy OR accuracies OR applicability OR precision OR repeatability OR reproducibility OR trueness OR sensitivity OR specificity OR specificities OR validation OR validity OR value OR agreement OR "spatial error *" OR "geometric error *" OR "dimensional error *" OR correctness OR exactness)
4. Search ((#1 and #2 and #3)) Filters: Publication date from 01/01/2005 to 13/05/2020

Initial screening of the titles and abstracts was independently performed by two investigators (O.Q. and J.E.). A list of the selected papers was compiled and compared, and any disagreements were discussed with a third investigator (K.A.) until a consensus was reached. Thereafter, the full text of the selected articles was reviewed to confirm the fulfilment of the inclusion criteria.

2.3. Data Extraction

Inclusion criteria and trial quality of included articles were assessed individually by two investigators (O.Q. and J.E.). The selected data were independently extracted and then cross-checked between the investigators and discrepancies were resolved by referring to a third investigator (K.A). Data collection, extraction and synthesis of the included studies was performed according to the following criteria:

- Sample size;
- model type;
- the 3D printing technology used;
- resolution (x,y) and layer thickness (z) used;
- materials and postprocessing protocol;
- accuracy of intraoral/lab scanner;
- accuracy assessment methodology;
- measurement of dimensional accuracy over time;
- presence of a study control;
- findings (accuracy); and
- limitations.

The authors of the included studies were not contacted to provide missing data not reported in their published studies.

2.4. Statistical Analysis and Risk of Bias (Quality) Assessment

A quality assessment of the methodology of the included studies was performed using the quality assessment of diagnostic accuracy-2 (QUADAS-2) [17] to assess their risk of bias and applicability concerns. Each domain was assessed and ranked as high risk, low risk or unclear.

3. Results

A total of 2209 studies were initially identified after the databases search (Figure 1). Screening of the titles and abstracts, and removing duplicates, resulted in 39 studies being selected. Six additional studies were identified through cross-referencing. Excluded studies either did not assess full-arch dental model [18–27] or were not published in English [28–30]. Three additional studies were later removed as they assessed and compared the accuracy of different intraoral scanners [5,31,32]. In addition, one study [33] was excluded as it was a published abstract. Finally, twenty-eight studies fulfilled the inclusion criteria and were further synthesised.

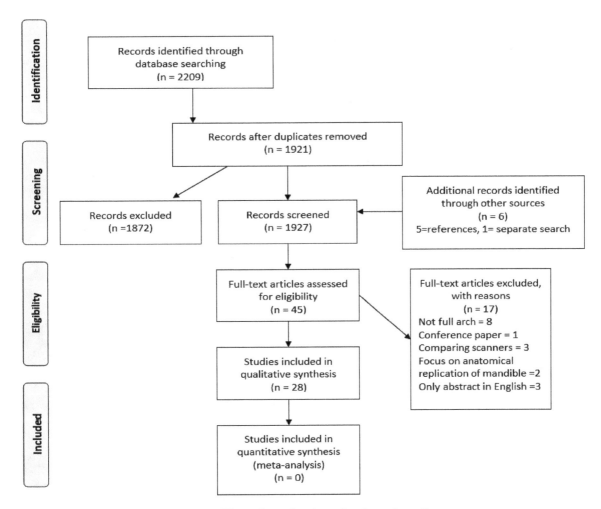

Figure 1. Flow chart for the selection of studies.

3.1. Study Characteristics

3.1.1. Sample Size and Reference Models

For this study, the sample size was determined based on the number of single dental arches manufactured by each printer. The majority of the studies ($n = 19/28$) assessed models of both maxillary and mandibular arches, and the remainder used either the maxillary ($n = 8$) or mandibular ($n = 1$) arches. The sample size ranged between one and sixty 3D printed single arch models per printer (Table 2).

Table 2. Details of studies included in the systematic review.

Authors/Date	3D printing Material	Model Data Source	Model Data Source	3D Printing System	3D Printer Details	Resolution x, y, z (µm)	Sample Size (Single Arch/Printer)	Assessment Method	Trueness (SD) (µm)	Precision (µm, ICC and IQR)
Aly and Mohsen, 2020 [34]	Photocurable polymer (liquid resin)	IOS scanned full dentate Typodont (Mx and Md)	IOS scanned Typodont	SLA	Projet 6000, 3D Systems	Unclear	10	Digital callipers Tooth: MD, CH Arch: IC, IM	190 (100)	Unclear
Bohner et al. 2019 [35]	Unclear	Typodont (Mx, 7–7) containing implants at sites of 21, 24 and 26	Typodont (maxillary)	SLA	Unclear, Envisiontec	Unclear	10	Surveying software Arch: IP, IM	19.7 (13.3)	Unclear
Brown, Currier, Kadioglu and Kierl, (2018) [36]	Unclear	Patient IOS and alginate impressions (Mx and Md, min 6–6) 30 cases	Patient IOS and alginate impressions 30 cases	DLP MJ	Juell 3D Flash OC, Park Dental Research; Objet Eden 260VS, Stratasys	z: 50, 100 z: 16	60	Digital callipers Arch: IC, IM, AD Tooth: MD, CH Occlusion: Unclear	70 80	Unclear
Burde et al. (2017) [37]	Poly-L-lactic acid wire Poly-L-lactic acid wire Grey light-curing resin	Patient stone model (Mx and Md) 10 cases. Unclear number of teeth present	Patient stone model 10 cases	FFF FFF SLA	Creatr HS, Leapfrog; Custom RepRap, (based on a PrusaI3 kit) Form 1+, Formlabs	z: 100 z: 100 z: 25	20	3D assessment Nominal ±11.51 Critical: ±230	156.2 (22.4) 128.3 (18.3) 207.9 (44.6)	Unclear
Camardella, de Vasconcellos Vilella and Breuning, (2017) [38]	Photopolymer resin Light-curing methacrylic resin (E-Denstone; Envisiontec)	Patient IOS 10 cases (Mx and Md, min 7–7)	Patient IOS 10 cases (mandibular)	MJ SLA	Objet Eden 260VS, Stratasys Ultra 3SP Ortho, Envisiontec	z: 16 z: 100	20	Surveying software Arch: IC, IP, IM Tooth: Unclear Occlusion: Unclear	Unclear	0.999ICC 0.998 ICC
Camardella, Vilella, van Hezel and Breuning, (2017) [39]	Light curing methacrylic resin (RC31, Envisiontec)	Patients IOS and impressions (Mx and Md, min 6–6) 28 cases	Patients IOS and impressions 28 cases	SLA	Ultra 3SP, Envisiontec	Unclear	56	Digital callipers Arch: IC, IM Tooth: MD, CH Occlusion: OJ, OB AND 3D assessment Nominal: ±50 Critical: ±500	579 (1050)	Unclear
Cho, Schaefer, Thompson and Guentsch, (2015) [40]	Unclear	Lab scanned fully dentate Typodont (Mx) with 5 prepared teeth (16, 15, 21, 23, 26)	Lab scanned Typodont (maxillary)	SLA	Unclear	Unclear	5	3D assessment Nominal: ±50 Critical: ±500	27 (7)	91 (10)
Choi, Ahn, Son and Huh, (2019) [4]	Photopolymer Photopolymer	Typodont (Mx, 7–7) with prepared teeth (16, 11, 24 and 26)	Typodont (maxillary)	SLA DLP	ZENITH U, Dentis DIOPROBO, DIO	z: 50 z: 50	10	3D assessment Nominal: ±50 Critical: ±500	85.2 (13.1) 105.5 (22.5)	49.6 (12.1) 53.8 (17.5)
Cuperus et al. (2012) [41]	Epoxy Resin	IOS Dry human skull (min 6–6, with max 1 missing or deciduous tooth per skull) 10 cases Intra-oral scanner	IOS Dry human skull 10 cases	SLA	Unclear	Unclear	20	Digital callipers Arch: IC, IM Tooth: MD Occlusion: Unclear	100	Unclear
Dietrich, Ender, Baumgartner and Mehl, (2017) [42]	Epoxy-based resin (Accura) photopolymer resins	Patient IOS 2 cases (Mx). Unclear number of teeth present	Patient IOS 2 cases (maxillary)	SLA MJ	Viper si2 SLA, 3D Systems Objet Eden 260, Stratasys	z: 100 at base and 50 at tooth level z: 16	10	3D assessment Nominal: ±20 Critical: ±100	92 (23) 62 (8)	20 (4) 38 (14)

Table 2. *Cont.*

Study	Material	Object (detailed)	Object	Technology	Printer	Layer thickness	n	Assessment	Result	Result
Favero et al. (2017) [43]	Grey photopolymer resin (FLGPGR02; Formlabs), Unclear	Typodont (Mx, 7–7)	Typodont (maxillary)	SLA / SLA / DLP / DLP / MJ	Form 2, Formlabs / Vector 3sp, Envisiontec / Juell 3D, Park Dental / Perfactory Desktop Vida, Envisiontec / Objet Eden 260V, Stratasys	z: 25, 50, 100 / z: 100 / z: 100 / z: 100 / z: 28	12	3D assessment, Nominal: ±20, Critical: ±250	64 / 79 / 44 / 56 / 85	Unclear
Hazeveld, Huddleston Slater and Ren, (2014) [44]	Unclear	Patient Stone model (Mx and Md, min 6–6), 6 cases	Patient Stone model 6 cases	DLP / BJ / MJ	Unclear, Envisiontec, / Unclear, Z-Corp / Unclear, Objet Geometries	Unclear	12	Digital callipers, Arch: Unclear, Tooth: MD, CH, Occlusion: Unclear	Unclear	Unclear
Jin, Jeong, Kim and Kim, (2018) [45]	Unclear	Lab scanned Typodont (Mx, 7–7)	Lab scanned Typodont (maxillary)	MJ / FFF	Projet 3500 HDMax, 3D Systems / Cube, 3D Systems	z: 31.97 (thickness measured after printing) / z: 123.71	10	3D assessment, Nominal: ±50, Critical: ±500	129.1 (7.8) / 149.0 (4.7)	44.6 (8.9) / 52.1 (10.9)
Jin, Kim, Kim and Kim, (2019) [6]	Photocurable liquid resin / Acrylic polymer	Lab scanned Typodont (Mx and Md, 7–7)	Lab scanned Typodont (maxillary)	SLA / MJ	Projet 6000, 3D Systems / Projet 3500 HD Max, 3D Systems	FMR / FMR	10	3D assessment, Nominal: ±50, Critical: ±500	114.3 (1.8) / 124 (3.7)	59.6 (8.2) / 41.0 (5.8)
Joda, Matthisson and Zitzmann, (2020) [7]	Light-curing polymer, (SHERAPrint-model plus "sand" UV, SHERA)	IOS Typodont (Mx, 7–7), with missing 25 and prepared 24 and 26)	IOS Typodont (maxillary)	SLA	P30, Straumann	Unclear	10	3D assessment, Nominal: unclear, Critical: unclear	3.3 (1.3)	Unclear
Kasparova et al. (2013) [46]	ABS plastic material, Clear resin	Patient stone model 10 cases. Unclear number of teeth present	Patient stone model 10 cases	FFF / MJ	RepRap, Unclear / ProJetHD3000, 3D Systems	x,y: 200, z: 0.35 / Unclear	20 / 2	Digital callipers, Tooth: CH, Arch: IC	Unclear / Unclear	Unclear / Unclear
Keating, Knox, Bibb and Zhurov, (2008) [47]	Hybrid epoxy-based resin	Patient stone model 15 cases. Unclear number of teeth present	Patient stone model 15 cases	SLA	SLA-250/40, 3D Systems	z: 150	30	Digital callipers, Tooth: CH, Arch: IC, IP, IM	150 (160)	Unclear
Kim et al. (2018) [19]	Unclear	Lab scanned Typodont (Mx and Md, 7–7)	Lab scanned Typodont	SLA: / DLP / MJ / FFF	ZENITH, Dentis / M-One, MAKEX Technology / Objet Eden 260VS, Stratasys / Cubicon 3DP-110F, HyVISION System	x,y: 50, z: 50 / x,y: 70, z: 75 / z: 16 / x,y: 100, z: 100	10	Surveying software, Tooth: MD, BL, CH, Arch: IC, IM	138 (79) / 446 (46) / 74 (39) / 307 (61)	88 (14) / 76 (14) / 68 (9) / 99 (14)
Kuo, Chen, Wong, Lu and Huang, (2015) [48]	Unclear	Patient IOS. Patient impressions poured, and lab scanned (Md, 7–7) 1 case	Patient IOS Patient impressions poured, and lab scanned 1 case	MJ	Connex 350, Stratasys	Unclear	1	3D assessment, Nominal: ±60, Critical: ±300	140	Unclear
Loflin et al. (2019) [49]	Grey photopolymer resin, (FLGPGR03; Formlabs)	Patient stone models (Mx and Md) 12 cases. Unclear number of teeth present	Patient stone model 12 cases	SLA	Form 2, Formlabs	z: 25, 50, 100	24	ABO tool, Tooth: marginal ridge, Occlusion: OJ, occlusal contacts	Unclear	Unclear

Table 2. *Cont.*

Study	Material	Object (cast/scan)	STL input	Technology	Printer/System	Resolution (µm)	Cases	Measurement method	Results	Accuracy
Nestler, Wesemann, Spies, Beuer and Bumann, (2020) [50]	Dental SG, Optiprint, Imprimo LC model, ABS, Polylactide	Cast in standard tessellation language (STL) format including 5 measuring cubes in areas 16, 26, 13, 23 and between 11 and 21	Maxillary cast in standard tessellation language (STL) format	SLA SLA DLP FFF FFF	Forms 2, Formlabs; Myrev140, Sisma; Asiga Max UV, Asiga M2, Makergear M2, Makerbot; Ultimaker 2+, Ultimaker	Unclear Unclear Xy: 62, Z: Unclear Unclear x,y: 12.5, z: Unclear	37 34 for Myrev140	Surveying software Arch: IC, IM, arch length	-80 (94) -175 (28) -16 (32) -55 (39) 12 (43)	134 28 47 55 56
Papaspyridakos et al., (2020) [51]	Photopolymer resin, dental model resin (Formlabs)	Lab scanned Patient stone model 1 case (Md) with 4 abutment-level implant analogs	Lab scanned Patient stone model 1 case (mandibular)	SLA	Form 2, Formlab	z: 25	25	3D assessment Nominal ±50 Critical: ±200	59 (16)	Unclear
Rebong, Stewart, Utreja and Ghoneima, (2018) [52]	Unclear	Patient stone models (Mx and Md, min 6-6) 12 cases	Patient stone model 12 cases	FFF SLA MJ	Makerbot Replicator, Makerbot Industries; Projet 6000, 3DSystems; Objet Eden 500V, Stratasys	z: 100 z: 50 z: 16	24	Digital calipers Arch: IC, IM Tooth: Unclear Occlusion: OJ, OB	110 (420) -20 (370) -190 (330)	Unclear
Rungrojwittayakul et al. (2020) [53]	Unclear	Lab scanned fully dentate Typodont (Mx.)	Lab scanned Typodont (maxillary)	CLIP DLP	Carbon M2, Carbon; MoonRay S100, SprintRay	Unclear	10	3D assessment Nominal: ±10 Critical: ±100	48 (44) 87 (57)	0.968 ICC 0.983 ICC
Saleh, Ariffin, Sherriff and Bister, (2015) [54]	Unclear	Lab scanned Typodont (Mx and Md, 7-7)	Lab scanned Typodont	MJ	Objet Eden 250, Stratasys	Unclear	8	Digital calipers Tooth: MD Arch: IC, IM Occlusion: OJ, OB	320 (156)	Unclear
Sherman, Kadioglu, Currier, Kierl and Li, (2020) [55]	Unclear	Patient IOS (Mx and Md, min 6-6) 15 cases	Patient IOS 15 cases	DLP	JUELL 3D Flash OC, Park Dental Research Corporation	z: 50, 100	30	Digital calipers Arch: IC, IM, AD Tooth: MD, CH Occlusion: Unclear	Unclear	Unclear
Wan Hassan, Yusoff and Mardi, 2017 [56]	High-performance composite (Zp151; 3D Systems).	Patient impression (Mx and Md, min 6-6) 10 cases	Patient impression 10 cases	BJ	Z Printer 450, 3D Systems	z: 89-102	30	Digital callipers Arch: IC, IP, IM Tooth: MD, CH, BL Occlusion: Unclear	-20	Unclear
Zhang, Li, Chu and Shen, (2019) [57]	Dental model resin (Formlabs); Model Ortho resin (Union Tec); Encashape, ENCA-Model resin; Light curing methacrylate resin; E-Denstone, EnvisionTEC	Patient IOS (Mx and Md, 7-7) 1 case	Patient IOS 1 case	SLA DLP DLP DLP	Form 2, Formlabs; EvoDent, UnionTec; EncaDent, Encashape; Vida HD, EnvisionTec	x,y: 140 z:25, 30,10; z: 50,100; x,y: 58; z: 20, 30, 50,100; x,y: 50; z: 50, 100	2	3D assessment Nominal: ±50 Critical: ±250	34.4 23.3 26.5 31.7	Unclear

Mx = maxillary, Mn = mandinular, CH = crown height, BL = buccolingual width, IC = intercanine width, MD = mesiodistal width, IP = interpremolar width, IM = intermolar width, OB = overbite, OJ = overjet, SLA = stereolithography, MJ = material jetting, BJ = binder jetting, DLP = digital light processing, CLIP = continuous liquid interface production, FFF = fused filament fabrication, IOS = intraoral scanner, ABO = American Board of Orthodontics.

3.1.2. Sample Details and Controls

The inclusion criteria for the studies that collected patient samples (digital or physical impressions or models) varied slightly with the majority ($n = 14/25$) being full arch dentate post-orthodontic models, including up to permanent first molars [36–39,42,44,46–49,52,55–57]. One of the studies [42] also used a model with a shortened dental arch. Another used an edentulous mandibular cast with four multi-unit abutments for implant prosthodontic rehabilitation [51].

Twenty-four studies included reference models as controls in their methodology design [6,7,34,36–53,55–57]. The controls included were a dental stone cast ($n = 8$), a digital STL image of a dental stone cast ($n = 3$), typodont digital STL image ($n = 7$), typodont ($n = 1$), prefabricated resin model digital STL image ($n = 2$), patient intraoral scan image (2) or a dry human skull ($n = 1$). In addition, there were four studies [4,35,47,54] that did not include a reference model as a control, rather compared various printing technologies against each other.

3.2. Additive Manufacturing

3.2.1. D printing Technologies Assessed and Printing Parameters

An array of additive manufacturing systems were assessed in the included studies with several investigating more than one type of technology, printer brand or parameter settings (Table 2). The majority of studies investigated SLA ($n = 20$), MJ ($n = 11$), DLP ($n = 9$) and, to a lesser extent, FFF ($n = 6$), BJ ($n = 2$) and CLIP ($n = 1$). With regards to printing parameters, one study reported following the manufacturers' recommendations [6], while others explicitly detailed the printing parameters used [4,19,36–38,42,43,45–47,49–52,55–57]. In contrast, the remainder of the studies did not provide clear details regarding the printing parameters used.

3.2.2. Layer Thickness

The specified printing layer thickness (z-axis resolution) substantially varied amongst studies and ranged from 25–150 μm for SLA, 20–100 μm for DLP, 16–32 μm for MJ, 100–150 μm for FFF and 89–102 μm for BJ. The study using CLIP technology did not specify the layer thickness used [53]. Most studies did not specify the printing resolution in the x- and y-axes. However, in those that did, the x-y plane resolution ranged from 50–140 μm for SLA, 50–70 μm for DLP and 12.5–200 μm for FFF.

3.2.3. Materials Used

The materials used by 3D printers are broadly classified based on their printing technologies. Vat polymerisation technologies (SLA, DLP and CLIP) used liquid photopolymers, including acrylates and epoxides, 3D material extrusion technology (FFF) used polylactic acid (PLA), or acrylonitrile butadiene styrene (ABS). MJ technology used photopolymers resins (acrylates) in liquid form and BJ technology used polylactic acid powder. Eleven studies did not specify the material used for the corresponding technology [19,35,36,40,44,45,48,52–55]. Within the studies assessing stone models, four used Type IV dental stone [6,35,40,45], one used Type III dental stone [4] and one did not specify the stone type utilised [34].

3.2.4. Base Designs and Filling Patterns

The three types of base designs used in the studies were horseshoe-shaped bases [4,34,36–39,41,43,49–51,55], regular American Board of Orthodontics (ABO) [35,38,44,46,47,49,52,54,57] and horseshoe-shaped with a transverse supporting bar [7,38,48,53]. Six studies did not specify their base design [6,19,40,42,45,56]. Filling patterns employed in these studies were predominantly solid; however, hollow shelled [53,55] and honeycomb [37] were also utilised.

3.2.5. Postprocessing Protocol

The majority of studies did not specify the postprocessing protocol ($n = 19/28$) [6,19,34–36,40,41,44–48,50–52,54–57]. Nine studies reported their post-curing protocol for vat polymerisation techniques [4,7,37–39,42,43,49,53] which included cleaning the models with isopropyl alcohol [37,43,49,53], or ethanol [4] to remove uncured resin followed by curing with UV light. Three studies only used UV light to post-process SLA models [38,39,42]. One study placed the SLA models in an ultrasonic bath followed by using light with wavelengths of 280–580 nm for post-curing [7]. Two studies reported that MJ and FFF did not require post-curing [37,38], and one study rinsed the MJ printed models in a bath of caustic soda to clean them [42]. Additionally, three studies specified removing the support structures from the models [37,42,57].

3.3. Assessment Methodology

The assessment of the accuracy of 3D printed models was performed using either 3D deviation analyses or 2D linear measurements. For the 3D assessment, step-height measurements through iterative point-cloud surface-matching followed by 3D deviation assessment were performed. For 2D linear measurements, reference points were selected and measured either directly onto the physical model using digital callipers or indirectly on the model's digital image using surveying software. The majority of studies relied on 3D assessment [4,6,7,37,39,40,42,43,45,48,51,53,57] followed by digital callipers [34,36,39,41,44,46,47,52,54–56] and surveying software measurements [19,35,38,50]. One study [49] used the ABO cast-radiograph evaluation tool.

3.3.1. Surface Matching and 3D Deviation Analyses

The studies which performed 3D assessment used min/max nominal values ranging between ±10 to ±60 µm and min/max critical values of ± 100 to ± 500 µm. Before superimposition, the 3D-printed models were scanned and converted to standard tessellation language (STL) format. The scanners included desktop/laboratory scanners ($n = 15$) [4,6,7,19,35,37,38,40,42,43,45,48,51,53,57], intraoral scanners ($n = 2$) [36,41], and computerised tomography scanner ($n = 1$) [38]. Two studies did not specify the details of image acquisition [34,50]. While most studies did not specify the accuracy of the scanners nor mentioned calibrating the scanners before scan acquisition, the remaining studies reported a scanning accuracy <20 µm [4,6,19,40,45,46,57].

3.3.2. Linear Measurements of Physical and Digital Models

Studies that utilised digital callipers with physical models or measuring software with digital models relied on various reference points to perform 2D linear measurements. The reported accuracy of all callipers was 10 µm, and the ABO tool was 100 µm. The selected reference points relied on varying tooth measurements (crown height, mesiodistal width, buccolingual width and marginal ridge width), arch measurements (intercanine width, interpremolar width and intermolar width) and occlusion measurements (overjet, overbite, occlusal contact and interarch sagittal relationships). Most studies used both tooth and arch measurements ($n = 10$) [19,34,36,39,41,43,46,47,55,56], while one study only used tooth measurements [44] and three studies only used arch measurements [35,38,40]. Moreover, five studies used occlusion measurements in addition to the arch measurements [19,39,49,52,54].

3.3.3. Time of Assessment

The time at which the 3D printed models were scanned or measured was reported by six studies [7,41,45–47,52]. Within those studies, five assessed the models after a week of printing [41,45–47,52] and one assessed the accuracy after one day, followed by weekly intervals for four consecutive weeks [7].

3.4. Outcomes Assessed

3.4.1. Clinical Acceptability

The clinically acceptable error defined in the studies varied widely from <100 μm [51,53], <200μm [6,45], <250 μm [43], <300 μm [44,48] and <500 μm [19,34–36,42,46,47,49,50,52,55–57]. One study [4] defined various acceptable ranges of error for different measurement points and seven studies did not define any clinically acceptable range [4,7,37,38,40,41,54]. From those, twelve assessed orthodontic models [19,36,39,42–44,47,49,52,55–57], five assessed fixed pros and implant models [6,34,35,51,53] and three did not specify [45,46,48].

3.4.2. Trueness

Overall, the mean deviations from the reference model across all studies ranged from 3.3 to 579 μm [7,39]. Studies which assessed the trueness of both 3D printed and stone models found that the mean error for the stone model was consistently lower than their 3D printed counterparts [4,6,34,35,40,45]. In contrast, one study [45] reported no statistical differences between stone and MJ models and another [6] found no statistical difference between SLA and stone. However, several studies did not fully report the details of the 3D printer/s used or their trueness results [38,40,41,44,46,49,55]. Nonetheless, six DLP printers, five SLA printers and one MJ printer had an error measurement of <100 μm for full-arch dental models, demonstrating high trueness (Figure 2). Similarly, the BJ printer (ZPrinter 450, 3D Systems, USA), CLIP printer (M2, Carbon, USA) and two FFF printers (Ultimaker 2+, Ultimaker B.V, Geldermalsen, The Netherlands; and M2, Makergear, USA) reported high trueness results (Table 2).

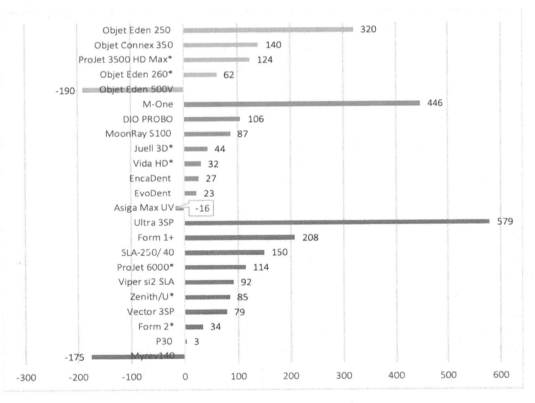

Figure 2. Reported trueness in microns for material jetting (MJ, green), digital light processing (DLP, orange) and stereolithography (SLA, blue) 3D printed full-arch dental models. * Asterisk denotes lowest mean error identified from different studies—other results in microns reported include: Form 2 = 59, 64 and −80; Zenith series = 138; Projet 6000 = 190; Juell 3D = 44, 70; Vida = 56; Objet Eden 260 series = 74, 80 and 85; Projet 3500 HD Max = 129. Data from studies that did not report details of 3D printer used or trueness data were not included in the figure.

All SLA printers consistently produced oversized 3D printed models compared to the control, excluding the Myrev 140 printer [50]. The P30 reported the lowest mean error of 3.3 μm [7] and the Form 2 printer followed with reported mean errors ranging between 34.4 to 64 μm [37,43,56]. The SLA Ultra 3SP demonstrated the highest mean error at 579 μm [39]. Similar results were found for DLP printers with the majority of printers producing oversized models, except the Asiga Max UV, which also reported the lowest mean error for DLP at—16 μm [50]. The Evodent was the second most accurate DLP printer with a 23.3 μm error, followed by the Encadent at 26.5 μm errors [50,57]. Furthermore, JUELL 3D FLASH OC, Vida HD and Vida had a reported mean error of 44 μm, 31.7 μm and 56μm, respectively [43,45,57]. The highest mean error for the DLP printing technology was the M-One printer with a mean error of 446 μm [19]. Within MJ printers, Objet Eden 260 series (V, VS) had the lowest mean errors ranging from 62 to 85 μm [19,36,42,43], whilst the highest mean error was 320 μm (Objet Eden 250) [54]. Ultimaker 2+ printer as FFF technology had the least deviation error of 12μm [50], while Cubicon 3DP 110F reported a mean error of 307 μm [19]. The two printers for BJ (Z printer 450 and unclear) and CLIP (Carbon M2) technologies had mean errors of—20 μm [56] and 48μm [53], respectively.

3.4.3. Precision

The precision of 3D printed models was assessed in 10 studies using either root mean square value (RMS) [4,6,19,40,42,45], the intraclass correlation coefficient (ICC) [38,53] and or interquartile range (IQR) [50]. The RMS value ranges for SLA, FFF, MJ and DLP were 23 to 91 μm, 52.1 to 99 μm, 38 to 68 μm and 53.8 to 76 μm, respectively. The range for ICC was 0.968 for CLIP and 0.999 for MJ. In addition, one study [50] reported IQR of 28 to 134 μm for SLA, 55 to 56 μm for FFF and 47 μm for DLP.

Two studies found 3D printed models to have equal or greater precision than conventional stone models [6,45]. By contrast, two studies [4,40] found conventional stone models to be more precise than the 3D printed models. Of note, studies that used ICC [38,53] to assess precision; demonstrated excellent reproducibility (>0.9 ICC value) of 3D printed models, according to the Koo and Li (2016) classification [58].

3.5. Statistical Analysis

The limited reporting, varying printing technologies, printing parameters, assessment methodology and statistical analysis employed in the included studies presented a heterogeneity that precluded from performing a meaningful meta-analysis.

3.6. Risk of Bias Assessment

The risk of bias and applicability concerns varied across the studies, which may have influenced the reliability of their results (Table 3). The reference standards used in almost all the studies had a low risk of bias and low concerns regarding applicability (27/28). The risk of the index test, however, was high for the majority of studies (21/28). This high risk was because the studies either did not use 3D superimposition, and therefore the mean error may not have been an accurate representation of the whole arch deviation, or the method of assessing the model's deviation introduced errors other than those arising from the CAM process. These errors include the use of full-arch intraoral scanning for data acquisition which may introduce scanner error in-addition to the 3D printing error. Similarly, lack of details of assessors and their calibration was a noted risk of bias in several studies. Finally, the majority of studies had a high risk of bias for sample selection. This high risk is attributed to the lack of details relating to sample size calculation, spectrum of selected samples and/or postprocessing protocol. However, most of the samples remained highly applicable with the measurement protocol employed in the studies appropriately described to allow the reviewer to answer the review question.

Table 3. Risk of bias and applicability concerns according to QUADAS-2 tool. Negative sign (−) denotes high risk of bias. Positive sign (+) denotes low risk of bias.

Study	Risk of Bias			Applicability Concerns		
	Patient (Sample) Selection	Index Test	Reference Standard	Patient (Sample) Selection	Index Test	Reference Standard
Aly and Mohsen, 2020 [34]	−	−	+	+	−	+
Bohner et al. 2019 [35]	−	−	+	−	−	+
Brown, Currier, Kadioglu and Kierl, 2018 [36]	−	−	+	+	−	+
Burde et al. 2017 [37]	−	+	+	+	+	+
Camardella, de Vasconcellos Vilella and Breuning, 2017 [38]	+	−	+	+	−	+
Camardella, Vilella, van Hezel and Breuning, (2017) [39]	−	−	+	+	−	+
Cho, Schaefer, Thompson and Guentsch, 2015 [40]	−	+	+	−	+	+
Choi, Ahn, Son and Huh, 2019 [4]	−	+	+	+	+	+
Cuperus et al. 2012 [41]	−	−	+	−	−	+
Dietrich, Ender, Baumgartner and Mehl, 2017 [42]	−	−	+	+	−	+
Favero et al. 2017 [43]	−	+	+	+	+	+
Hazeveld, Huddleston Slater and Ren, 2014 [44]	−	−	+	−	−	+
Jin, Jeong, Kim and Kim, 2018 [45]	−	+	+	+	+	+
Jin, Kim, Kim and Kim, 2019 [6]	−	+	+	+	+	+
Joda, Matthisson and Zitzmann, 2020 [7]	−	−	+	+	−	+
Kasparova et al. 2013 [46]	−	−	+	+	−	+
Keating, Knox, Bibb and Zhurov, 2008 [47]	−	−	+	+	−	+
Kim et al. 2018 [19]	−	+	+	+	+	+
Kuo, Chen, Wong, Lu and Huang, 2015 [48]	−	−	+	+	−	+
Loflin et al. 2019 [49]	−	−	+	+	−	+
Nestler, Wesemann, Spies, Beuer and Bumann, 2020 [50]	−	-	+	+	−	+
Papaspyridakos et al., 2020 [51]	+	−	+	+	−	+
Rebong, Stewart, Utreja and Ghoneima, 2018 [52]	−	−	+	+	−	+
Rungrojwittayakul et al. 2020 [53]	−	−	+	+	−	+
Saleh, Ariffin, Sherriff and Bister, 2015 [54]	−	−	+	+	−	+
Sherman, Kadioglu, Currier, Kierl and Li, 2020 [55]	−	−	+	+	−	+
Wan Hassan, Yusoff and Mardi, 2017 [56]	+	−	+	+	−	+
Zhang, Li, Chu and Shen, 2019 [57]	−	−	+	+	−	+

4. Discussion

Given 3D printing's promising potential and increased use in dentistry, it is essential to evaluate the accuracy of 3D printed dental models. This is the first systematic review, to the authors' knowledge, investigating the accuracy of dental models manufactured using 3D printing technology. The selection criteria for the included reference standards were high, subsequently the risk of bias and applicability concerns were low according to the QUADAS-2 tool. The findings of this review support the use of 3D printing for the fabrication of dental models and deem them as clinically acceptable with the majority of included studies ($n = 20/28$) establishing a clinically acceptable error range of <100 to 500 μm. 3D printed models were found to be a valid alternative to stone models when taking precision into account. Nonetheless, the study by Wan Hassan (2019) was an outlier which found BJ 3D printed models not clinically acceptable due to their discrepancy of >500 μm. It is, however, worth noting the included studies which used orthodontic models [19,34,36,42,46,47,49,50,52,55,57] had more relaxed thresholds for clinical acceptability (up to 500 μm), compared to those intended for prosthodontic applications (up to 200 μm) [6,51,53]. Indeed, in orthodontics, a measurement difference of <300 μm between orthodontic casts and 3D printed models has been reported to be clinically acceptable [59–61]. On the other hand, in prosthodontics, the accuracy needs of dental models for the fabrication of dental prostheses is generally considered higher. A recent study concluded that three-unit fixed partial dentures fabricated using 3D printed models, whilst demonstrating inferior fit when compared to those fabricated using stone casts [27], the detected marginal gaps remained within the clinically accepted threshold of 120 μm reported in the literature [62]. Such clinically relevant thresholds become more critical in complex prosthodontic treatment modalities. Implant-supported complete dental prostheses or hybrid bridges have a maximum acceptable threshold of fit between the prostheses platform and the dental implants ranging between 59–150 μm [63–65]. Accordingly, the choice of 3D printing technology must be determined by its intended application. Hence, it is reasonable to conclude that 3D printed models which are clinically acceptable for orthodontic purposes may not necessarily be acceptable for the prosthodontic workflow or other dental applications requiring high accuracy.

The most common 3D printing technology investigated by the included studies was SLA with the findings demonstrating that SLA and DLP achieved the best accuracy for full-arch models. Amongst the

SLA printers, Form 2 by Formlabs was investigated the most, and consistently produced clinically acceptable models. Although a wider range of mean errors was observed amongst SLA printed models, the Form 2 SLA desktop printer [43,49,51,57] also consistently produced models more accurate than MJ printers and was more cost-effective [43,44]. Moreover, the SLA printer P30 reported the most accurate models amongst all studies, followed by the DLP Asiga Max UV [7,50]. Additionally, SLA printers produced acceptable results regardless of their layer thickness, and therefore the layer thickness of 100 μm may be considered as an optimal thickness that balances accuracy and printing time when compared to 25 and 50 μm layers [49,57]. Moreover, it was suggested that a hollow or honeycomb infill could be indicated to reduce printing time and material-use with study models. Although no studies assessed the effect of using different resins with the same printer, using the manufacturer recommended resin was advised. In contrast, only one study assessed CLIP technology and used the Carbon M2 printer, which printed 3D models with deviations as small as 48 μm [53]. This study also concluded that the accuracy of 3D printed models was affected by the printing technique regardless of the base design. However, due to the limited studies that assessed the accuracy of BJ [56] and CLIP technologies [53], further investigation of these techniques is required to validate the viability of these printers. It is worth mentioning that some studies did not provide details of the sample size calculation, resin materials and/or post-curing protocols (Table 3), exposing them to high risk of bias and applicability concerns with regards to sample selection. As a result, no conclusions were drawn based on these parameters, other than those studies that reported using the manufacturer's recommendations.

The two studies which examined the Ultra printer by EnvisionTEC [38,39] reported that the SLA models with horseshoe bases were not accurate nor clinically acceptable due to contraction in the transversal dimension during the post-curing protocol. However, as the horseshoe base is favoured for appliance fabrication and reduces material use, the inclusion of a posterior connection bar was suggested to prevent this significant dimensional reduction in the posterior region of the SLA model [37,38]. Nevertheless, several studies assessing other SLA printers [4,34,37,41,43,50,51] contradicted these findings and concluded that models printed by SLA with a horseshoe base to be clinically acceptable.

When assessing DLP technology, apart from the M-One printer used by Kim et al. (2018), all other printers had accuracies comparable to SLA and MJ. The Asiga Max UV printer produced the lowest mean error (−16 μm) [50]. In addition, Sherman et al. (2020) and Zhang et al. (2019) assessed the accuracy of DLP printed models with various layer thicknesses ranging from 20–100 μm and suggested that all the printed models were clinically acceptable. Thus, similar to SLA printers, it can be inferred that a layer thickness of 100 μm can still produce models with clinically acceptable accuracies for DLP printers. In addition to layer thicknesses, two studies assessed different filling patterns for DLP printed models [53,55]. Altering the filling pattern from solid to hollow reduced material wastage, build time and cost with no statistically significant difference in mean error.

Most MJ printers could reproduce models with high levels of trueness and precision, regardless of their base design [38]. From those, Objet Eden 260 series [19,36,42,43], was the most commonly investigated printer and consistently produced models with the highest accuracies due to its smaller layer thickness of 16 μm followed by the Projet3500 HDMax [6,45]. These printers were used due to their relatively affordable price and ability to print in smaller layer thicknesses. It is worth mentioning that although the reduction in layer height resulted in smoother surface finish and greater detail, the printing time increased [43].

FFF desktop printers, albeit considered the most affordable printers [46,50], provided models with acceptable accuracy. The most accurate models were created by the Ultimaker 2+ printer (12 μm) [50]. Although the materials used by FFF printers, namely PLA or ABS were inexpensive; the resultant models had inferior surface properties compared to acrylates and epoxides which were used for vat polymerisation technologies (SLA, DLP and CLIP). Similar to SLA and DLP, studies assessing FFF suggested a layer thickness of 100 μm to be clinically acceptable. Moreover, Burde et al. (2017) printed

FFF models with a honeycomb pattern to reduce print time, material and cost with the resultant models deemed clinically acceptable.

There were very limited data to compare the results from 3D assessment to linear measurements for the same printers. However, it is worth noting that the highest risk of bias and applicability concerns for index test were recorded for studies that used linear measurements. This was reflective of the limited measuring points provided by those studies in comparison to a full arch deviation measurement by 3D superimposition. Additionally, some of the studies had a high risk of bias as human error may have been introduced by performing physical linear measurements with no information provided on the calibration of the examiners [19,49,50,53]. Furthermore, for 3D superimposition techniques, the risk of bias and applicability concerns were low for most studies as high accuracy desktop scanners were utilised and CAM was the only identified source of error. Nevertheless, studies that used intraoral scanners, made conventional impressions with or without pouring casts had a higher risk of bias due to the additional stages that may have introduced their own set of errors.

The Projet 6000 printed models were assessed using different methods [6,34]. The mean error calculated using full arch 3D superimposition (114.3 μm) was smaller than the intermolar width error measured by a surveying software (190 μm). Similarly, two studies assessed the Juell 3D printer [36,43], and the mean error calculated by full arch superimposition (44 μm) was smaller than the digital calliper measurements for the intermolar width (70 μm). On the other hand, two studies [19,36] assessed the Objet Eden 260VS model, using two different linear measurement methods. The mean errors calculated using surveying software and digital calliper were very similar (74 and 80 μm, respectively). These findings do highlight the need for a standardised measuring protocol to facilitate comparison of results across studies given the noted discrepancy between the different assessment techniques.

A potential limitation of this review is the assessment findings of the included studies in relevance to the measurement time of the 3D printed models. This limitation is due to the possible dimensional changes exhibited by printed models over time, with only six of the included studies identifying the time of model measurement. Joda et al. (2020) [7] assessed the effect of time on the accuracy of the printed models and was the solely identified study that reported assessing the models for more than one week. The results suggested that the accuracy of SLA printed models was time-dependent due to a statistically significant change in their dimensions after three weeks of storage, suggesting the use of SLA 3D printed models as single-use products with definitive prosthetic reconstructions. The lack of standardised reporting in included studies is also a limitation that may have resulted in a high risk of bias in terms of index test and sample selection.

Consequently, the evident heterogeneity of the included studies with varying techniques, manufacturing parameters, materials and assessment protocols, a meta-analysis was not feasible. It is also worth noting the limitations present in the literature which need to be addressed in future studies. Investigation of different layer thicknesses for FFF, MJ, BJ and CLIP printing technologies, the effect of time and storage conditions on the accuracy of different 3D printed models, as well as clinical patient outcomes, remain lacking. A standardised accuracy assessment protocol for 3D printing of dental models is also necessary to facilitate performance comparison. Future studies should also involve a standardised reporting protocol that details all printing parameters, materials used, postprocessing protocol and time of assessment.

5. Conclusions

The findings of this study support the use of 3D printed dental models, especially as orthodontic study models. Irrespective of the 3D printing technology, certain printers were able to demonstrate low errors and hence can be recommended for dental applications that require high accuracy models. Other factors such as layer thickness, base design, postprocessing and storage can equally influence the accuracy of the resultant 3D printed models. Nonetheless, the high risk of bias with regards to the lack of standardised testing of accuracy warrants careful interpretation of the findings.

Author Contributions: Y.E.-S.; methodology, writing—original draft, writing—review and editing, project administration. O.B.Q.; methodology, validation, formal analysis, investigation, writing—review and editing. J.E.; methodology, validation, formal analysis, investigation, writing—review and editing. F.A.-S.; methodology, writing—review and editing, supervision. K.E.A.; conceptualization, methodology, writing—original draft, writing—review and editing, project administration, supervision. All authors have read and agreed to the published version of the manuscript.

References

1. Dawood, A.; Marti, B.M.; Sauret-Jackson, V. 3D printing in dentistry. *Br. Dent. J.* **2015**, *219*, 521–529. [CrossRef]
2. Ender, A.; Mehl, A. Accuracy of complete-arch dental impressions: A new method of measuring trueness and precision. *J. Prosthet. Dent.* **2013**, *109*, 121–128. [CrossRef]
3. Ahmed, K.E.; Whitters, J.; Ju, X.; Pierce, S.G.; MacLeod, C.N.; Murray, C.A. A Proposed Methodology to Assess the Accuracy of 3D Scanners and Casts and Monitor Tooth Wear Progression in Patients. *Int. J. Prosthodont.* **2016**, *29*, 514–521. [CrossRef]
4. Choi, J.-W.; Ahn, J.-J.; Son, K.; Huh, J.-B. Three-Dimensional Evaluation on Accuracy of Conventional and Milled Gypsum Models and 3D Printed Photopolymer Models. *Materials* **2019**, *12*, 3499. [CrossRef]
5. Patzelt, S.B.; Bishti, S.; Stampf, S.; Att, W. Accuracy of computer-aided design/computer-aided manufacturing–generated dental casts based on intraoral scanner data. *J. Am. Dent. Assoc.* **2014**, *145*, 1133–1140. [CrossRef]
6. Jin, S.-J.; Kim, D.-Y.; Kim, J.-H.; Kim, W.-C. Accuracy of Dental Replica Models Using Photopolymer Materials in Additive Manufacturing: In Vitro Three-Dimensional Evaluation. *J. Prosthodont.* **2018**, *28*, e557–e562. [CrossRef] [PubMed]
7. Joda, T.; Matthisson, L.; Zitzmann, N.U. Impact of Aging on the Accuracy of 3D-Printed Dental Models: An In Vitro Investigation. *J. Clin. Med.* **2020**, *9*, 1436. [CrossRef] [PubMed]
8. Oberoi, G.; Nitsch, S.; Edelmayer, M.; Janjić, K.; Müller, A.S.; Agis, H. 3D Printing—Encompassing the Facets of Dentistry. *Front. Bioeng. Biotechnol.* **2018**, *6*, 172. [CrossRef] [PubMed]
9. Alifui-Segbaya, F. Biomedical photopolymers in 3D printing. *Rapid Prototyp. J.* **2019**, *26*, 437–444. [CrossRef]
10. Ligon, S.C.; Liska, R.; Stampfl, J.; Gurr, M.; Mülhaupt, R. Polymers for 3D Printing and Customized Additive Manufacturing. *Chem. Rev.* **2017**, *117*, 10212–10290. [CrossRef] [PubMed]
11. Stansbury, J.W.; Idacavage, M.J. 3D printing with polymers: Challenges among expanding options and opportunities. *Dent. Mater.* **2016**, *32*, 54–64. [CrossRef] [PubMed]
12. Quan, H.; Zhang, T.; Xu, H.; Luo, S.; Nie, J.; Zhu, X. Photo-curing 3D printing technique and its challenges. *Bioact. Mater.* **2020**, *5*, 110–115. [CrossRef] [PubMed]
13. International Organization for Standardization. *Accuracy (Trueness and Precision) of Measurement Methods and Results—Part 1: General Principles and Definitions (ISO 5725-1)*; International Organization for Standardization: Geneva, Switzerland, 1994; Available online: https://www.iso.org/standard/11833.html (accessed on 25 July 2020).
14. Sayers, A. Tips and tricks in performing a systematic review. *Br. J. Gen. Pract.* **2008**, *58*, 136. [CrossRef] [PubMed]
15. Moher, D.; Liberati, A.; Tetzlaff, J.; Altman, D.G. Preferred reporting items for systematic reviews and meta-analyses: The PRISMA statement. *J. Clin. Epidemiol.* **2009**, *62*, 1006–1012. [CrossRef] [PubMed]
16. McGowan, J.; Sampson, M.; Salzwedel, D.M.; Cogo, E.; Foerster, V.; Lefebvre, C. PRESS Peer Review of Electronic Search Strategies: 2015 Guideline Statement. *J. Clin. Epidemiol.* **2016**, *75*, 40–46. [CrossRef]
17. Whiting, P.F.; Rutjes, A.W.; Westwood, M.E.; Mallett, S.; Deeks, J.J.; Reitsma, J.B.; Leeflang, M.M.; Sterne, J.A.; Bossuyt, P.M.M. QUADAS-2: A Revised Tool for the Quality Assessment of Diagnostic Accuracy Studies. *Ann. Intern. Med.* **2011**, *155*, 529–536. [CrossRef]
18. Jeong, Y.-G.; Lee, W.-S.; Lee, K.-B. Accuracy evaluation of dental models manufactured by CAD/CAM milling method and 3D printing method. *J. Adv. Prosthodont.* **2018**, *10*, 245–251. [CrossRef] [PubMed]
19. Kim, S.-Y.; Shin, Y.-S.; Jung, H.-D.; Hwang, C.-J.; Baik, H.-S.; Cha, J.-Y. Precision and trueness of dental models manufactured with different 3-dimensional printing techniques. *Am. J. Orthod. Dentofac. Orthop.* **2018**, *153*, 144–153. [CrossRef]
20. Al-Imam, H.; Gram, M.; Benetti, A.R.; Gotfredsen, K. Accuracy of stereolithography additive casts used in a digital workflow. *J. Prosthet. Dent.* **2018**, *119*, 580–585. [CrossRef]

21. Budzik, G.; Bazan, A.; Turek, P.; Burek, J. Analysis of the Accuracy of Reconstructed Two Teeth Models Manufactured Using the 3DP and FDM Technologies. *Strojniški Vestnik J. Mech. Eng.* **2016**, *62*. [CrossRef]

22. Ishida, Y.; Miyasaka, T. Dimensional accuracy of dental casting patterns created by 3D printers. *Dent. Mater. J.* **2016**, *35*, 250–256. [CrossRef] [PubMed]

23. Arnold, C.; Monsees, D.; Hey, J.; Schweyen, R. Surface Quality of 3D-Printed Models as a Function of Various Printing Parameters. *Materials* **2019**, *12*, 1970. [CrossRef] [PubMed]

24. Park, M.-E.; Shin, S.-Y. Three-dimensional comparative study on the accuracy and reproducibility of dental casts fabricated by 3D printers. *J. Prosthet. Dent.* **2018**, *119*, 861.e1–861.e7. [CrossRef] [PubMed]

25. Ayoub, A.; Rehab, M.; O'Neil, M.; Khambay, B.; Ju, X.; Barbenel, J.; Naudi, K. A novel approach for planning orthognathic surgery: The integration of dental casts into three-dimensional printed mandibular models. *Int. J. Oral Maxillofac. Surg.* **2014**, *43*, 454–459. [CrossRef]

26. Hatz, C.; Msallem, B.; Aghlmandi, S.; Brantner, P.; Thieringer, F.M. Can an entry-level 3D printer create high-quality anatomical models? Accuracy assessment of mandibular models printed by a desktop 3D printer and a professional device. *Int. J. Oral Maxillofac. Surg.* **2020**, *49*, 143–148. [CrossRef]

27. Jang, Y.; Sim, J.-Y.; Park, J.-K.; Kim, W.-C.; Kim, H.-Y.; Kim, J.-H. Accuracy of 3-unit fixed dental prostheses fabricated on 3D-printed casts. *J. Prosthet. Dent.* **2020**, *123*, 135–142. [CrossRef]

28. Zhang, H.-R.; Yin, L.-F.; Liu, Y.-L.; Yan, L.-Y.; Wang, N.; Liu, G.; An, X.-L.; Liu, B. Fabrication and accuracy research on 3D printing dental model based on cone beam computed tomography digital modeling. *West China J. Stomatol.* **2018**, *36*, 156–161.

29. Xiao, N.; Sun, Y.C.; Zhao, Y.J.; Wang, Y. A method to evaluate the trueness of reconstructed dental models made with photo-curing 3D printing technologies. *Beijing Da Xue Xue Bao Yi Xue Ban* **2019**, *51*, 120–130.

30. Zeng, F.-H.; Xu, Y.-Z.; Fang, L.; Tang, X.-S. Reliability of three dimensional resin model by rapid prototyping manufacturing and digital modeling. *Shanghai Kou Qiang Yi Xue Shanghai J. Stomatol.* **2012**, *21*, 53–56.

31. AlShawaf, B.; Weber, H.-P.; Finkelman, M.; El Rafie, K.; Kudara, Y.; Papaspyridakos, P. Accuracy of printed casts generated from digital implant impressions versus stone casts from conventional implant impressions: A comparative in vitro study. *Clin. Oral Implant. Res.* **2018**, *29*, 835–842. [CrossRef]

32. Dostálová, T.; Kasparova, M.; Kriz, P.; Halamova, S.; Jelinek, M.; Bradna, P.; Mendricky, J. Intraoral scanner and stereographic 3D print in dentistry—Quality and accuracy of model—New laser application in clinical practice. *Laser Phys.* **2018**, *28*, 125602. [CrossRef]

33. Burde, A.V.; VarvarĂ, M.; Dudea, D.; Câmpian, R.S. Quantitative evaluation of accuracy for two rapid prototyping systems in dental model manufacturing. *Clujul Med.* **2015**, *88*, S44.

34. Aly, P.; Mohsen, C. Comparison of the Accuracy of Three-Dimensional Printed Casts, Digital, and Conventional Casts: An In Vitro Study. *Eur. J. Dent.* **2020**, *14*, 189–193. [CrossRef] [PubMed]

35. Bohner, L.; Hanisch, M.; Canto, G.D.L.; Mukai, E.; Sesma, N.; Neto, P.T.; Tortamano, P. Accuracy of Casts Fabricated by Digital and Conventional Implant Impressions. *J. Oral Implant.* **2019**, *45*, 94–99. [CrossRef] [PubMed]

36. Brown, G.B.; Currier, G.F.; Kadioglu, O.; Kierl, J.P. Accuracy of 3-dimensional printed dental models reconstructed from digital intraoral impressions. *Am. J. Orthod. Dentofac. Orthop.* **2018**, *154*, 733–739. [CrossRef] [PubMed]

37. Burde, A.V.; Gasparik, C.; Baciu, S.; Manole, M.; Dudea, D.; Câmpian, R.S. Three-Dimensional Accuracy Evaluation of Two Additive Manufacturing Processes in the Production of Dental Models. *Key Eng. Mater.* **2017**, *752*, 119–125. [CrossRef]

38. Camardella, L.T.; Vilella, O.D.V.; Breuning, H. Accuracy of printed dental models made with 2 prototype technologies and different designs of model bases. *Am. J. Orthod. Dentofac. Orthop.* **2017**, *151*, 1178–1187. [CrossRef] [PubMed]

39. Camardella, L.T.; Vilella, O.V.; Van Hezel, M.M.; Breuning, K.H. Accuracy of stereolithographically printed digital models compared to plaster models Genauigkeit von stereolitographisch gedruckten digitalen Modellen im Vergleich zu Gipsmodellen. *J. Orofac. Orthop. Fortschritte Kieferorthopädie* **2017**, *40*, 162–402. [CrossRef]

40. Cho, S.-H.; Schaefer, O.; Thompson, G.A.; Guentsch, A. Comparison of accuracy and reproducibility of casts made by digital and conventional methods. *J. Prosthet. Dent.* **2015**, *113*, 310–315. [CrossRef]

41. Cuperus, A.M.R.; Harms, M.C.; Rangel, F.A.; Bronkhorst, E.M.; Schols, J.G.; Breuning, K.H. Dental models made with an intraoral scanner: A validation study. *Am. J. Orthod. Dentofac. Orthop.* **2012**, *142*, 308–313. [CrossRef]

42. Dietrich, C.A.; Ender, A.; Baumgartner, S.; Mehl, A. A validation study of reconstructed rapid prototyping models produced by two technologies. *Angle Orthod.* **2017**, *87*, 782–787. [CrossRef]

43. Favero, C.S.; English, J.D.; Cozad, B.E.; Wirthlin, J.O.; Short, M.M.; Kasper, F.K. Effect of print layer height and printer type on the accuracy of 3-dimensional printed orthodontic models. *Am. J. Orthod. Dentofac. Orthop.* **2017**, *152*, 557–565. [CrossRef] [PubMed]

44. Hazeveld, A.; Slater, J.J.H.; Ren, Y. Accuracy and reproducibility of dental replica models reconstructed by different rapid prototyping techniques. *Am. J. Orthod. Dentofac. Orthop.* **2014**, *145*, 108–115. [CrossRef]

45. Jin, S.-J.; Jeong, I.-D.; Kim, J.-H.; Kim, W.-C. Accuracy (trueness and precision) of dental models fabricated using additive manufacturing methods. *Int. J. Comput. Dent.* **2018**, *21*, 107–113. [PubMed]

46. Kasparova, M.; Grafova, L.; Dvorak, P.; Dostalova, T.; Prochazka, A.; Eliasova, H.; Prusa, J.; Kakawand, S. Possibility of reconstruction of dental plaster cast from 3D digital study models. *Biomed. Eng. Online* **2013**, *12*, 49. [CrossRef]

47. Keating, A.P.; Knox, J.; Bibb, R.; Zhurov, A.I. A comparison of plaster, digital and reconstructed study model accuracy. *J. Orthod.* **2008**, *35*, 191–201. [CrossRef]

48. Kuo, R.-F.; Chen, S.-J.; Wong, T.-Y.; Lu, B.-C.; Huang, Z.-H. Digital Morphology Comparisons between Models of Conventional Intraoral Casting and Digital Rapid Prototyping. In Proceedings of the 5th International Conference on Biomedical Engineering in Vietnam, Ho Chi Minh, Viet Nam, 16–18 June 2014; Springer International Publishing: Cham, Switzerland, 2015.

49. Loflin, W.A.; English, J.D.; Borders, C.; Harris, L.M.; Moon, A.; Holland, J.N.; Kasper, F.K. Effect of print layer height on the assessment of 3D-printed models. *Am. J. Orthod. Dentofac. Orthop.* **2019**, *156*, 283–289. [CrossRef] [PubMed]

50. Nestler, N.; Wesemann, C.; Spies, B.C.; Beuer, F.; Bumann, A. Dimensional accuracy of extrusion- and photopolymerization-based 3D printers: In vitro study comparing printed casts. *J. Prosthet. Dent.* **2020**. [CrossRef]

51. Papaspyridakos, P.; Chen, Y.-W.; AlShawaf, B.; Kang, K.; Finkelman, M.; Chronopoulos, V.; Weber, H.-P. Digital workflow: In vitro accuracy of 3D printed casts generated from complete-arch digital implant scans. *J. Prosthet. Dent.* **2020**. [CrossRef]

52. Rebong, R.E.; Stewart, K.T.; Utreja, A.; Ghoneima, A.A. Accuracy of three-dimensional dental resin models created by fused deposition modeling, stereolithography, and Polyjet prototype technologies: A comparative study. *Angle Orthod* **2018**, *88*, 363–369. [CrossRef]

53. Rungrojwittayakul, O.; Kan, J.Y.; Shiozaki, K.; Swamidass, R.S.; Goodacre, B.J.; Goodacre, C.J.; Lozada, J.L. Accuracy of 3D Printed Models Created by Two Technologies of Printers with Different Designs of Model Base. *J. Prosthodont.* **2019**, *29*, 124–128. [CrossRef] [PubMed]

54. Saleh, W.K.; Ariffin, E.; Sherriff, M.; Bister, D. Accuracy and reproducibility of linear measurements of resin, plaster, digital and printed study-models. *J. Orthod.* **2015**, *42*, 301–306. [CrossRef] [PubMed]

55. Sherman, S.L.; Kadioglu, O.; Currier, G.F.; Kierl, J.P.; Li, J. Accuracy of digital light processing printing of 3-dimensional dental models. *Am. J. Orthod. Dentofac. Orthop.* **2020**, *157*, 422–428. [CrossRef] [PubMed]

56. Hassan, W.W.; Yusoff, Y.; Mardi, N.A. Comparison of reconstructed rapid prototyping models produced by 3-dimensional printing and conventional stone models with different degrees of crowding. *Am. J. Orthod. Dentofac. Orthop.* **2017**, *151*, 209–218. [CrossRef]

57. Zhang, Z.-C.; Li, P.-L.; Chu, F.-T.; Shen, G. Influence of the three-dimensional printing technique and printing layer thickness on model accuracy. *J. Orofac. Orthop. Fortschritte Kieferorthopädie* **2019**, *80*, 194–204. [CrossRef]

58. Koo, T.K.; Li, M.Y. A Guideline of Selecting and Reporting Intraclass Correlation Coefficients for Reliability Research. *J. Chiropr. Med.* **2016**, *15*, 155–163. [CrossRef]

59. Hirogaki, Y.; Sohmura, T.; Satoh, H.; Takahashi, J.; Takada, K. Complete 3-D reconstruction of dental cast shape using perceptual grouping. *IEEE Trans. Med. Imaging* **2001**, *20*, 1093–1101. [CrossRef]

60. Bell, A.; Ayoub, A.F.; Siebert, P. Assessment of the accuracy of a three-dimensional imaging system for archiving dental study models. *J. Orthod.* **2003**, *30*, 219–223. [CrossRef]

61. Naidu, D.; Freer, T.J. Validity, reliability, and reproducibility of the iOC intraoral scanner: A comparison of tooth widths and Bolton ratios. *Am. J. Orthod. Dentofac. Orthop.* **2013**, *144*, 304–310. [CrossRef]

62. McLean, J.W.; Von Fraunhofer, J.A. The estimation of cement film thickness by an in vivo technique. *Br. Dent. J.* **1971**, *131*, 107–111. [CrossRef]

63. Jemt, T.; Book, K. Prosthesis misfit and marginal bone loss in edentulous implant patients. *Int. J. Oral Maxillofac. Implant.* **1996**, *11*, 620–625.

64. Jemt, T. In vivo measurements of precision of fit involving implant-supported prostheses in the edentulous jaw. *Int. J. Oral Maxillofac. Implant.* **1996**, *11*, 151–158.

65. Papaspyridakos, P.; Chen, C.-J.; Chuang, S.-K.; Weber, H.-P.; Gallucci, G.O. A systematic review of biologic and technical complications with fixed implant rehabilitations for edentulous patients. *Int. J. Oral Maxillofac. Implant.* **2012**, *27*, 102–110.

5

Digital Undergraduate Education in Dentistry

Nicola U. Zitzmann *, Lea Matthisson, Harald Ohla and Tim Joda

Department of Reconstructive Dentistry, University Center for Dental Medicine Basel, University of Basel, 4058 Basel, Switzerland; lea.matthisson@unibas.ch (L.M.); h.ohla@unibas.ch (H.O.); tim.joda@unibas.ch (T.J.)
* Correspondence: n.zitzmann@unibas.ch

Abstract: The aim of this systematic review was to investigate current penetration and educational quality enhancements from digitalization in the dental curriculum. Using a modified PICO strategy, the literature was searched using PubMed supplemented with a manual search to identify English-language articles published between 1994 and 2020 that reported the use of digital techniques in dental education. A total of 211 articles were identified by electronic search, of which 55 articles were selected for inclusion and supplemented with 27 additional publications retrieved by manual search, resulting in 82 studies that were included in the review. Publications were categorized into five areas of digital dental education: Web-based knowledge transfer and e-learning, digital surface mapping, dental simulator motor skills (including intraoral optical scanning), digital radiography, and surveys related to the penetration and acceptance of digital education. This review demonstrates that digitalization offers great potential to revolutionize dental education to help prepare future dentists for their daily practice. More interactive and intuitive e-learning possibilities will arise to stimulate an enjoyable and meaningful educational experience with 24/7 facilities. Augmented and virtual reality technology will likely play a dominant role in the future of dental education.

Keywords: dental education; digital dentistry; augmented reality (AR); virtual reality (VR)

1. Introduction

The implementation of digital technologies in dental curricula has started globally and reached varying levels of penetration depending on local resources and demands. One of the biggest challenges in digital education is the need to continuously adapt and adjust to the developments in technology and apply these to dental practice [1]. Most dental offices in Europe are equipped with software solutions for managing patients' records, agenda and recall reminders; recording provided services, including working time schedules; ordering materials; and managing the maintenance contracts of medical devices. These systems incorporate medical histories, digital radiographs, intraoral photographs, medicine lists, and correspondences. The systems also enable easy access to detailed odontograms showing fillings per tooth surface, restorations and carious lesions, periodontal status with visualization of the attachment level, probing pocket depth, and recession [2].

The introduction of intraoral optical scanning (IOS) allows the current anatomic situation to be digitized, enabling chairside or laboratory fabrication of restorations, to plan oral rehabilitations with a set-up [3], and/or to superimpose the situation with 3-dimensional (3D) radiography (e.g., for guided implant placement) [4]. While the penetration of these scanners in dental offices is still limited (present in an estimated 20%–25% of European dental offices) [5], laboratory scanners are presumably used by more than two-thirds of dental laboratories. The dental technician uses the 3D model files derived from IOS by the clinician or from scanned conventional casts to facilitate the fabrication of restorations. Compared to waxing, the digital design offers several advantages for quality control, such as providing data about material thickness and values of connector cross sections. While the main shortcomings of lost wax casting were erroneous castings or shrinkage cavities, with a digital workflow the laboratory benefits from improved material properties when industrially manufactured products can be used with subtractive milling or additive printing processes [6].

3D education programs have been introduced to enhance students' spatial ability, their interactivity, critical thinking, and clinical correlations with the integration of multiple dental disciplines. Augmented reality in 3D visualization allows insights in tooth morphology, and also facilitates treatment planning with fixed or removable partial denture (RPD) programs [7]. Digital technologies also include the 3D printing of virtual teeth, which has been suggested to enhance transparency for all students due to the identical setups [8].

A recent review on the application of augmented reality (AR) and virtual reality (VR) in dental medicine demonstrated that the use of AR/VR technologies for educational motor skill training and clinical testing of maxillofacial surgical protocols is increasing [9]. It was concluded that these digital technologies are valuable in dental undergraduate and postgraduate education, offering interactive learning concepts with 24/7 access and objective evaluation. A recent scoping review analyzed the application of VR in pre-clinical dental education and identified four educational thematic areas (simulation hardware, realism of simulation, scoring systems, and validation), highlighting the need for a better evidence base for the utility of VR in dental education [10]. In communicating with dental professionals, medical doctors, dental technicians, and insurance providers, dental students have to be prepared to manage digitized data, ensure patient safety, and understand the benefits and limitations of conventional and digital processes.

Overall, digitalization seems to have had a major impact on dental education, addressing various aspects, such as e-learning and Web-based knowledge transfer, but also related to diagnostics using 3D imaging and digital radiography, and practically oriented trainings in terms of dental simulator motor skills including IOS with 3D printing, prototyping, and digital surface mapping. Digital applications can provide additional opportunities to evaluate and improve education, implementing evidence-based surveys related to the penetration and acceptance of digital education.

The aim of this systematic review was: (i) to investigate the current level of implementation of digital technology in dental education; and (ii) to outline the educational quality enhancements that result from digitalization in main focus areas within the dental curriculum.

2. Materials and Methods

This systematic review was conducted in accordance with the guidelines of Preferred Reporting Items of Systematic Reviews and Meta-Analyses (PRISMA) [11]. A systematic electronic search of PubMed was performed, limited to English-language articles published between 1 January 1994 and 15 April 2020. A modified PICO search was defined for Population/TOPIC, Intervention/METHOD, and Outcome/INTEREST; whereas Comparison was omitted. The search syntax used was: ((students[MeSH]) AND (education, dental[MeSH] OR teaching[MeSH] AND digital)) AND (dentistry[MeSH] OR dental medicine). In addition, the bibliographies of all full texts selected from the electronic search were manually searched, and an extensive search of articles published in the *Journal of Dental Education* and the *European Journal of Dental Education* was conducted.

This systematic review focused on randomized controlled trials, cohort studies, case–control studies, observational trials, and descriptive studies that investigated the application of digital technologies in dental education. Reports without an underlying study design and studies not involving dental students were not included. Furthermore, the vast body of literature about the transition from glass to digital slide microscopy was also excluded. Four reviewers (N.U.Z., T.J., L.M., H.O.) independently screened the titles, abstracts, and the full texts of the identified articles to select those for inclusion in the review. Disagreements were resolved by discussion. Duplicates or preliminary reports that were followed by original publications were excluded.

3. Results

A total of 211 titles were identified by the electronic search (Figure 1). After screening of the titles, abstracts, and full-text articles, 55 publications were included that reported a digital application in dental education. The manual search retrieved 27 additional publications, resulting in the inclusion of 82 studies (Annex S1 and Annex S2).

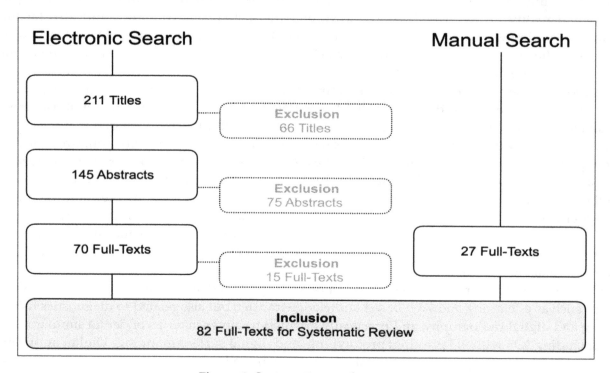

Figure 1. Systematic search strategy.

The publications were categorized into six areas of digital dental education:

- Web-based knowledge transfer/e-learning (22 studies);
- Digital surface mapping (20 studies);
- Dental simulator motor skills including IOS (23 studies);
- 3D printing and prototyping (2 studies);
- Digital radiography (5 studies); and
- Surveys related to the penetration and acceptance of digital education (10 studies).

3.1. Web-Based Knowledge Transfer/e-Learning

Fifteen studies reported the use of Web-based learning tools in the dental curriculum, comprising orthodontics [12,13], tooth anatomy [14–16], oral pathogens and immunology [17], dental radiology [18,19], oral surgery [20] or implant dentistry [21], prosthetic dentistry [22], caries detection [23,24], in growth and development [25], and the general use of Web-based learning tools [26] (Table 1). Three additional studies reported on the use of video illustrations of clinical procedures with behavior management in pediatric dentistry [27], intraoral suturing [28], or tooth preparation [29]. Practicing history-taking and decision-making in periodontology with a Web-based database application, where students used free text communication on the screen to interact with patient data, improved their capability and empathy during the first patient contact [30]. One other study described the introduction of portable digital assistants for undergraduate students in a primary dental care clinic to access a virtual learning environment; these tools proved to be a convenient and versatile method for accessing online education [31]. Mobile devices were found to support learning by offering the opportunity to personalize digital learning materials by making comments, underlining, annotating images, and making drawings [32]. The availability of free 3D viewer software favored the planning of RPD designs on 3D virtual model situations [33]. Online access to digital tools without time restrictions was identified as a major benefit in dental education, and Web-based instructional modules facilitated students' individual learning approach and accommodated varying learning paces. While an initial effort was required to prepare online educational material, faculty time was reduced in the long term.

Table 1. Web-based knowledge transfer / e-learning ($n = 22$).

Study (Year)	Study Design	Theory/Practice	Participants	Materials and Methods	Results
Komolpis et al. 2002 [12]	RCT	P	99	Compared effectiveness (exam scores and time spent) in clinical orthodontic diagnosis in test group (50 students with web-based digital records) and control group (49 students provided with traditional records) with study models, panoramic and cephalometric radiograph, facial and intraoral photographs.	Test and control group performed similar in the exam with no difference in test time; positive feedback about the web-based learning module, students benefit from convenient access to study material on the computer without time constrictions.
Schultze-Mosgau et al. 2004 [20]	OT	T	82	Evaluated a web-based course with a concluding online examination. Feed-back by questionnaire.	Course gradings excellent or good were given for accessibility independent of time (89%), for access independent of location (83%), for objectification of knowledge transfer (67%), and for use of videos for surgical techniques (91%).
Schittek Janda et al. 2004 [30]	RCT	P	39	Compared the effect of a web-based virtual learning environment (VLE) on students' performance in history interview. Both groups underwent standard instruction in professional behavior, history taking, clinical decision making and treatment planning. Test group worked with the virtual periodontal patient for 1 week prior to their first patient contact; control group was first allowed to use the virtual patient after their first patient contact. Time spent, type and order of questions and professional behavior were analyzed.	Test group asked more relevant questions, spent more time on patient issues, and performed a more complete history interview than control. The use of the virtual patient and the process of writing questions in working with the virtual patient stimulated students to organize their knowledge and resulted in more confident behavior towards the patient.
Boynton et al. 2006 [27]	CS	P	108	Explored students' behaviors management in pediatric dentistry using portable video instructions; test group: 11 students reviewing video lecture material on a portable device (iPod) supplementing conventional pediatric behavior management lecture; additional 6 students (intermediate) used audio versions or video on the computer; control group: 91 students without digital learning material; exam on student comprehension.	Test group performed significantly better on the examination (mean 9.3) than control (7.9) or intermediate group (7.8); portable format was preferred.
Reynolds et al. 2007 [31]	CS	P	12	Investigated students' educational use of portable digital assistants (PDA) to access a Virtual Learning Environment in a primary dentalcare clinic and at home; cross over trial with 6 students with / 6 without for 12 weeks.	PDA was frequently used for online education; over 90% wanted PDA as part of their dental kit.
Kingsley et al. 2009 [17]	CS	P	78	Examined students' ability to use web-based online technologies to find recently published online citations and to answer clinically relevant questions (oral pathogens and immunology course); technology skills analyzed: ability to locate online library resources, understand how information is organized within the library system, access online databases, interpret and evaluate research materials within the context of a specific discipline; students were provided with a review article of vaccines against caries from 2001.	100% of students had correct responses to the content-specific or technology-independent portions; 46% had correct responses to the information literacy or technology-dependent portions; as web-based technologies grow more prevalent in the digital era, information literacy and technology-dependent, applied research assignments should be integrated into graduate-level curricula.
Weaver et al. 2009 [28]	RCT	P	12	Evaluated performance in intraoral suturing after digital multimedia instruction; control group: written information; test group: plus teaching tool; suturing performed on a model situation, evaluated by 10 grading criteria.	Test group performed better than control; video addressed common mistakes made by novice students, improved long-term understanding of the basic suture principles.

Table 1. *Cont.*

Study (Year)	Study Design	Theory/Practice	Participants	Materials and Methods	Results
Wright et al. 2009 [14]	OT	T	235	Determined whether dental students used an interactive DVD-tooth atlas as a study aid and perceived the 3D interactive tooth atlas as a value-added learning experience.	14% students downloaded the DVD voluntarily prior to adding atlas-related exam questions as incentives; after adding incentives 43% downloaded the material; financial concerns and overly sophisticated content were deemed responsible for the low acceptance.
Curnier 2010 [16]	OT	P	26	Assessed VR integration into teaching of dental anatomy, feedback by questionnaire	70% of the students were satisfied/very satisfied with IT integration in the curriculum.
Bains et al. 2010 [13]	RCT	T	90	Compared effectiveness and attitudes toward e-learning (EL, online tutorial without teacher), face-to-face learning (F2FL, led by teacher) and blended learning (BL) subdivided in BL1 (EL first then F2FL) and BL2 (F2FL first then EL) among 4th year students. Groups received cephalometric tutorial in the allocated mode, answered an MCQ (Multiple Choice Questionnaire).	F2FL and BL resulted in similar test results; EL alone was less effective. BL was the most and F2FL was the least accepted method, EL was significantly less preferred, the order B1 or 2 had no effect.
Mitov et al. 2010 [15]	CS	T	36	Testing an e-learning software (morphoDent) to prepare for an anatomy exam. 3D models with description and x-rays of permanent human teeth were available for viewing and interaction on the learning platform. Practical dental morphology exam was compared to virtual tooth anatomy exam. Evaluation of students' perceptions in a questionnaire.	Similar exam scores in traditional and online exam. Majority felt the software helped them learning dental morphology, despite of difficulties in operating the program.
Vuchkova et al. 2012 [19]	CS	P	88	Evaluated interactive digital versus conventional radiology textbook (course radiographic anatomy), outcome was radiographic interpretation test and survey feedback.	95% perceived positive enhancement of learning and interpretation.
Smith et al. 2012 [29]	OT	P	26	Compared the use of online video-clips with traditional live demonstrations with one-to-one supervision; students exam scores before and after the video introduction were compared. Feed-back by questionnaire.	76% preferred video-clips to live demonstrations, 57% reviewed DVD at home; 57% felt one-to-one supervision more effective developing their competence in tooth preparation.
Qi et al. 2013 [21]	RCT	P	95	Comparison of active versus passive approaches in using 3D virtual scenes in dental implant cases. Students were exposed to educational materials about implant restoration on three types of webpages: traditional 2D (group 1); active-controlling 3D (group 2); passive-controlling 3D (group 3). After reviewing their webpages, students were asked to complete a posttest to assess the relative quality of information acquisition. Before study exposure, students performed a standardized test of spatial ability (mental rotations test, MRT).	Posttest scores were highest in group 3 (passive control) and lowest in group 2 (active control). Higher MRT scores were associated with better posttest performances in all three groups. Individuals with low spatial ability did not benefit from 3D interactive virtual reality, while passive control produced higher learning effects compared to active control.
Reissmann et al. 2015 [22]	OT	T	71	Creation of a blended learning model; e-learning modules covered fundamental principles, additional information, and learning tests (tests were repeated until passed and the next video sequence unlocked); modules comprised (i) tooth preparation, placement of post and core, and provisional crown; (ii) with preparation, manufacturing and insertion of a FDP (Fixed Dental Prosthesis). Students rated the course on a questionnaire, comparison to previous courses without e-learning.	Significantly higher satisfaction among students enrolled in the e-learning modules compared to the years prior to integration of the e-learning modules. Results suggest that instructor-based practical demonstrations in preclinical courses in prosthetic dentistry could be successfully replaced by e-learning applications provided that course content is structured according to specific predefined learning goals and procedures.
Luz et al. 2015 [24]	RCT	P	39	Evaluated the effect of a digital learning tool on students' caries detection in 12 pediatric patients (3.4 per student) using ICDAS (International Caries Detection & Assessment System) (1264 dental surfaces). 2 weeks after first exam students were split into 3 training groups: Group 1: ICDAS e-learning program; group 2: plus digital learning tool; group 3: no learning strategy; students reassessed the same patients 2 weeks, and results compared.	After training group 1 and 2 had improved with significantly higher sensitivity; group 2 showed significant increase in sensitivity at the D2 and D3 thresholds as a result of the digital learning tool.

Table 1. *Cont.*

Study (Year)	Study Design	Theory/Practice	Participants	Materials and Methods	Results
Gonzales et al. 2016 [18]	OT	T	40	Implementation social media (Twitter) in a dental radiology course and evaluated students' use and perception by a questionnaire.	95% (38) had not used Twitter prior to the course; 53% (21) created an account during the course to view radiographic examples and stay informed; overall Twitter had a positive impact with improved accessibility to the instructor.
Jackson et al. 2018 [25]	OT	P	80	Evaluated dental students study patterns using self-directed web-based learning modules with scheduled self-study time instead of lectures; web-based module access (date and time) was recorded for four courses in the growth & development curriculum; scheduled access time was 8 am to 5 pm.	Frequency of module access (at least once) varied among the four courses (10–64%); only three students had > 20% of their total accesses taking place during designated self-study times. For all courses the proportion of module access was significantly higher 0–2 days before an exam compared to 3–7 or >7 days before final exam; no association between module access during scheduled times and course performance.
Alves et al. 2018 [23]	RCT	P	64	Evaluated the effect of a digital learning tool on students' caries detection in 80 teeth using ICDAS; Group 1 (21 students): ICDAS e-learning program; group 2 (22 students): plus digital learning tool; group 3 (21 students): no training; reassessment of the 80 teeth 2 weeks after training.	After training group 1 and 2 had improved with significantly higher sensitivity and specificity; group 3 had increased sensitivity at the D2 thresholds; ICDAS e-learning with or without digital learning tool improved occlusal caries detection.
Botelho et al. 2019 [26]	OT	T	40	Surveyed dental students' perception of cloud-based practice records (documenting clinical progression) compared to traditional paper record.	Cloud based records were rated significantly better in terms of usefulness, ease of use, and learning, satisfaction.
Pyörälä et al. 2019 [32]	OT	T	176	Investigated perception of mobile devices for study use among 124 medical, 52 dental students provided with iPads and followed from 1st to 5th year; feed-back by questionnaire.	Note taking was the most frequent application of the mobile device in the 1st–5th year; students personalized digital learning materials by making comments, underlining, marking images and drawings. Students retrieved their notes anytime when studying for examinations and treating patients in clinical practice.
Mahrous et al. 2019 [33]	RCT	P	77	Compared virtual 3D casts with 2D paper-based exercise in planning removable partial denture design; group 1 ($n = 39$) planned RPD in Kennedy class IV in virtual 3D and Kennedy class II in traditional 2D format, group 2 (=38) planned class IV traditional and class II virtual; survey lines and undercut positions were drawn on virtual 3D casts or given in written descriptions (2D); students planned design (with rests, clasp type, retention location, guide plane) was scored; feed-back by questionnaire.	Similar scores for 3D and 2D exercises; majority favored virtual 3D casts because of improved understanding of relevant parameters and spatial visualization. Currently, physical casts are still required to practice surveying and drawing on the cast.

RCT = Randomized Controlled Trial; CT = Controlled Trial; CS = Cohort Study; CCS = Case-Control-Study; OT = Observational Study.

3.2. Digital Surface Mapping

Visual inspection of students' work is known to have shortcomings in inter- and intra-examiner reliability, whereas standardized digital surface mapping of abutment tooth preparations facilitates objective evaluation and feedback (Table 2) [34–46]. In the preclinical training of dental students, the use of software that can match the student's scanned preparation with an ideal tooth preparation has been proven to be a helpful tool in the evaluation of preparation form, taper, and substance removal. High intra-rater agreement was also found for the repeated digital grading of wax-ups in the undergraduate curriculum [47], and students' initial self-assessment was overrated compared to the digital grading [48]. Limitations of digital assessments have been found for intracoronal cavity preparations, due to the restricted analysis of cavity depth [49,50]. With specified software skills, successful application was documented for class II mesio-occlusal-distal (MOD) cavity assessments, class III composite preparations, and mesio-occlusal (MO) onlay preparations [51–53]. These studies of digital surface mapping clearly demonstrate the tremendous development of this technology since 2006, which now enables a thorough and consistent analysis of several preparation parameters, with freely available open-source comparison tools.

Table 2. Digital surface mapping ($n = 20$).

Study (Year)	Study Design	Theory/Practice	Participants	Materials and Methods	Results
Esser et al. 2006 [35]	CS	P	36	Compared conventional visual examination by faculty with digital analysis ("Prep Assistant") of students' preparation of a central incisor for a metal-ceramic crown; preparations were scanned; before the exam preparation, students had received theoretical and practical exercises.	Digital measuring technique was superior for convergence angle, occlusal reduction and width of shoulder; low correlation between visual and digital was observed for the assessments of chamfer, path of insertion, width of bevel and basic form; calibration of evaluators benefit from digital analysis tool.
Hamil et al. 2014 [37]	OT	P	81	Evaluated dental students' opinion about a new grading software program (E4D Compare with surface mapping technology) for their self-assessment and as faculty-grading tool in a preclinical course to evaluate crown preparations. Software was introduced (one-hour lecture and three-hour hands-on laboratory session) and applied for self-assessment during one semester; questionnaire about students' perception.	Students preferred digital grading system over traditional hand-grading 95% reported on feedback inconsistencies among different faculty members, 72% reported on inconsistencies from the examiner; 85% agreed or strongly agreed that E4D Compare provided more consistent grading than faculty; 79% responded that the software provided more feedback, 90% found the software helping them to understand their deficiencies; 89% agreed or strongly agreed that E4D Compare grading helped them be better clinicians.
Mays et al. 2014 [49]	CT	P	25	Compared students' visual self-assessment, students' digital (CAD/CAM) self-assessment, faculty visual assessment, and faculty digital assessment. Students prepared mesial-occlusal amalgam cavity, used standardized grading sheets for visual self-assessment, scanned their preparation, used design tool of Cerec software for digital self-assessment.	Moderate agreement between faculty visual and digital evaluation for occlusal and proximal shape, orientation and definition; poor agreement between student visual and digital evaluation for occlusal shape, and fair for proximal shape, orientation and definition; slight to poor agreement between students visual and faculty visual evaluation, and digital assessment did not improve student/faculty agreement.
Kwon et al. 2014 [47]	OT	P	60	Compared conventional visual faculty grading of wax-ups to digital assessment in dental anatomy course; 30 faculty wax-ups, 15 student wax-ups and 15 dentoform teeth; visual grading was performed by two experienced faculty members, digital grading by one operator, both gradings were repeated after 1 week; maxillary 1st molar wax-up (from faculty) with highest scores from visual grading was used as master model for digital grading.	Modest intra-rater reliability for visual scoring with similar rating between the two trials (0.7); low inter-rater agreement between the two faculty raters; digital grading showed high intra-rater agreement for the repeated assessment (ICC 0.9); modest correlation between visual and digital grading.
Garrett et al. 2015 [48]	CCS	P	57	Evaluated E4D software (Planmeca) to assess incisor and molar wax-ups of 57 students, who used digital images for self-assessment, and compare to faculty members; based on five assessment criteria (arch alignment, proximal contacts, proximal contour and embrasures, facial contour, lingual contour) and applying 300, 400, and 500 μm level of tolerance in E4D.	Students' self-assessment of the maxillary incisor wax-up was higher than faculty and E4D300, but lower than E4D 400 and 500. For the molar wax-up, self-assessment was not different to faculty, but higher than E4D300. E4D500 evaluations were sig. superior than other assessments.

Table 2. *Cont.*

Study (Year)	Study Design	Theory/Practice	Participants	Materials and Methods	Results
Callan et al. 2015 [34]	CCS	P	82	Validated E4D software (Planmeca) to assess molar crown preparation of 82 students and compare to calibrated faculty members based on four criteria (occlusal reduction, proximal reduction, facial/lingual reduction, margins and draw). Agreement in rankings between faculty scores and E4D Compare scores was measured with Spearman's correlation coefficient (SCC) at five different tolerance levels (0.1–0.5 mm).	SCC values for practical exams varied between 0.20 and 0.56. None of the upper 95% confidence limits reached the for strong correlation. SCC values indicated only weak to moderate agreement in ranks between practical exam scores and scores obtained with E4D Compare. When ranked from lowest to highest, the results from the conventional grading by the faculty did not correlate within an acceptable range to E4D Compare software data.
Mays et al. 2016 [42]	CCS	P	50	Validated E4D software (Planmeca) to assess occlusal convergence (TOC) of 50 molar crown preparations from students and compared to traditional faculty assessment.	Digital software could distinguish differences in TOC, which were grouped as minimum taper (mean 11°), moderate (mean 23°), or excessive (mean 47°). Digital TOC evaluation was more objective compared to faculty visual scoring.
Gratton et al. 2016 [45]	RCT	P	80	Compared effect of access to digital systems in addition to conventional preparation instructions; CEREC prepCheck (n = 20), E4D Compare (n=20), and control without access to digital system (n = 40); incisor and molar crown preparations were assessed by the students, by 3 faculties and by E4D Compare at 0.30 mm tolerance.	All groups had similar preparation scores. Visual and digital assessment scores showed modest correlation.
Gratton et al. 2017 [46]	RCT	P	79	Compared digital systems Compare (n = 42) and prepCheck (n = 37) as additional evaluation tool assessing their crown preparations (maxillary central incisor and mandibular molar); all preparations were graded by faculty Compare and prepCheck; feed-back with post-course questionnaire.	Both groups had similar technical scores; both systems had modest correlation with faculty scores and strong correlation with each other. 55.3% of students felt unfavorable about learning digital evaluation protocols, while 62.3% felt favorable about the integration of the tools into the curriculum.
Park et al. 2017 [44]	OT	P	36	Evaluated prepCheck for self-assessment, students performed ceramo-metal crown preparation (maxillary molar during formative exercise, mandibular molar during summative exam); five learning tools were used for assessments: reduction, margin width, surface finish, taper, undercut; tools were rated for usefulness, user-friendliness, and frequency of use (scale from 1 = lowest to 5 = highest). Faculty members graded tooth preparations as pass (P), marginal-pass (MP), or fail (F).	Tools assessing undercut and taper received highest scores for usefulness, user-friendliness, and frequency of use. Students' performance was 38.8% P, 30.6% MP and 30.6% F. Failing students had the highest score (4.4) on usefulness.
Kateeb et al. 2017 [38]	OT	P	96	Compared digital assessment software of students' crown preparation with traditional visual inspection; four examiners; sample of 20 preparations were reassessed for intra-rater reliability.	Intra-rater reliability (ICC) was 0.73–0.78 and 0.99 for the digital grading system; inter-rater reliability among the four examiners was good (0.76); agreement between examiners and digital ratings were low to moderate; digital grading was more consistent.
Sly et al. 2017 [50]	OT	P	98	Compared E4D software (Planmeca) to assess students intracoronal Class I preparation with traditional visual inspection; four examiners.	Similar results for grading of isthmus width and remaining marginal ridge, while pulpal floor depth was assessed more precisely with visual inspection; results indicate that software has limitations for intracoronal cavity assessment but offers a self-assessment tool to improve psychomotor skills with independent and immediate feedback.
Kunkel et al. 2018 [40]	OT	P	69	Compared prepCheck with visual faculty assessment of taper in students' crown preparation of typodont teeth, 10 experienced course instructors.	Instructor gradings were overrated compared to digital prepCheck grades, prepCheck facilitates evaluation instantly and exactly by students and examiners.

Table 2. *Cont.*

Study (Year)	Study Design	Theory/Practice	Participants	Materials and Methods	Results
Kozarovska & Larsson 2018 [39]	RCT	P	57	Evaluated a digital preparation validation tool (PVT) for students' self-assessment of crown preparation (tooth 11 and 21); group A ("prep-and-scan") self-assessed and scanned three preparations; group B ("best-of-three") self-assessed the three attempts, chose the best for scanning; questionnaire about students' and teachers' experiences with PVT.	Group A showed an increase in agreement of self-assessment and feedback from PVT, while group B showed low level agreement with PVT. Bucco-incisal reduction, reduction of the tuberculum surface and presence of undercuts were difficult to correctly identify by the students. Questionnaire feedback revealed need for PVT to develop skills, to ease assessment, while critical aspects were PVT's time efficiency and the need for verbal feedback. Teachers observed the PVT as a motivation during skills laboratory training, while verbal feedback were still deemed necessary.
Wolgin et al. 2018 [53]	RCT	P	47	Investigated digital self-assessment concept (prepCheck software) for students in the phantom course preparing a three surface (MOD) class II amalgam cavity; intervention group (IG): compared a 3D image of their preparation against master preparation with PrepCheck; control group (CG): received verbal feedback from supervisor based on pre-defined criteria.	Test and control groups performed similar and self-assessment learning tool was deemed equivalent to conventional supervision.
Lee et al. 2018 [51]	OT	P	69	Compared students' self-assessment (conventional and digital with Cerec software) with assessment (conventional and digital) by faculty members for class II amalgam preparations (C2AP) and Class III composite preparations (C3CP).	Students overestimated their performance (positive S-F gap) in both the C2AP and C3CP preparation exercises in conventional (11% and 5%) and digital assessments (8% and 2%); in conventional assessments, preclinical performance was negatively correlated with student-faculty gap (r = −0.47, $p <$ 0.001); particularly students in the bottom quartile sig. improved their self-assessment accuracy using digital self-assessments over conventional assessments.
Nagy et al. 2018 [52]	RCT	P	36	Investigated the effect of a digital feedback (test group) for mesio-occlusal onlay preparation by a 3D visualization of the cavity (Dental Teacher software, KaVo), while verbal feedback from supervisor was given to control group. Following feedbacks, 2nd corrective preparations were conducted and improvements measured. Parameters: occlusal cavity depth (OD), approximal depth (AD), extent of cusp reduction on the mesiobuccal cusp (CR), width of shoulder preparation around the mesiobuccal cusp (SW), cavity width at two different points in the occlusal box (OW).	Test group improved in all parameter and showed significantly smaller deviations of mean OD, AD and mean SW; in control group, parameter deviations were similar during 1st and 2nd preparation.
Liu et al. 2018 [41]	RCT	P	66	Evaluated the effectiveness of preclinical training on ceramic crown preparation using digital training system compared with traditional training method; test group: trained with digital method with Online Peer-Review System (OPRS) and Real-time Dental Training and Evaluation System (RDTES); control group: traditional method with instructor demonstration and evaluation; central incisor crown preparation.	Five of 15 assessed items were significantly better in test group; 96.97% of test students agreed or strongly agreed that using digital training system could better improve the practical ability than traditional method.
Greany et al. 2019 [36]	OT	P	67	Compared conventional visual faculty inspection of wax-ups to digital assessment; six examiners evaluated 67 students' wax-ups of maxillary first molar, reevaluation after 1 week; scan with IOS, STL files imported to free available open source data cloud comparison utility (Cloud Compare.org), digital evaluation by two examiners.	Visual inspection had low inter-examiner precision (ICC 0.332) and accuracy; intra-examiner precision for reevaluation was low; inter-examiner precision of digital exam was high (ICC 0.866) with high accuracy.

Table 2. *Cont.*

Study (Year)	Study Design	Theory/Practice	Participants	Materials and Methods	Results
Miyazone et al. 2019 [43]	OT	P	100	Compared prepCheck with visual faculty assessment of students' crown preparation of typodont teeth (mandibular first molar as crown abutment, maxillary 2nd premolar and 2nd molar as FDP abutments), assess inter- and intra-grader agreement of five experienced examiners conducting visual and digital exam; scoring repeated three times; parameters for crown abutments: axial tissue removal, margin width, undercut, occlusal reduction, cusp tips, occlusal anatomy; for FDP abutments: path of insertion.	Intra-grader agreement was better with prepCheck than visual assessment for all parameters except cusp tip and occlusal anatomy; inter-grader agreement for path of insertion was questionable with visual, but good with digital assessment. Inter-grader disagreement was greater in visual than digital assessment. Overestimation of tooth reduction in visual grading was eliminated by digital analysis.

RCT = Randomized Controlled Trial; CT = Controlled Trial; CS = Cohort Study; CCS = Case-Control-Study; OT = Observational Study; ICC = Inter-Class Correlation; STL = Standard Tessellation Language.

3.3. Dental Simulator Motor Skills Including Intraoral Optical Scanning

A high level of interest and acceptance was documented among undergraduate students for simulator training in cavity preparations [54–56], or in surgical interventions such as apicoectomies (Table 3) [57]. A trend toward improved technical skills and ergonomics was documented when simulator training with real-time feedback was added to traditional instructions [58–60]. Training with a VR-based simulator improved students' preparation of class I occlusal cavities [61], and of abutments for porcelain-fused-to-metal crowns [62]. In evaluating the manual dexterity of students, professionals, and non-professionals, the simulator scoring algorithm showed a high reliability to differentiate between non-professionals and dental students or dentists [63]. Instruction time from faculty for teaching cavity and crown preparations was significantly reduced when virtual reality computer-assisted simulation systems were used compared to contemporary non-computer-assisted simulation systems [64]. Preparation performance on VR units with continuous evaluations and advice from clinical instructors led to better preparation quality than real-time feedback from the virtual dental unit. Self-paced learning and the immediate software feedback were beneficial with the VR unit, and it was perceived as adjunct, but not replacing faculty instructions [65]. Students requested software improvements with more realistic force feedback during interaction with different tissues in the virtual oral environment including the maxilla, mandible, gum, tongue, cheek, enamel, dentine, pulp, cementum, etc. [66]. Recent advancements of simulators enabled variations in force feedback accounting for varying hardness of the virtual material, cut speed gain, and push force [67].

Improved student performance in crown digitization and framework design was observed when CAD/CAM (Computer-Aided Design/Computer-aided manufacturing) courses were introduced in dental education [68]. While students enjoyed designing a full crown using CAD as compared to traditional waxing, limits of the technology in representing anatomic contours and excursive occlusion were identified [69]. Viewing their scanned crown preparations magnified on the screen improved students' understanding of the finishing line [70]. The application of IOS in the simulation training showed that even inexperienced dental students were capable of acquiring the skills needed to use digital tools, and students preferred IOS over conventional impressions [71,72]. Furthermore, students' work time was shorter with IOS than with conventional impression [72,73], although more teaching time was required for digital scanning than for conventional impression techniques [74]. Applying digital complete denture treatment (AvaDent; AvaDent Digital Dental Solutions, Scottsdale, AZ, USA) in the student clinics resulted in restorations with superior gradings that were preferred by both students and patients [75]. Using an intraoral camera increased patients' consent for crown treatment, and was positively perceived by students and patients, while faculty members were neutral [76].

Table 3. Dental simulator motor skills incl. IOS ($n = 23$).

Study (Year)	Study Design	Theory / Practice	Participants	Materials and Methods	Results
Quinn et al. 2003 [65]	RCT	P	20	Compared students' performance in preparing class I amalgam cavity on a VR-based training unit; test group had virtual real-time feedback and software evaluation, control group had clinical instructor available during preparation. Anonymous scoring by 2 faculties, criteria: outline form, retention form, smoothness, cavity depth and cavity margin angulation. Questionnaire feed-back in test group.	Similar results for retention and wall angulation, while outline form, smoothness and cavity depth scored better in control. Test group assessed software as superior for immediate feed-back, self-paced learning, consistency of evaluation, encouraging independent work and more thorough assessment, while conventional training was superior for increasing confidence in cavity preparation. VR-based training should be used as adjunct but not replacing conventional training methods.
Jasinevicius et al. 2004 [64]	CT	P	28	Compared students' performance in amalgam and crown preparations on typodont teeth either with a contemporary non-computer-assisted simulation system (CS), or with a virtual reality computer-assisted simulation system (VR). Both groups were provided with presentations describing preparations, CS group received handouts, VR group had preparation criteria available on the computer. Student-faculty (S-F) interaction time was logged.	Preparation quality did not differ between CS and VR. CS required 2.8 h, VR 0.5 h S-F. CS received five times more instructional time from faculty than VR.
LeBlanc et al. 2004 [60]	RCT	P	68	Compared students' technical skills in preclinical operative dentistry after standard traditional laboratory-based instructions (over 110 h) and additional virtual reality simulator-enhanced training (test group with 20 students) Simulator (DentSim, DenX) provided real-time feedback, training conducted during 6–10 h in 3 blocks over 8 months.	While all students improved in the 4 tests during the year, test students tended to better scores in the final exam. Virtual reality simulators can be implemented in the traditional training of future dentists.
Rees et al. 2007 [54]	CT	P	16	Evaluated simulator training (DentSim, DenX) by undergraduate students for Class I and II preparations (time, marks, number of evaluations), students spent 6 h cutting an unlimited number of Class I cavities and Class II cavities; feedback by questionnaire.	Class I preparations obtained a mean mark of 66.8, preparation time was 12.5 min, with 6.7 evaluations; Class II had a mark of 26.5, time 18 min, with 7.0 evaluations. Class II was more difficult to cut. Students appreciated easy change of teeth, working at their own pace and examine the cavity in a cross-section.
Welk et al. 2008 [55]	OT	P/T	80	Evaluated students' performance in operative dentistry after training with computer-assisted dental simulator (DentSim, DenX), feedback by questionnaire.	Students indicated high interest in simulator training, high acceptance and response to additional elective training time in the computer assisted simulation lab. The shift in curriculum and instructional goals has to be optimized continuously.
Urbankova et al. 2010 [58]	RCT	P	75	Evaluated adjunctive computerized dental simulator (CDS; DentSim) training (8 h) in operative dentistry (Class I and II preparations): either before ($n = 26$) or after 1st exam ($n = 13$); control group ($n = 36$) with traditional preclinical dental training alone (110 h).	CDS-trained students performed better than control in the 1st and 2nd exam, no difference between pre-exam and post-exam groups. In the 3rd exam (end of the year) CDS group had higher, but not significantly different scores than control.
Pohlenz et al. 2010 [57]	CT	P	53	Evaluated VR training (Voxel-Man) for virtual apicoectomy; questionnaire about simulated force feedback, spatial 3D perception, resolution and integration of further pathologic conditions.	92.7% recommended the virtual simulation as additional modality in dental education, 81.1% reported the simulated force feedback as good or very good, 86.8% evaluated 3D spatial perception as good or very good; 100% recommended integration of further pathologies.

Table 3. *Cont.*

Study (Year)	Study Design	Theory / Practice	Participants	Materials and Methods	Results
Gottlieb et al. 2011 [59]	CT	T	202	Evaluated VR simulation training (DentSim, Image Navigation Ltd.) in operative preparations and restorations, 60 h VR training, laboratory course was reduced to 234 h (instead of traditional 304h). 13 experienced faculties assessed 97 non-VR students (1st year, control) and 105 students with 1 semester VR experience (test); survey about students' abilities in ergonomics, confidence level, performance, preparation, and self-assessment.	Faculty expected greater psychomotor skills and ability to prepare teeth in VR, abilities were lower than anticipated but numerically higher than in non-VR students. Faculty members perceived students' ergonomics in the test group better than in control.
Ben-Gal et al. 2011 [56]	CT	P	33	Evaluated use of VR simulator (IDEA Dental) for dental instruction, self-practice, and student evaluation. 21 experienced dental educators, 12 randomly selected experienced dental students (5th year) performed 5 drilling tasks using the simulator, feed-back by questionnaire.	Both groups found that the simulator could provide significant benefits in teaching and self-learning of manual dental skills.
Ben-Gal et al. 2013 [63]	CT	P	106	Evaluated potential of VR training simulator (IDEA Dental) to assess manual dexterity in 63 dental students, 28 dentists, 14 non-dentists, performed virtual drilling tasks in different geometric shapes: time to completion, accuracy, number of trials to successful completion, score provided by the simulator.	Simulator scoring algorithm showed high reliability in all parameters and was able to differentiate between non-professionals and dental students or non-professionals and dentists.
Lee & Gallucci 2013 [73]	CT	P	30	Compared digital (IOS) to conventional impression for single implant restorations, evaluated efficiency, difficulty and students' preference.	Mean total treatment time, preparation time and working time were significantly longer for conventional than for IOS; conventional impressions were assessed as more difficult than IOS; 60% preferred IOS, 7% conventional, 33% either techniques
Kikuchi et al. 2013 [62]	RCT	P	43	Compared VR simulator (DentSim) training with or without instructor feedback for preparation of porcelain fused to metal (PFM) crown preparation. 43 students (5th year). randomly divided into: 1. VR group with instructor's feedback (DSF; n = 15); 2. VR without instructor's feedback (DS; n = 15); 3. neither VR simulator training nor faculty feedback (NDS; n = 13); preparation time and scores of 4 crown preparations (1week for 4 weeks).	DSF and DS had significantly higher total scores than NDS. Similar results in DSF and DS, but shortened preparation time with instructors' feed-back (DSF) at early stages.
Douglas et al. 2014 [69]	CT	P	50	Compared students' performance in traditional waxing vs. computer-aided crown designing (IOS with CEREC 3D, Sirona Dental Systems), faculty grading of occlusal contacts and anatomic form, feed-back by questionnaire.	Similar gradings for wax design (79.1) and crown design (78.3); more occlusal contacts with CAD; students enjoyed designing a full contour crown using CAD and required less time with CAD. Students recognized limits of CAD technology in representing anatomic contours and excursive occlusion compared to conventional wax techniques.
Wang et al. 2015 [66]	CT	P	20	Compared VR simulator (iDental with Phanotm Omni, SensAble Tech. Inc.) in novice group (graduate students with less than 3 years clinical practice experience) and resident group (with 3–0 years clinical practice); assessment of caries removal, pulp chamber opening, time and amount of removed healthy/unhealthy tissue; feed-back by a questionnaire.	No differences in time and amount of tissue removal between groups; residents spend slightly more time than students; both groups suggested improvements in spatial registration precision, more realistic model with material properties and force feedback of different tissues, improvement of the depth of the virtual space.
Schwindling et al. 2015 [68]	CT	P	56	Evaluated a CAD/CAM hands-on course (test) compared to video-supported lecture only (control); written exam about cast digitizing and zirconia crown designing.	Test group performed significantly better than controls (16.8/20 vs. 12.5/20 correct answers); interest of students in CAD/CAM was higher after hands-on course.
Kattadiyil et al. 2015 [75]	CCS	P	15	Compared clinical treatment outcomes, patient satisfaction, and dental student preferences for digital (AvaDent, two appointments) and conventional (five appointments) complete dentures (CD) in 15 patients, 15 dental students fabricated two sets of CDs for each patient. Faculty and patient ratings, patient and student preferences, perceptions, treatment time was analyzed.	Digital process was equally effective and more time-efficient than conventional; faculty scored digital better than conventional dentures; patients and students preferred digital dentures.

Table 3. *Cont.*

Study (Year)	Study Design	Theory / Practice	Participants	Materials and Methods	Results
Zitzmann et al. 2017 [72]	RCT	P	50	Investigated performance (time recording) and perception (questionnaire feedback) of IOS and conventional implant impression after video teaching.	Students rated conventional impressions as more difficult (VAS 46) than IOS (VAS 70), with greater patient-friendliness of IOS (VAS 83) compared to conventional impressions (VAS 36); 76% preferred digital, 88% felt most effective with IOS; total work time of all steps was significantly shorter with 301 sec. for IOS and 723 sec. for conventional impressions.
Wegner et al. 2017 [70]	OT	P	108	Evaluated students' perception (questionnaire feedback) of IOS (Lava Cos Training, 3M Espe), scanning of 3 typodont tooth preparations.	63.9% positive opinion, 60.2% considered scanning process as manageable, 55.6% profited from magnified view of their preparation to understand chamfer finish lines.
Marti et al. 2017 [74]	RCT	P	25	Analyzed time to instruct IOS (DS; LAVA C.O.S. digital impression system) and conventional impression technique (CI; polyvinyl siloxane) with video lecture, investigator led demonstration, and independent impression exercise: time recording and questionnaire about familiarity and student's expectations.	Teaching DS required significantly more time than CI for video lecture (16 vs. 10 min), demonstration time (9 vs 5 min) and impression time (18 vs. 9 min). Initially students were more familiar with CI (3.96) than DS (1.96) technique. After instructions and practice, CI technique proved significantly easier than expected. Manageability of DS was not influenced by the instruction and practice experience. 96% expressed an expectation that DS will become their predominant impression technique.
dc Boer et al. 2019 [67]	RCT	P	126	Investigated skill transfer between various levels of force feedback (FFB) using Simodont dental trainer (Moog) for cross-figure preparations as manual dexterity exercise. Assessment of students' satisfaction by questionnaire.	Longer practice time was correlated with test performance: students passing at different FFB levels had mean of 300h, those passing in one FFB level had 271 h, failing students had 224 h. Skill transfer from one level of FFB to another was feasible with sufficient training.
Schott et al. 2019 [71]	OT	P	31	Evaluated dental students' perception of IOS compared to conventional alginate impression; survey after basic training and self-practicing.	77% (24) students were overall "very" or "rather satisfied" with the handling of IOS; 58% preferred IOS from the dentist's perspective, no significant difference from the patient's perspective but reduced comfort related to the impression tray.
Murbay et al. 2020 [61]	RCT	P	32	Incorporated VR with Moog Simodont dental trainer in preclinical training; students performed an occlusal preparation on typodont teeth and had previous exposure to VR (group 1) or no VR exposure (group 2); assessment was conducted (satisfactory / unsatisfactory) by manual approach or digital (Magic 19.01 64-bit).	VR use improved preparation significantly with 75% (12/16) satisfactory preparations in group 1 and 44% (7/16) in group 2. Manual and digital evaluation methods did not differ significantly.
Murrell et al. 2019 [76]	OT	P	288	Evaluated completion of posterior crown planning with or without presenting the situation to the patient by intraoral camera use; 51 students completed 198 surveys, 35 faculty members with 64 surveys, 202 patient surveys, survey was voluntary and camera use optional.	Positive perception of intraoral camera use by students and patients, while faculty was neutral; significantly higher completion rate when intraoral camera was used.

RCT = Randomized Controlled Trial; CT = Controlled Trial; CS = Cohort Study; CCS = Case-Control-Study; OT = Observational Study; DSF = VR group with instructor feedback; DS = VR group without instructor feedback; NDS = Neither VR simulator training nor faculty feedback; VAS = Visual Analog Scale; IDEA = International Dental Education Association.

3.4. 3D Rapid Prototyping

Two studies evaluated training models created by 3D rapid prototyping [77,78]. Such methods can supplement teaching on human teeth or even replace it, and educational needs can easily be adapted to students' skills (Table 4).

Table 4. Group 4: 3D printing and prototyping (*n* = 2).

Study (Year)	Study Design	Theory/Practice	Participants	Materials and Methods	Results
Soares et al. 2013 [77]	OT	T	40	Cavity preparation was taught with conventional teaching materials with 2D schematic illustration and photographs. New didactic material with virtual 3D (videos of the preparations) and magnified nylon prototyped models was introduced. Evaluation by questionnaire.	Improvement of teaching quality when combining 3D virtual technology with real models.
Kröger et al. 2016 [78]	OT	P	22	3D printed simulation models based on real patient situations were used for hands-on practice. Models simulated realistic tooth positions and wide variability of dental cases and procedures. Students removed a crown from tooth 16, detected and removed caries, did a build-up filling and crown preparation within 3 h. Students' feedback on a VAS questionnaire.	Students evaluated models based on real patient situations as good training possibilities. The lack of gingiva was disturbing.

RCT = Randomized Controlled Trial; CT = Controlled Trial; CS = Cohort Study; CCS = Case-Control-Study; OT = Observational Study.

3.5. Digital Radiography

Four studies dealt with diagnosing radiographic changes [79–81] or detecting positional errors on panoramic radiographs [82] (Table 5). Senior students showed a poor ability for approximal caries detection on both conventional and digital radiographs when compared to histo-pathologic analysis from sectioned teeth [80]. One study demonstrated that digital learning supported the development of students' diagnostic skills [81]. Another study showed that the accuracy of radiographic caries detection was improved by a computer-assisted learning calibration program, which provided feedback illustrating the actual tooth surface condition [79]. In one study, two digital systems for endodontic tooth length measurements were compared, and students' positive attitudes towards digital radiography were documented [83].

Table 5. Group 5: Digital Radiology (*n* = 5).

Study (Year)	Study Design	Theory/Practice	Participants	Materials and Methods	Results
Mileman et al. 2003 [79]	RCT	P	67	Investigated computer-assisted learning (CAL) calibration program to improves dental students' accuracy in dentin caries detection from bitewing radiographs; experimental (*n* = 33) group: used CAL with feedback for self-calibration control (*n* = 34) group.	CAL improved students' diagnostic performance; true positive ratio (sensitivity) for caries detection was significantly higher in test 76.3% than control with 66.9%, while false positive ratio (specificity) was similar (28.1 and 28.7%); diagnostic odds ratio was sig. higher in test (12.4) than in control (8.8).
Wenzel et al. 2004 [83]	RCT	P	31	Compared 2 digital systems (RVG-ui CCD sensor, Digora PSP plate system) for radiographic examination; after education in digital radiography one student group started with CCD, one with PSP and both completed endodontic treatment of single-rooted extracted tooth; groups switched radiography system and treated a 2nd tooth. True tooth length (TTL) and root filling length (RFL) were measured with the software and compared to manual measurement; feed-back questionnaire after each treatment.	Using CCD sensor required less time than PSP; positioning the tooth was easier with PSP plate; positive attitudes towards digital radiography; lengths measured on the digital images from both digital systems were slightly larger than true tooth lengths with no difference in ratio TTL/RFL between systems.

Table 5. *Cont.*

Study (Year)	Study Design	Theory/Practice	Participants	Materials and Methods	Results
Minston et al. 2013 [80]	CT	P	20	Investigated students' diagnostic performance on approximal caries detection with analog and digital radiographs from 46 extracted human premolars and molars, compared diagnostic accuracy; teeth were sectioned and histopathologically analyzed (gold standard)	Students ability for caries detection was poor, no difference between analog and digital radiographs.
Busanello et al. 2015 [81]	CCS	P	62	Evaluated digital learning object to improve skills in diagnosing radiographic dental changes (Visual Basic Application software); test group used the digital tool, control group: conventional imaging diagnosis course; diagnosis test after 3 weeks.	Test group performed significantly better, females were better than males.
Kratz et al. 2018 [82]	CT	P	169	Evaluated students' ability to identify positional errors (tongue position, head rotation, chin position) in panoramic radiographs of edentulous patients, students in 2nd year (*n* = 84) and 3rd–4th year (*n* = 85)	2nd year students identified significantly more positional errors than 3rd and 4th students. Students were more experienced at identifying radiographic findings compared to positional errors.

RCT = Randomized Controlled Trial; CT = Controlled Trial; CS = Cohort Study; CCS = Case-Control-Study; OT = Observational Study; CCD = Charged Couple Device; PSP = Photostimulable Phosphor.

3.6. Surveys Related to the Penetration and Acceptance of Digital Education

Six surveys evaluated students' perception and acceptance of digital technologies (Table 6) [84–89]. The more recent studies reflected that digital technologies have become established teaching tools, particularly in the field of digital radiography and microscopy, and the use of textbooks decreased; simulation training was preferred [86,87].

Table 6. Surveys related to digital education (*n* = 10).

Study (Year)	Study Design	Theory/Practice	Participants	Materials and Methods	Results
Scarfe et al. 1996 [88]	OT	T	277	Investigated the effects of instructions in intraoral digital radiology on dental students' knowledge, attitudes and beliefs; 174 from a university with formal instruction on digital dental radiography, and 103 from a university without instructions.	Students with instructions knew significantly more than students without; 93% wanted digital radiology to be included in the dental curriculum.
McCann et al. 2010 [85]	OT	T	366	Surveyed student's (dental and dental hygiene) preferences for e-teaching and learning, using an online questionnaire in 2008 related to computer experience, use and effectiveness of e-resources, preferences for various environments, need for standardization, and preferred modes of communication.	64% preferred printed text over digital and 74% wanted e-materials to supplement but not replace lectures; 71% preferred buying traditional textbooks, 11% preferred electronic versions; among e-resources virtual microscopy (69%), digital skull atlas (68%), and digital tooth atlas (64%) were reported as most effective; e-materials would enhance learning, in particular e-lectures (59%), clinical videos (54%), and podcasts (45%). E-resources should not replace interactions with faculty; students wanted lectures and clinical procedures recorded.
Jathanna et al. 2014 [84]	OT	T	186	Surveyed the perception of Indian dental students toward usefulness of digital technologies in improving dental practice, willingness to use digital and electronic technologies, perceived obstacles to use digital and electronic technologies in dental care setups, and their attitudes toward internet privacy issues.	Students indicated that digital technology increases patient satisfaction and practice efficiency, improves record quality, doctor-doctor communication, case diagnosis and treatment planning; obstacles to the wide adoption of these technologies were cost and dentists' lack of knowledge and comfort with technology.
Chatham et al. 2014 [90]	OT	T	11	Surveyed the penetration of digital technologies in UK dental schools (11/16 responded).	45% did not teach digital technologies (36% because it was not part of the curriculum, or in 95% due to the lack of technical expertise or support); half of those teaching digital technologies did so with lectures or demonstrations, the other half allowed practical involvement.

Table 6. *Cont.*

Study (Year)	Study Design	Theory/Practice	Participants	Materials and Methods	Results
Brownstein et al. 2015 [91]	OT	T	33	Surveyed the penetration of emerging dental technologies into the curricula at US dental schools (62 eligible schools were contacted); academic Deans answered 19 questions related to 12 dental topics; 19 schools had <100 students/class; 14 had >100 students.	Highest penetration was in preclinical didactic courses (62%) and lowest was in preclinical laboratory (36%); most common specific technologies were digital radiography (85%) and rotary endodontics (81%), least common were CAD/CAM denture fabrication (20%) and hard tissue lasers (24%); the bigger the class sizes (>100 students) and the older the school, the lower the incorporation of newer technologies.
Bhardwaj et al. 2015 [92]	OT	T	54	Surveyed faculties' opinion (15 dental, 42 medical faculty members in Melaka, Malaysia) toward the existing e-learning activities, and to analyze the extent of adopting and integration of e-learning into their traditional teaching methods; questionnaire with socio-demographic profile, skills and aptitude on the use of computer, knowledge and use of existing e-learning technology (e.g., MOODLE), experiences and attitudes towards e-learning, faculty opinion on novel e-learning techniques, and initiatives to be adopted for optimization of existing e-learning facilities.	65.4% of faculty was positive towards e-learning; formal training required to support e-learning that enables smooth transition of the faculty from traditional teaching into blended approach; traditional instructor centered teaching is shifting to learner centered model facilitating students to control their own learning. Popular e-learning education tools: Virtual Learning Environment systems such as WebCT™.
Ren et al. 2017 [86]	OT	T	389	Questionnaire assessed students' attitudes towards digital simulation technologies and teaching methods, how students compare digital technologies with traditional training methods; four categories: digital microscope, virtual pathology slides, digital radiology, virtual simulation training.	Most students accepted digital technologies as stimulating tool for self-learning; digital X-ray images were used to study oral radiology and preferred to conventional X-rays. Dental simulation training was most preferred technology (54.6%), 16.7% preferred digital microscopy, 15.0% virtual pathology slides, 13.7% digital x-ray images. 76% used the virtual simulation training machine to study oral clinical skills; 61% felt that the simulator would be a useful addition to current pre-clinical training; 66% felt that the simulator provided a realistic virtual environment.
Roberts et al. 2019 [87]	OT	T	282 (in 2015) 129 (in 2017)	Surveyed the use of student-managed online technologies in collaborative e-learning; comparison of web-based applications and other study methods (survey in 2015 focused on Google Doc/survey in 2017 focused on all e-learning technologies).	Significant decrease in Google Docs overall usage in 2017 (95%) compared to 2015 (99%), but significantly increased frequency of use in all courses from 36% (2015) to 71.6% (2017). The use of textbooks dropped significantly from 25% (2015) to 15% (2017). Only 4% reported that textbooks were worth the cost. 52% would not use textbooks to study even when placed at disposal. In 2017 52% spent study time with social media (Twitter or Facebook), 66% "sometimes" questioned the validity of information posted by others in collaborative documents. To collaboratively study with peers, Google Docs and personal contacts were the top choices in 2017.
Prager & Liss 2019 [2]	OT	T	54	Surveyed the extent of teaching digital modalities and use for patient care in dental schools (54 out of 76 dental schools in U.S. and Canada responded) in February 2019.	93% used CAD/CAM digital scanning, IOS was performed exclusively in 55%, extraoral model scan was used as sole technique in 8%, intra- and extraoral scanning in 37% of the schools. IOS was applied for crowns (100%), inlays/onlays (77%), implant crowns (52%), fixed partial denture (34%), complete denture (2%), but none of the schools indicated to use IOS always for crowns. 59% had a digital workflow established to deliver same-day restorations. 34% had at least 10% of faculty proficient in IOS, 66% had 10% or less.
Turkyilmaz et al. 2019 [89]	OT	T	255	Surveyed students' perception of e-learning impact on dental education, response rate of 22.6% (255 out of 1130 electronically distributed 14-question surveys to 2nd–4th year students).	48.6% preferred traditional lecture mixed with online learning, 18.4% online classes only, 18.0% traditional lecture style only; greatest impact on learning had YouTube, Bone Box, and Google. 60% spent between 1 and >4 h per day on electronic resources for academic performance. E-learning had a significant perceived effect on didactic and clinical understanding. Students observed that faculties estimated <50 years of age were more likely to incorporate e-learning into courses and more likely to use social media for communication.

RCT = Randomized Controlled Trial; CT = Controlled Trial; CS = Cohort Study; CCS = Case-Control-Study; OT = Observational Study.

Four surveys analyzed the penetration of and attitudes towards digital technologies at dental schools in the UK [90], U.S. [91], North America [2], or among the faculty staff at a dental school in Malaysia [92]. According to the most recent survey, CAD/CAM technologies were taught in most dental schools in North America (93%), while other digital modalities showed less penetration [2].

Despite a high acceptance of digital technologies in dental education by faculty [92] and students [86], it was concluded that e-resources should not replace interactions with faculty; students wanted lectures and clinical procedures recorded [85].

4. Discussion

The systematic review aimed to investigate current penetration and educational quality enhancements from digitalization in the dental curriculum. Heterogeneous study types addressing various fields of digital applications were found. While a meta-analysis was not feasible, a descriptive approach for identified publications was conducted.

Digitalization in dental education is frequently used to enhance the accessibility and exchange of documents and to facilitate the collaboration and communication among students, teachers, and administrative staff. Digitalization enables cloud-based records, evaluation, and feedback, as well as the provision of e-learning modules [23]. Students today, particularly the Millennials, expect services instantly, expect to be able to download their grades, course schedules, and other information automatically, and to be able to get assistance 24 h a day. In order to satisfy these expectations, it is necessary to promote a change of mindset of the dental faculty and provide instructors with training in e-learning and e-teaching to enable theoretical and practical knowledge transfer [85]. The coronavirus disease (Covid-19) pandemic that started in 2019 caused dental schools around the world to close, and highlighted the need for alternative channels for education (e.g., Web-based learning platforms) [93]. Scheduled webinars can provide a structure for students' theoretical learning. Additional applications of digital features include educational videos illustrating clinical exams or therapeutic steps, interactive systems, adaptive systems that monitor students' ability and adjust teaching accordingly, online collaborative tools, etc. The use of pictograms instead of scripts in educational videos facilitates a language-independent application in several countries.

Especially in the field of motor skills training, digital software tools can be used to evaluate the manual abilities of potential candidates for the dental curriculum, to analyze students' preclinical preparations, to enable self-assessment, and to enhance the quality of education. The objective and exact nature of these digital evaluations helps to improve students' visualization, provides immediate feedback, and enhances instructor evaluation and student self-evaluation and self-correction [43,94]. Students can learn to self-assess their work with self-reflection and faculty guidance in conjunction with a specially designed digital evaluation tool [48]. IOS and digital impression techniques can be included early in the dental curriculum to help familiarize students with ongoing development in the computer-assisted technologies used in oral rehabilitation [3,72].

While undergraduate students today have to be prepared for digital dentistry, they still need to acquire the knowledge of conventional treatment strategies and processes. Growing up in the digital world, they will easily adapt to digital features. Digital dentistry offers several options for an objective standardized evaluation of students' performance, which should be used for quality enhancement. It is currently a "teaching transition time", and new standards have to be defined for dental education in general. Open questions remain, such as: (i) in which phase of the dental curricula should digital technologies be introduced as the routine tool; (ii) which analog techniques can be omitted; and iii) which digital content should be taught in which disciplines?

Several studies indicated that personal instruction and feedback from faculty cannot be replaced by simulator training and feedback [39,65,85]. In this context, faculty should be aware of their responsibility in teaching young dentists, who are treating individuals with individual needs requiring empathy and an informed consent for any treatment decision. Digitalization cannot replace all educational lessons or courses, and the role-model function of faculty is important when supervising students during patient treatment in the clinical courses.

It should be emphasized that there are still no uniform standards in dental education with regard to the digital tools applied. Such standards are essential to ensure uniformity in teaching, which is particularly important for an international exchange. Society as well as dentistry is currently undergoing a digital transformation. It is necessary to clarify learning contents, to what extent conventional workflows should still be taught, and what can be done digitally. While digital tools and applications in knowledge transfer are a general challenge for undergraduate education in all disciplines, the field of dentistry with its high degree of practical training units is specifically demanding. Just because training units are designed digitally does not mean that students learn on their own. Continuous training with supervision and feed-back is still the key to good dental education. In this context, digitization is certainly a great opportunity to convey the learning content with more joy and newly awakened enthusiasm.

Following the rule, "you can only teach what you are able to perform yourself", a highly motivated faculty is needed that is willing to embrace the latest digital technologies. Besides personal motivation, the financial aspect of implementing the various digital tools and applications has to be managed at dental universities. Collaborations with industry would be helpful here. This is a classic "win–win situation"—the dental school would be equipped with the latest products and updates, and the industry would get access to the youngest target group of potential customers. In the event of such collaborations, it is vital that universities maintain their objectivity by offering a variety of products from diverse companies; otherwise, there is a risk of unduly influencing dental students and biasing them towards one particular technological option. The rapid pace of change in dental technology must also be considered. Dental technology companies are constantly introducing new products and workflows. While this provides exciting opportunities for dental research, to test and analyze those new developments, it complicates the implementation of digital workflows in dental education programs. New job descriptions are also necessary at dental schools in order to maintain the technical infrastructures required for these new technologies and to guarantee a smooth operation in clinical practice. In future, the best dental schools will be ranked according to their digital infrastructure combined with the level of innovation of the teaching faculty.

5. Conclusions

Digital tools and applications are now widespread in routine dental care. Therefore, this trend towards digitization and ongoing developments must be considered in dental curricula in order to prepare future dentists for their daily work-life. There is a need to establish generally accepted digital standards of education—at least among the different dental universities within individual countries. Digitalization offers the potential to revolutionize the entire field of dental education. More interactive and intuitive e-learning possibilities will arise that motivate students and provide a stimulating, enjoyable, and meaningful educational experience with convenient access 24 h a day.

At present, digital dental education encompasses several areas of teaching interests, including Web-based knowledge transfer and specific technologies such as digital surface mapping, dental simulator motor skills including IOS, and digital radiography. Furthermore, it is assumed that AR/VR-technology will play a dominant role in the future development of dental education.

Author Contributions: Conceptualization, Methodology, and Writing—Original Draft Preparation, N.U.Z. and T.J.; Writing—Review and Editing, N.U.Z., T.J., L.M., and H.O.; Supervision, N.U.Z. and T.J.; Project Administration, T.J. All authors have read and agreed to the published version of the manuscript.

References

1.   Fernandez, M.A.; Nimmo, A.; Behar-Horenstein, L.S. Digital Denture Fabrication in Pre- and Postdoctoral Education: A Survey of U.S. Dental Schools. *J. Prosthodont.* **2016**, *25*, 83–90. [CrossRef] [PubMed]

2.   Prager, M.C.; Liss, H. Assessment of Digital Workflow in Predoctoral Education and Patient Care in North American Dental Schools. *J. Dent. Educ.* **2019**. [CrossRef]

3.   Joda, T.; Lenherr, P.; Dedem, P.; Kovaltschuk, I.; Bragger, U.; Zitzmann, N.U. Time efficiency, difficulty, and operator's preference comparing digital and conventional implant impressions: A randomized controlled trial. *Clin. Oral Implant. Res.* **2017**, *28*, 1318–1323. [CrossRef] [PubMed]

4.   Joda, T.; Ferrari, M.; Bragger, U.; Zitzmann, N.U. Patient Reported Outcome Measures (PROMs) of posterior single-implant crowns using digital workflows: A randomized controlled trial with a three-year follow-up. *Clin. Oral Implant. Res.* **2018**, *29*, 954–961. [CrossRef] [PubMed]

5.   Muhlemann, S.; Sandrini, G.; Ioannidis, A.; Jung, R.E.; Hammerle, C.H.F. The use of digital technologies in dental practices in Switzerland: A cross-sectional survey. *Swiss Dent. J.* **2019**, *129*, 700–707.

6.   Joda, T.; Zarone, F.; Ferrari, M. The complete digital workflow in fixed prosthodontics: A systematic review. *BMC Oral Health* **2017**, *17*, 124. [CrossRef]

7.   Goodacre, C.J. Digital Learning Resources for Prosthodontic Education: The Perspectives of a Long-Term Dental Educator Regarding 4 Key Factors. *J. Prosthodont.* **2018**, *27*, 791–797. [CrossRef]

8.   De Boer, I.R.; Wesselink, P.R.; Vervoorn, J.M. The creation of virtual teeth with and without tooth pathology for a virtual learning environment in dental education. *Eur. J. Dent. Educ.* **2013**, *17*, 191–197. [CrossRef]

9.   Joda, T.; Gallucci, G.O.; Wismeijer, D.; Zitzmann, N.U. Augmented and virtual reality in dental medicine: A systematic review. *Comput. Biol. Med.* **2019**, *108*, 93–100. [CrossRef]

10.   Towers, A.; Field, J.; Stokes, C.; Maddock, S.; Martin, N. A scoping review of the use and application of virtual reality in pre-clinical dental education. *Br. Dent. J.* **2019**, *226*, 358–366. [CrossRef]

11.   Moher, D.; Liberati, A.; Tetzlaff, J.; Altman, D.G.; Group, P. Preferred reporting items for systematic reviews and meta-analyses: The PRISMA statement. *Ann. Intern. Med.* **2009**, *151*, 264–269. [CrossRef]

12.   Komolpis, R.; Johnson, R.A. Web-based orthodontic instruction and assessment. *J. Dent. Educ.* **2002**, *66*, 650–658. [PubMed]

13.   Bains, M.; Reynolds, P.A.; McDonald, F.; Sherriff, M. Effectiveness and acceptability of face-to-face, blended and e-learning: A randomised trial of orthodontic undergraduates. *Eur. J. Dent. Educ.* **2011**, *15*, 110–117. [CrossRef] [PubMed]

14.   Wright, E.F.; Hendricson, W.D. Evaluation of a 3-D interactive tooth atlas by dental students in dental anatomy and endodontics courses. *J. Dent. Educ.* **2010**, *74*, 110–122. [PubMed]

15.   Mitov, G.; Dillschneider, T.; Abed, M.R.; Hohenberg, G.; Pospiech, P. Introducing and evaluating MorphoDent, a Web-based learning program in dental morphology. *J. Dent. Educ.* **2010**, *74*, 1133–1139. [PubMed]

16.   Curnier, F. Teaching dentistry by means of virtual reality—The Geneva project. *Int. J. Comput. Dent.* **2010**, *13*, 251–263.

17.   Kingsley, K.V.; Kingsley, K. A case study for teaching information literacy skills. *BMC Med. Educ.* **2009**, *9*, 7. [CrossRef]

18.   Gonzalez, S.M.; Gadbury-Amyot, C.C. Using Twitter for Teaching and Learning in an Oral and Maxillofacial Radiology Course. *J. Dent. Educ.* **2016**, *80*, 149–155.

19.   Vuchkova, J.; Maybury, T.; Farah, C.S. Digital interactive learning of oral radiographic anatomy. *Eur. J. Dent. Educ.* **2012**, *16*, e79–e87. [CrossRef]

20.   Schultze-Mosgau, S.; Zielinski, T.; Lochner, J. Web-based, virtual course units as a didactic concept for medical teaching. *Med. Teach.* **2004**, *26*, 336–342. [CrossRef]

21.   Qi, S.; Yan, Y.; Li, R.; Hu, J. The impact of active versus passive use of 3D technology: A study of dental students at Wuhan University, China. *J. Dent. Educ.* **2013**, *77*, 1536–1542. [PubMed]

22.   Reissmann, D.R.; Sierwald, I.; Berger, F.; Heydecke, G. A model of blended learning in a preclinical course in prosthetic dentistry. *J. Dent. Educ.* **2015**, *79*, 157–165. [PubMed]

23.   Alves, L.S.; de Oliveira, R.S.; Nora, A.D.; Cuozzo Lemos, L.F.; Rodrigues, J.A.; Zenkner, J.E.A. Dental Students' Performance in Detecting In Vitro Occlusal Carious Lesions Using ICDAS with E-Learning and Digital Learning Strategies. *J. Dent. Educ.* **2018**, *82*, 1077–1083. [CrossRef] [PubMed]

24. Luz, P.B.; Stringhini, C.H.; Otto, B.R.; Port, A.L.; Zaleski, V.; Oliveira, R.S.; Pereira, J.T.; Lussi, A.; Rodrigues, J.A. Performance of undergraduate dental students on ICDAS clinical caries detection after different learning strategies. *Eur. J. Dent. Educ.* **2015**, *19*, 235–241. [CrossRef] [PubMed]

25. Jackson, T.H.; Zhong, J.; Phillips, C.; Koroluk, L.D. Self-Directed Digital Learning: When Do Dental Students Study? *J. Dent. Educ.* **2018**, *82*, 373–378. [CrossRef]

26. Botelho, J.; Machado, V.; Proenca, L.; Rua, J.; Delgado, A.; Joao Mendes, J. Cloud-based collaboration and productivity tools to enhance self-perception and self-evaluation in senior dental students: A pilot study. *Eur. J. Dent. Educ.* **2019**, *23*, e53–e58. [CrossRef]

27. Boynton, J.R.; Johnson, L.A.; Nainar, S.M.; Hu, J.C. Portable digital video instruction in predoctoral education of child behavior management. *J. Dent. Educ.* **2007**, *71*, 545–549.

28. Weaver, J.M.; Lu, M.; McCloskey, K.L.; Herndon, E.S.; Tanaka, W. Digital multimedia instruction enhances teaching oral and maxillofacial suturing. *J. Calif. Dent. Assoc.* **2009**, *37*, 859–862.

29. Smith, W.; Rafeek, R.; Marchan, S.; Paryag, A. The use of video-clips as a teaching aide. *Eur. J. Dent. Educ.* **2012**, *16*, 91–96. [CrossRef]

30. Schittek Janda, M.; Mattheos, N.; Nattestad, A.; Wagner, A.; Nebel, D.; Farbom, C.; Le, D.H.; Attstrom, R. Simulation of patient encounters using a virtual patient in periodontology instruction of dental students: Design, usability, and learning effect in history-taking skills. *Eur. J. Dent. Educ.* **2004**, *8*, 111–119. [CrossRef]

31. Reynolds, P.A.; Harper, J.; Dunne, S.; Cox, M.; Myint, Y.K. Portable digital assistants (PDAs) in dentistry: Part II—Pilot study of PDA use in the dental clinic. *Br. Dent. J.* **2007**, *202*, 477–483. [CrossRef] [PubMed]

32. Pyorala, E.; Maenpaa, S.; Heinonen, L.; Folger, D.; Masalin, T.; Hervonen, H. The art of note taking with mobile devices in medical education. *BMC Med. Educ.* **2019**, *19*, 96. [CrossRef] [PubMed]

33. Mahrous, A.; Schneider, G.B.; Holloway, J.A.; Dawson, D.V. Enhancing Student Learning in Removable Partial Denture Design by Using Virtual Three-Dimensional Models Versus Traditional Two-Dimensional Drawings: A Comparative Study. *J. Prosthodont.* **2019**, *28*, 927–933. [CrossRef]

34. Callan, R.S.; Haywood, V.B.; Cooper, J.R.; Furness, A.R.; Looney, S.W. The Validity of Using E4D Compare's "% Comparison" to Assess Crown Preparations in Preclinical Dental Education. *J. Dent. Educ.* **2015**, *79*, 1445–1451. [PubMed]

35. Esser, C.; Kerschbaum, T.; Winkelmann, V.; Krage, T.; Faber, F.J. A comparison of the visual and technical assessment of preparations made by dental students. *Eur. J. Dent. Educ.* **2006**, *10*, 157–161. [CrossRef]

36. Greany, T.J.; Yassin, A.; Lewis, K.C. Developing an All-Digital Workflow for Dental Skills Assessment: Part I, Visual Inspection Exhibits Low Precision and Accuracy. *J. Dent. Educ.* **2019**, *83*, 1304–1313. [CrossRef]

37. Hamil, L.M.; Mennito, A.S.; Renne, W.G.; Vuthiganon, J. Dental students' opinions of preparation assessment with E4D compare software versus traditional methods. *J. Dent. Educ.* **2014**, *78*, 1424–1431.

38. Kateeb, E.T.; Kamal, M.S.; Kadamani, A.M.; Abu Hantash, R.O.; Abu Arqoub, M.M. Utilising an innovative digital software to grade pre-clinical crown preparation exercise. *Eur. J. Dent. Educ.* **2017**, *21*, 220–227. [CrossRef]

39. Kozarovska, A.; Larsson, C. Implementation of a digital preparation validation tool in dental skills laboratory training. *Eur. J. Dent. Educ.* **2018**, *22*, 115–121. [CrossRef]

40. Kunkel, T.C.; Engelmeier, R.L.; Shah, N.H. A comparison of crown preparation grading via PrepCheck versus grading by dental school instructors. *Int. J. Comput. Dent.* **2018**, *21*, 305–311.

41. Liu, L.; Li, J.; Yuan, S.; Wang, T.; Chu, F.; Lu, X.; Hu, J.; Wang, C.; Yan, B.; Wang, L. Evaluating the effectiveness of a preclinical practice of tooth preparation using digital training system: A randomised controlled trial. *Eur. J. Dent. Educ.* **2018**, *22*, e679–e686. [CrossRef]

42. Mays, K.A.; Crisp, H.A.; Vos, P. Utilizing CAD/CAM to Measure Total Occlusal Convergence of Preclinical Dental Students' Crown Preparations. *J. Dent. Educ.* **2016**, *80*, 100–107.

43. Miyazono, S.; Shinozaki, Y.; Sato, H.; Isshi, K.; Yamashita, J. Use of Digital Technology to Improve Objective and Reliable Assessment in Dental Student Simulation Laboratories. *J. Dent. Educ.* **2019**, *83*, 1224–1232. [CrossRef] [PubMed]

44. Park, C.F.; Sheinbaum, J.M.; Tamada, Y.; Chandiramani, R.; Lian, L.; Lee, C.; Da Silva, J.; Ishikawa-Nagai, S. Dental Students' Perceptions of Digital Assessment Software for Preclinical Tooth Preparation Exercises. *J. Dent. Educ.* **2017**, *81*, 597–603. [CrossRef] [PubMed]

45. Gratton, D.G.; Kwon, S.R.; Blanchette, D.; Aquilino, S.A. Impact of Digital Tooth Preparation Evaluation Technology on Preclinical Dental Students' Technical and Self-Evaluation Skills. *J. Dent. Educ.* **2016**, *80*, 91–99. [PubMed]

46. Gratton, D.G.; Kwon, S.R.; Blanchette, D.R.; Aquilino, S.A. Performance of two different digital evaluation systems used for assessing pre-clinical dental students' prosthodontic technical skills. *Eur. J. Dent. Educ.* **2017**, *21*, 252–260. [CrossRef] [PubMed]

47. Kwon, S.R.; Restrepo-Kennedy, N.; Dawson, D.V.; Hernandez, M.; Denehy, G.; Blanchette, D.; Gratton, D.G.; Aquilino, S.A.; Armstrong, S.R. Dental anatomy grading: Comparison between conventional visual and a novel digital assessment technique. *J. Dent. Educ.* **2014**, *78*, 1655–1662.

48. Garrett, P.H.; Faraone, K.L.; Patzelt, S.B.; Keaser, M.L. Comparison of Dental Students' Self-Directed, Faculty, and Software-Based Assessments of Dental Anatomy Wax-Ups: A Retrospective Study. *J. Dent. Educ.* **2015**, *79*, 1437–1444.

49. Mays, K.A.; Levine, E. Dental students' self-assessment of operative preparations using CAD/CAM: A preliminary analysis. *J. Dent. Educ.* **2014**, *78*, 1673–1680.

50. Sly, M.M.; Barros, J.A.; Streckfus, C.F.; Arriaga, D.M.; Patel, S.A. Grading Class I Preparations in Preclinical Dental Education: E4D Compare Software vs. the Traditional Standard. *J. Dent. Educ.* **2017**, *81*, 1457–1462. [CrossRef]

51. Lee, C.; Kobayashi, H.; Lee, S.R.; Ohyama, H. The Role of Digital 3D Scanned Models in Dental Students' Self-Assessments in Preclinical Operative Dentistry. *J. Dent. Educ.* **2018**, *82*, 399–405. [CrossRef] [PubMed]

52. Nagy, Z.A.; Simon, B.; Toth, Z.; Vag, J. Evaluating the efficiency of the Dental Teacher system as a digital preclinical teaching tool. *Eur. J. Dent. Educ.* **2018**, *22*, e619–e623. [CrossRef] [PubMed]

53. Wolgin, M.; Grabowski, S.; Elhadad, S.; Frank, W.; Kielbassa, A.M. Comparison of a prepCheck-supported self-assessment concept with conventional faculty supervision in a pre-clinical simulation environment. *Eur. J. Dent. Educ.* **2018**, *22*, e522–e529. [CrossRef] [PubMed]

54. Rees, J.S.; Jenkins, S.M.; James, T.; Dummer, P.M.; Bryant, S.; Hayes, S.J.; Oliver, S.; Stone, D.; Fenton, C. An initial evaluation of virtual reality simulation in teaching pre-clinical operative dentistry in a UK setting. *Eur. J. Prosthodont. Restor. Dent.* **2007**, *15*, 89–92.

55. Welk, A.; Maggio, M.P.; Simon, J.F.; Scarbecz, M.; Harrison, J.A.; Wicks, R.A.; Gilpatrick, R.O. Computer-assisted learning and simulation lab with 40 DentSim units. *Int. J. Comput. Dent.* **2008**, *11*, 17–40.

56. Gal, G.B.; Weiss, E.I.; Gafni, N.; Ziv, A. Preliminary assessment of faculty and student perception of a haptic virtual reality simulator for training dental manual dexterity. *J. Dent. Educ.* **2011**, *75*, 496–504.

57. Pohlenz, P.; Grobe, A.; Petersik, A.; von Sternberg, N.; Pflesser, B.; Pommert, A.; Hohne, K.H.; Tiede, U.; Springer, I.; Heiland, M. Virtual dental surgery as a new educational tool in dental school. *J. Cranio-Maxillofac. Surg.* **2010**, *38*, 560–564. [CrossRef]

58. Urbankova, A. Impact of computerized dental simulation training on preclinical operative dentistry examination scores. *J. Dent. Educ.* **2010**, *74*, 402–409.

59. Gottlieb, R.; Lanning, S.K.; Gunsolley, J.C.; Buchanan, J.A. Faculty impressions of dental students' performance with and without virtual reality simulation. *J. Dent. Educ.* **2011**, *75*, 1443–1451.

60. LeBlanc, V.R.; Urbankova, A.; Hadavi, F.; Lichtenthal, R.M. A preliminary study in using virtual reality to train dental students. *J. Dent. Educ.* **2004**, *68*, 378–383.

61. Murbay, S.; Neelakantan, P.; Chang, J.W.W.; Yeung, S. Evaluation of the introduction of a dental virtual simulator on the performance of undergraduate dental students in the pre-clinical operative dentistry course. *Eur. J. Dent. Educ.* **2019**. [CrossRef] [PubMed]

62. Kikuchi, H.; Ikeda, M.; Araki, K. Evaluation of a virtual reality simulation system for porcelain fused to metal crown preparation at Tokyo Medical and Dental University. *J. Dent. Educ.* **2013**, *77*, 782–792.

63. Ben-Gal, G.; Weiss, E.I.; Gafni, N.; Ziv, A. Testing manual dexterity using a virtual reality simulator: Reliability and validity. *Eur. J. Dent. Educ.* **2013**, *17*, 138–142. [CrossRef] [PubMed]

64. Jasinevicius, T.R.; Landers, M.; Nelson, S.; Urbankova, A. An evaluation of two dental simulation systems: Virtual reality versus contemporary non-computer-assisted. *J. Dent. Educ.* **2004**, *68*, 1151–1162. [PubMed]

65. Quinn, F.; Keogh, P.; McDonald, A.; Hussey, D. A study comparing the effectiveness of conventional training and virtual reality simulation in the skills acquisition of junior dental students. *Eur. J. Dent. Educ.* **2003**, *7*, 164–169. [CrossRef]

66. Wang, D.; Zhao, S.; Li, T.; Zhang, Y.; Wang, X. Preliminary evaluation of a virtual reality dental simulation system on drilling operation. *Biomed. Mater. Eng.* **2015**, *26* (Suppl. 1), S747–S756. [CrossRef]

67. de Boer, I.R.; Lagerweij, M.D.; Wesselink, P.R.; Vervoorn, J.M. The Effect of Variations in Force Feedback in a Virtual Reality Environment on the Performance and Satisfaction of Dental Students. *Simul. Healthc.* **2019**, *14*, 169–174. [CrossRef]

68. Schwindling, F.S.; Deisenhofer, U.K.; Porsche, M.; Rammelsberg, P.; Kappel, S.; Stober, T. Establishing CAD/CAM in Preclinical Dental Education: Evaluation of a Hands-On Module. *J. Dent. Educ.* **2015**, *79*, 1215–1221.

69. Douglas, R.D.; Hopp, C.D.; Augustin, M.A. Dental students' preferences and performance in crown design: Conventional wax-added versus CAD. *J. Dent. Educ.* **2014**, *78*, 1663–1672.

70. Wegner, K.; Michel, K.; Seelbach, P.H.; Wostmann, B. A questionnaire on the use of digital denture impressions in a preclinical setting. *Int. J. Comput. Dent.* **2017**, *20*, 177–192.

71. Schott, T.C.; Arsalan, R.; Weimer, K. Students' perspectives on the use of digital versus conventional dental impression techniques in orthodontics. *BMC Med. Educ.* **2019**, *19*, 81. [CrossRef] [PubMed]

72. Zitzmann, N.U.; Kovaltschuk, I.; Lenherr, P.; Dedem, P.; Joda, T. Dental Students' Perceptions of Digital and Conventional Impression Techniques: A Randomized Controlled Trial. *J. Dent. Educ.* **2017**, *81*, 1227–1232. [CrossRef] [PubMed]

73. Lee, S.J.; Gallucci, G.O. Digital vs. conventional implant impressions: Efficiency outcomes. *Clin. Oral Implant. Res.* **2013**, *24*, 111–115. [CrossRef]

74. Marti, A.M.; Harris, B.T.; Metz, M.J.; Morton, D.; Scarfe, W.C.; Metz, C.J.; Lin, W.S. Comparison of digital scanning and polyvinyl siloxane impression techniques by dental students: Instructional efficiency and attitudes towards technology. *Eur. J. Dent. Educ.* **2017**, *21*, 200–205. [CrossRef] [PubMed]

75. Kattadiyil, M.T.; Jekki, R.; Goodacre, C.J.; Baba, N.Z. Comparison of treatment outcomes in digital and conventional complete removable dental prosthesis fabrications in a predoctoral setting. *J. Prosthet. Dent.* **2015**, *114*, 818–825. [CrossRef]

76. Murrell, M.; Marchini, L.; Blanchette, D.; Ashida, S. Intraoral Camera Use in a Dental School Clinic: Evaluations by Faculty, Students, and Patients. *J. Dent. Educ.* **2019**, *83*, 1339–1344. [CrossRef]

77. Soares, P.V.; de Almeida Milito, G.; Pereira, F.A.; Reis, B.R.; Soares, C.J.; de Sousa Menezes, M.; de Freitas Santos-Filho, P.C. Rapid prototyping and 3D-virtual models for operative dentistry education in Brazil. *J. Dent. Educ.* **2013**, *77*, 358–363.

78. Kroger, E.; Dekiff, M.; Dirksen, D. 3D printed simulation models based on real patient situations for hands-on practice. *Eur. J. Dent. Educ.* **2017**, *21*, e119–e125. [CrossRef]

79. Mileman, P.A.; van den Hout, W.B.; Sanderink, G.C. Randomized controlled trial of a computer-assisted learning program to improve caries detection from bitewing radiographs. *Dentomaxillofac. Radiol.* **2003**, *32*, 116–123. [CrossRef]

80. Minston, W.; Li, G.; Wennberg, R.; Nasstrom, K.; Shi, X.Q. Comparison of diagnostic performance on approximal caries detection among Swedish and Chinese senior dental students using analogue and digital radiographs. *Swed. Dent. J.* **2013**, *37*, 79–85.

81. Busanello, F.H.; da Silveira, P.F.; Liedke, G.S.; Arus, N.A.; Vizzotto, M.B.; Silveira, H.E.; Silveira, H.L. Evaluation of a digital learning object (DLO) to support the learning process in radiographic dental diagnosis. *Eur. J. Dent. Educ.* **2015**, *19*, 222–228. [CrossRef]

82. Kratz, R.J.; Nguyen, C.T.; Walton, J.N.; MacDonald, D. Dental Students' Interpretations of Digital Panoramic Radiographs on Completely Edentate Patients. *J. Dent. Educ.* **2018**, *82*, 313–321. [CrossRef]

83. Wenzel, A.; Kirkevang, L.L. Students' attitudes to digital radiography and measurement accuracy of two digital systems in connection with root canal treatment. *Eur. J. Dent. Educ.* **2004**, *8*, 167–171. [CrossRef]

84. Jathanna, V.R.; Jathanna, R.V.; Jathanna, R. The awareness and attitudes of students of one Indian dental school toward information technology and its use to improve patient care. *Educ. Health (Abingdon)* **2014**, *27*, 293–296. [CrossRef] [PubMed]

85. McCann, A.L.; Schneiderman, E.D.; Hinton, R.J. E-teaching and learning preferences of dental and dental hygiene students. *J. Dent. Educ.* **2010**, *74*, 65–78. [PubMed]

86. Ren, Q.; Wang, Y.; Zheng, Q.; Ye, L.; Zhou, X.D.; Zhang, L.L. Survey of student attitudes towards digital simulation technologies at a dental school in China. *Eur. J. Dent. Educ.* **2017**, *21*, 180–186. [CrossRef] [PubMed]

87. Roberts, B.S.; Roberts, E.P.; Reynolds, S.; Stein, A.F. Dental Students' Use of Student-Managed Google Docs and Other Technologies in Collaborative Learning. *J. Dent. Educ.* **2019**, *83*, 437–444. [CrossRef] [PubMed]

88. Scarfe, W.C.; Potter, B.J.; Farman, A.G. Effects of instruction on the knowledge, attitudes and beliefs of dental students towards digital radiography. *Dentomaxillofac. Radiol.* **1996**, *25*, 103–108. [CrossRef]

89. Turkyilmaz, I.; Hariri, N.H.; Jahangiri, L. Student's Perception of the Impact of E-learning on Dental Education. *J. Contemp. Dent. Pract.* **2019**, *20*, 616–621. [CrossRef]

90. Chatham, C.; Spencer, M.H.; Wood, D.J.; Johnson, A. The introduction of digital dental technology into BDS curricula. *Br. Dent. J.* **2014**, *217*, 639–642. [CrossRef]

91. Brownstein, S.A.; Murad, A.; Hunt, R.J. Implementation of new technologies in U.S. dental school curricula. *J. Dent. Educ.* **2015**, *79*, 259–264.

92. Bhardwaj, A.; Nagandla, K.; Swe, K.M.; Abas, A.B. Academic Staff Perspectives Towards Adoption of E-learning at Melaka Manipal Medical College: Has E-learning Redefined our Teaching Model? *Kathmandu Univ. Med. J. (KUMJ)* **2015**, *13*, 12–18. [CrossRef]

93. Meng, L.; Hua, F.; Bian, Z. Coronavirus Disease 2019 (COVID-19): Emerging and Future Challenges for Dental and Oral Medicine. *J. Dent. Res.* **2020**. [CrossRef]

94. Greany, T.J.; Yassin, A.; Lewis, K.C. Developing an All-Digital Workflow for Dental Skills Assessment: Part II, Surface Analysis, Benchmarking, and Grading. *J. Dent. Educ.* **2019**, *83*, 1314–1322. [CrossRef]

6

Impact of Aging on the Accuracy of 3D-Printed Dental Models: An In Vitro Investigation

Tim Joda *[ID], Lea Matthisson and Nicola U. Zitzmann[ID]

Department of Reconstructive Dentistry, University Center for Dental Medicine Basel, University of Basel, 4058 Basel, Switzerland; lea.matthisson@unibas.ch (L.M.); n.zitzmann@unibas.ch (N.U.Z.)
* Correspondence: tim.joda@unibas.ch

Abstract: The aim of this in vitro study was to analyze the impact of model aging on the accuracy of 3D-printed dental models. A maxillary full-arch reference model with prepared teeth for a three-unit fixed dental prosthesis was scanned ten times with an intraoral scanner (3Shape TRIOS Pod) and ten models were 3D printed (Straumann P-Series). All models were stored under constant conditions and digitized with a desktop scanner after 1 day; 1 week; and 2, 3, and 4 weeks. For accuracy, a best-fit algorithm was used to analyze the deviations of the abutment teeth (GFaI e.V Final Surface®). *Wilcoxon Rank Sum Tests* were used for comparisons with the level of significance set at $\alpha = 0.05$. Deviation analysis of the tested models showed homogenous intragroup distance calculations at each timepoint. The most accurate result was for 1 day of aging (3.3 ± 1.3 μm). A continuous decrease in accuracy was observed with each aging stage from day 1 to week 4. A time-dependent difference was statistically significant after 3 weeks ($p = 0.0008$) and 4 weeks ($p < 0.0001$). Based on these findings, dental models should not be used longer than 3 to 4 weeks after 3D printing for the fabrication of definitive prosthetic reconstructions.

Keywords: rapid prototyping; 3D printing; accuracy; dental materials science; digital workflow

1. Introduction

Digitalization is en vogue: *#WhatCanBeDigitalWillBe*. Therefore, it is not surprising that the demands of clinicians and patients are also changing in the field of dentistry. Scan technology has opened the possibility to digitize the patient's dental situation: either lab-side scanning of conventional gypsum casts or directly chairside with an intraoral scanning device (IOS). With both methods, the patient-specific situation can be captured optically and stored as a three-dimensional (3D) surface file, namely a standard tessellation language (STL) file [1]. Scan technology is currently of great interest in all dental disciplines, in particular in prosthodontics for the manufacturing of fixed dental prostheses (FDP) [2].

IOS enables fully digital chairside workflows, incorporating computer-aided-design and computer-aided-manufacturing (CAD/CAM) without any physical models [3]. IOS meets the ubiquitous trend of digitalization in the society, supports more convenient treatments [4], and will successively displace conventional impression taking in dentistry [5]. Whenever possible, complete digital workflows will be used in dental medicine in the future [6].

The typical IOS domain has been single-unit restorations. Complete digital workflows have been proven for tooth- and implant-supported monolithic single-unit restorations, especially in posterior sites [7,8]. From an economic point of view, clinical and technical protocols for single crowns can be streamlined to achieve time-efficient therapy outcomes with a reasonable cost–benefit ratio and a high quality of CAD/CAM-processed restorations [9,10].

At present, not all prosthetic indications can be addressed with model-free workflows, i.e., manually veneered multi-unit FDPs. Even though technical progress is rapid and the combination of IOS and laser-melting seems to be promising for CAD/CAM processing of frameworks of removable partial dentures (RPD), a dental model is still required for the finalization of the RPD [11,12]. With the increase in performance of IOS devices, however, the desire to expand the range of indications from single crowns to more complex prosthetic reconstructions including removable restorations with edentulous mucosal tissues has grown [13]. Clinical and technical protocols (combining IOS and dental model fabrication) are required to cover such complex indications in a digital workflow. Rapid prototyping is a technique to construct and build any geometry using 3D printing [14]. The 3D printing process is a promising solution to generate dental models out of polymers based on lab-side or intraorally acquired STL files [15]. Dental models reconstructed by 3D printing were considered clinically acceptable in terms of accuracy and reproducibility compared to classical stone casts [16]; while compared to CAD/CAM milling, 3D-printed models demonstrated even higher accuracy [17].

Three-dimensional printing is a relatively new technique in dentistry, and consequently, detailed information on the dimensional accuracy and stability of 3D printed models with regard to time and storage is not available [18]. Initial laboratory studies evaluated the accuracy of 3D-printed full-arch dental models [19–22] but did not consider the impact of aging of the models.

Therefore, this in vitro study aimed to investigate the impact of model aging on the dimensional stability of 3D-printed dental models. The hypothesis was that the period of storage time has no significant influence on the accuracy of printed models.

2. Experimental Section

2.1. Study Setup

A maxillary full-arch reference model (Model ANA-4, Frasaco GmbH, Tettnang, Germany) with abutment tooth preparation for a three-unit FDP in positions 24–26 was scanned ten times using an IOS device (TRIOS Pod, version 19.2.4, 3Shape, Copenhagen, Denmark). All IOSs were performed by an experienced single operator. The IOS system was calibrated prior to each scan, and the scan strategy followed the manufacturer's instructions. Scan data were directly exported as STL data sets ($n = 10$).

Afterwards, TRIOS STL files were converted into 3D printable data sets using the built-in model builder tool of the desktop scanner (Netfabb, version 2020.2, Institut Straumann AG, Basel, Switzerland). Standardized parameters were defined for 3D-printed models with a base height of 4 mm and a thickness of 3 mm with two stabilizing bars. A base plate with hexagonal cell design with a height of 2 mm, wall thickness of 0.8 mm, and cell size of 1.5 mm was selected for all models (Figure 1).

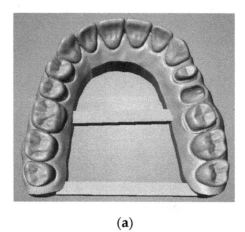
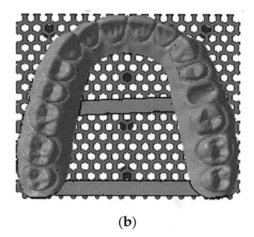

(a)   (b)

Figure 1. Conversion of TRIOS standard tessellation language (STL) files into 3D printable data sets with (**a**) model builder software including two stabilizing bars (**b**) virtual preparation for 3D printing using a base plate with hexagonal cell design.

Based on each of these IOS data sets from the TRIOS STL files, ten dental models were 3D printed (P 30, version 2019.2.11, Institut Straumann AG, Basel, Switzerland) using a light-curing 3D printing material with 385-nm wavelength technology (SHERAPrint-model plus "sand" UV, SHERA, Lemförde, Germany). This polymer is specifically formulated for the production of high-precision dental models. The printing model platform was cleaned with isopropanol and placed in the 3D printer. Afterwards, the models were removed from the platform and placed in an ultrasonic bath for cleaning. The models were then blown dry with compressed air, checked for excess material, cleaned again if required, and left to rest for 30 min before further processing. Finally, the models were exposed to a burst of light with wavelengths of 280–580 nm to cure the polymer.

The 3D-printed models were stored under constant conditions at 20° C and 50% humidity without direct light exposure and successively digitized with laboratory desktop scanner (Series 7, version 13.1.3.33179, Institut Straumann AG, Basel, Switzerland) after storage periods of 1 day, 1 week, 2 weeks, 3 weeks, and 4 weeks.

2.2. Accuracy Analysis

A total of 50 STL files (ten 3D-printed dental models scanned at five timepoints) were evaluated for accuracy by means of trueness (means) and precision (standard deviations). For accuracy measurements, the original maxillary full-arch reference model was digitized using the same laboratory desktop scanner that was used to digitize the 3D-printed models after aging. Based on the manufacturer's information, the power of the laser diode is 5 mW with a laser wavelength of 660 nm and the accuracy is specified with 7 μm.

The STL file of the reference model was imported into a 3D analysis software and matched pairwise with the 50 STL files of the 3D-printed models (Final Surface® version 2019.0, GFaI e.V., Berlin, Germany). A best-fit algorithm of the 3D analysis software was applied for accuracy testing of the superimposed model pairings using a 2D distance analysis of the abutment teeth in areas 24 and 26 at indexed landmarks at the finishing lines. For visualization, a color mapping function of the 3D analysis software was used with a graduate scale in μm (Figure 2).

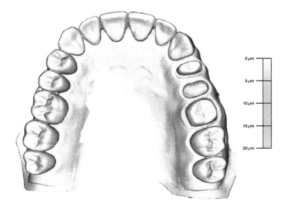

Figure 2. Visualization of the superimposed 3D-printed model with the reference by means of color mapping (Final Surface® version 2019.0, GFaI e.V., Berlin, Germany).

2.3. Statistical Analysis

Statistical analysis was carried out to evaluate the impact of aging on the accuracy of the 3D-printed dental models. Descriptive statistics were calculated for means with standard deviations (SD) including minimum and maximum values. *Wilcoxon Rank Sum Tests* were used for all comparisons. The level of significance was set at $\alpha = 0.05$. Calculations were made with the open-source software "GraphPad Software" (http://www.graphpad.com).

3. Results

The descriptive statistics are shown in Table 1. The deviation analysis of the 3D-printed models #01–#10 compared to the reference model demonstrated overall homogenous intragroup results for distance calculations at each isolated timepoint. Taking into account the entire investigation period, the range of mean deviations was very close for all tested 3D-printed models, revealing minimum to maximum distance values of 1 to 12 μm.

Table 1. Deviation (in μm) of the 3D-printed models #01–#10 from the reference model after aging of 1 day; 1 week; and 2, 3, and 4 weeks (SD = standard deviation, Min = minimum, and Max = maximum).

	1 Day	1 Week	2 Weeks	3 Weeks	4 Weeks
#01	2	2	3	5	6
#02	1	2	2	3	5
#03	2	3	2	7	8
#04	2	2	3	4	9
#05	4	3	6	6	9
#06	4	6	5	7	10
#07	5	7	6	8	12
#08	5	5	7	7	9
#09	3	4	7	8	9
#10	5	6	8	9	12
Mean	3.3	4.0	4.9	6.4	8.9
SD	1.3	1.9	2.2	1.9	2.2
Min	1	2	2	3	5
Max	5	7	8	9	12

Considering the factor of aging of the 3D-printed models, the most accurate result was for 1 day with a mean deviation of 3.3 ± 1.3 μm. A continuous decrease in accuracy was observed with each further aging stage of the tested 3D-printed models from 1 day up to 4 weeks (Figure 3). The time-dependent difference was statistically significant after 3 weeks ($p = 0.0008$) and 4 weeks ($p < 0.0001$), respectively, when comparing with 1 day.

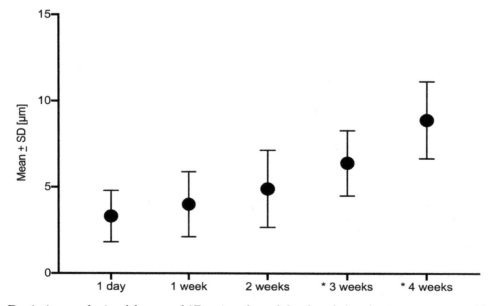

Figure 3. Deviation analysis of the tested 3D-printed models after defined aging represented by the five timepoints for mean values including standard deviations (SD) in micrometer (μm) with significant differences after * 3 weeks ($p = 0.0008$) and * 4 weeks ($p < 0.0001$).

4. Discussion

This in vitro investigation aimed to analyze the impact of aging on the dimensional stability of 3D-printed dental models. The present findings revealed a time-dependent significant change in dimensions after 3 and 4 weeks of aging. Therefore, the hypothesis that the period of storage time has no significant influence on the accuracy of 3D printed models had to be rejected.

The present study setup was carried out with an exemplary tooth-supported three-unit FDP in regions 24 to 26 for deviation analysis of the prepared abutment teeth. For fabrication of a manually veneered FDP, the overall time required-comprising the sum of clinical and technical work steps, including impression taking, try-in, potential adjustments, and seating of the reconstruction, is approximately 2–3 weeks [23]. During this period of time, the dental technician must rely on the dimensional stability of the dental cast. Based on this supposed working schedule, the present investigation considered five timepoints up to 4 weeks of aging for accuracy analysis of 3D-printed models.

The focus of the present study was to investigate the dimensional changes of the 3D-printed models related to the prepared abutment teeth representing short-span analysis rather than full-arch comparisons. The obtained results for accuracy during aging up to 4 weeks were very consistent for intragroup comparisons at each isolated timepoint. Analyzing longer spans, i.e., cross-arch reconstructions, the accuracy testing might reveal different results for intra- as well as intergroup comparisons. Even though significant differences of the 3D-printed models were observed after 3 and 4 weeks of aging, examination of the distance analysis revealed negligible changes of 1 to 12 μm for minimum to maximum values. Therefore, the question of clinical relevance remains, provided that the prosthetic reconstruction can be completed on the model within 3 or 4 weeks and that the models have been properly stored during this time (constant conditions at 20 °C and 50% humidity without direct light exposure). It must be critically emphasized that the dimensional changes of the 3D-printed models were small and comparable to investigations analyzing the accuracy of dental stone casts obtained from classical impression taking [24,25].

Ideally, dental master casts for the manufacturing of retrievable prosthetic reconstructions, such as screw-retained implant-supported FDPs or removable dental prostheses, can be reused in case of a potential emergency in the future. Tested 3D-printed models demonstrated a continuous decrease of dimensional stability. We cannot extrapolate beyond the 4-week duration of this study; therefore, it is not possible to predict with certainty whether these changes will continue or stabilize somehow over time. Thus, 3D-printed dental master models should be considered as single-use product, at least for the manufacturing of definitive prosthetic reconstructions. Nevertheless, the existing digital data sets can be stored and reused for the production of "fresh" dental models if necessary.

The bottleneck of accuracy is the process chain of STL files. The interface management guaranteeing a loss-free data transfer from the IOS device to the software of the virtual model builder and to the 3D printer is the key for success. The findings are therefore only representative for the combination of the equipment and materials used in this investigation and cannot be transferred to workflows of other manufacturers. Further investigations are necessary to analyze different setups of IOS > software > 3D printer including materials used and additional prosthetic indications. The following has to be considered: what are the impacts of the polymer and the 3D-printing technology, or is it a combination of both?

In general, the translation of laboratory findings into clinical (routine) protocols must proceed with caution. In the present study, the in vitro study setting can only be transferred with digital impressions in the upper jaw. It must be taken into account that in vivo digital impressions are different considering the localization. In contrast to the maxilla, the mandible exhibits characteristic inherent mobility during dynamic movements, in particular during mouth opening. The transfer of laboratory results from full-arch scans to an in vivo patient situation is difficult, specifically in the mandible.

While in the past, conventional workflows with classical impression techniques and plaster model production have been continuously optimized, there are still no explicit recommendations for digital workflows with IOS, further STL processing, and consecutive fabrication of 3D-printed dental models. Due to the various commercially available 3D printers with different quality levels and the diverse light-curing polymers in the material segment, the field of digitally produced dental models is very complex and subject to constant change without generally defined standards [15,26]. Kim et al. (2018) reported on significant differences for the analysis of full-arch dental models manufactured with different 3D printing techniques [27]. In addition, Nestler et al. (2020) have shown that inexpensive 3D printers were no less accurate than more expensive ones [19]. However, the authors did not clarify what is the meaning of "inexpensive" compared to "expensive", especially when a global market is considered. Three-dimensional printing generates not only enthusiasm but also great uncertainty. Therefore, future research must focus on the definition and establishment of evidenced-based standards in the field of 3D printing techniques in dentistry. Otherwise it is not possible for both dental technicians and dentists to distinguish which workflows with which equipment and material combination can deliver reliable results [28].

5. Conclusions

Three-dimensionally printed dental models for the production of three-unit FDPs demonstrated very accurate results. However, a significant decrease in dimensional stability of the models was observed after 3 weeks of aging under constant conditions. Based on these findings, it can be concluded that 3D-printed dental master models should not be used for the fabrication of definitive prosthetic reconstructions more than 3 to 4 weeks after 3D printing. Nevertheless, the changes observed due to aging in this study were small and comparable to the variation seen in conventional plaster cast models that are used in routine practice today.

Author Contributions: Conceptualization and methodology, T.J.; software; validation, formal analysis, and investigation, T.J. and L.M.; resources, T.J. and N.U.Z.; data curation, T.J. and L.M.; writing—original draft preparation, T.J.; writing—review and editing, T.J. and N.U.Z.; visualization, supervision, and project administration, T.J.; funding acquisition, n/a. All authors have read and agreed to the published version of the manuscript.

Acknowledgments: The authors express their gratitude to Isabell Wiestler for lab-side digitalization of the 3D-printed models at the different timepoints and to James Ashman for proofreading the final manuscript.

References

1. Chiu, A.; Chen, Y.W.; Hayashi, J.; Sadr, A. Accuracy of CAD/CAM Digital Impressions with Different Intraoral Scanner Parameters. *Sensors* **2020**, *20*, 1157. [CrossRef] [PubMed]

2. Joda, T.; Bornstein, M.M.; Jung, R.E.; Ferrari, M.; Waltimo, T.; Zitzmann, N.U. Recent Trends and Future Direction of Dental Research in the Digital Era. *Int. J. Environ. Res. Public Health* **2020**, *17*, 1987. [CrossRef] [PubMed]

3. Blatz, M.B.; Conejo, J. The Current State of Chairside Digital Dentistry and Materials. *Dent. Clin. N. Am.* **2019**, *63*, 175–197. [CrossRef] [PubMed]

4. Joda, T.; Bragger, U. Patient-centered outcomes comparing digital and conventional implant impression procedures: A randomized crossover trial. *Clin. Oral Implant. Res.* **2016**, *27*, e185–e189. [CrossRef]

5. Guo, D.N.; Liu, Y.S.; Pan, S.X.; Wang, P.F.; Wang, B.; Liu, J.Z.; Gao, W.H.; Zhou, Y.S. Clinical Efficiency and Patient Preference of Immediate Digital Impression after Implant Placement for Single Implant-Supported Crown. *Chin. J. Dent. Res.* **2019**, *22*, 21–28.

6. Joda, T.; Zarone, F.; Ferrari, M. The complete digital workflow in fixed prosthodontics: A systematic review. *BMC Oral Health* **2017**, *17*, 124. [CrossRef]

7. Joda, T.; Bragger, U. Time-efficiency analysis of the treatment with monolithic implant crowns in a digital workflow: A randomized controlled trial. *Clin. Oral Implant. Res.* **2016**, *27*, 1401–1406. [CrossRef]

8. Joda, T.; Ferrari, M.; Bragger, U. Monolithic implant-supported lithium disilicate (LS2) crowns in a complete digital workflow: A prospective clinical trial with a 2-year follow-up. *Clin. Implant Dent. Relat. Res.* **2017**, *19*, 505–511. [CrossRef]

9.   Joda, T.; Bragger, U. Time-Efficiency Analysis Comparing Digital and Conventional Workflows for Implant Crowns: A Prospective Clinical Crossover Trial. *Int. J. Oral Maxillofac. Implant.* **2015**, *30*, 1047–1053. [CrossRef]

10. Joda, T.; Bragger, U. Digital vs. conventional implant prosthetic workflows: A cost/time analysis. *Clin. Oral Implant. Res.* **2015**, *26*, 1430–1435. [CrossRef]

11. Almufleh, B.; Emami, E.; Alageel, O.; de Melo, F.; Seng, F.; Caron, E.; Nader, S.A.; Al-Hashedi, A.; Albuquerque, R.; Feine, J.; et al. Patient satisfaction with laser-sintered removable partial dentures: A crossover pilot clinical trial. *J. Prosthet. Dent.* **2018**, *119*, 560–567. [CrossRef] [PubMed]

12. Gintaute, A.; Straface, A.; Zitzmann, N.U.; Joda, T. Removable Dental Prosthesis 2.0: Digital from A to Z? *Swiss Dent. J.* **2020**, *130*, 229–235. [PubMed]

13. Joda, T.; Ferrari, M.; Gallucci, G.O.; Wittneben, J.G.; Bragger, U. Digital technology in fixed implant prosthodontics. *Periodontology 2000* **2017**, *73*, 178–192. [CrossRef] [PubMed]

14. Alharbi, N.; Wismeijer, D.; Osman, R.B. Additive Manufacturing Techniques in Prosthodontics: Where Do We Currently Stand? A Critical Review. *Int. J. Prosthodont.* **2017**, *30*, 474–484. [CrossRef]

15. Quan, H.; Zhang, T.; Xu, H.; Luo, S.; Nie, J.; Zhu, X. Photo-curing 3D printing technique and its challenges. *Bioact. Mater.* **2020**, *5*, 110–115. [CrossRef]

16. Hazeveld, A.; Huddleston Slater, J.J.; Ren, Y. Accuracy and reproducibility of dental replica models reconstructed by different rapid prototyping techniques. *Am. J. Orthod. Dentofac. Orthop.* **2014**, *145*, 108–115. [CrossRef]

17. Jeong, Y.G.; Lee, W.S.; Lee, K.B. Accuracy evaluation of dental models manufactured by CAD/CAM milling method and 3D printing method. *J. Adv. Prosthodont.* **2018**, *10*, 245–251. [CrossRef]

18. Zhang, Z.C.; Li, P.L.; Chu, F.T.; Shen, G. Influence of the three-dimensional printing technique and printing layer thickness on model accuracy. *J. Orofac. Orthop.* **2019**, *80*, 194–204. [CrossRef]

19. Nestler, N.; Wesemann, C.; Spies, B.C.; Beuer, F.; Bumann, A. Dimensional accuracy of extrusion- and photopolymerization-based 3D printers: In vitro study comparing printed casts. *J. Prosthet. Dent.* **2020**. [CrossRef]

20. Rungrojwittayakul, O.; Kan, J.Y.; Shiozaki, K.; Swamidass, R.S.; Goodacre, B.J.; Goodacre, C.J.; Lozada, J.L. Accuracy of 3D Printed Models Created by Two Technologies of Printers with Different Designs of Model Base. *J. Prosthodont.* **2020**, *29*, 124–128. [CrossRef]

21. Sim, J.Y.; Jang, Y.; Kim, W.C.; Kim, H.Y.; Lee, D.H.; Kim, J.H. Comparing the accuracy (trueness and precision) of models of fixed dental prostheses fabricated by digital and conventional workflows. *J. Prosthodont. Res.* **2019**, *63*, 25–30. [CrossRef] [PubMed]

22. Dietrich, C.A.; Ender, A.; Baumgartner, S.; Mehl, A. A validation study of reconstructed rapid prototyping models produced by two technologies. *Angle Orthod.* **2017**, *87*, 782–787. [CrossRef] [PubMed]

23. Muhlemann, S.; Benic, G.I.; Fehmer, V.; Hammerle, C.H.F.; Sailer, I. Randomized controlled clinical trial of digital and conventional workflows for the fabrication of zirconia-ceramic posterior fixed partial dentures. Part II: Time efficiency of CAD-CAM versus conventional laboratory procedures. *J. Prosthet. Dent.* **2019**, *121*, 252–257. [CrossRef] [PubMed]

24. Valente Vda, S.; Zanetti, A.L.; Feltrin, P.P.; Inoue, R.T.; de Moura, C.D.; Padua, L.E. Dimensional accuracy of stone casts obtained with multiple pours into the same mold. *ISRN Dent.* **2012**, *2012*, 730674. [CrossRef]

25. Vitti, R.P.; da Silva, M.A.; Consani, R.L.; Sinhoreti, M.A. Dimensional accuracy of stone casts made from silicone-based impression materials and three impression techniques. *Braz. Dent. J.* **2013**, *24*, 498–502. [CrossRef]

26. Barazanchi, A.; Li, K.C.; Al-Amleh, B.; Lyons, K.; Waddell, J.N. Additive Technology: Update on Current Materials and Applications in Dentistry. *J. Prosthodont.* **2017**, *26*, 156–163. [CrossRef]

27. Kim, S.Y.; Shin, Y.S.; Jung, H.D.; Hwang, C.J.; Baik, H.S.; Cha, J.Y. Precision and trueness of dental models manufactured with different 3-dimensional printing techniques. *Am. J. Orthod. Dentofac. Orthop.* **2018**, *153*, 144–153. [CrossRef]

28. Jockusch, J.; Ozcan, M. Additive manufacturing of dental polymers: An overview on processes, materials and applications. *Dent. Mater. J.* **2020**. [CrossRef]

7

Dental Practice Integration into Primary Care: A Microsimulation of Financial Implications for Practices

Sung Eun Choi [1,*], **Lisa Simon** [2,3], **Jane R. Barrow** [2], **Nathan Palmer** [4], **Sanjay Basu** [5,6,7] and **Russell S. Phillips** [5]

1   Department of Oral Health Policy and Epidemiology, Harvard School of Dental Medicine, Boston, MA 02115, USA
2   Office of Global and Community Health, Harvard School of Dental Medicine, Boston, MA 02115, USA; Lisa_Simon@hms.harvard.edu (L.S.); Jane_Barrow@hsdm.harvard.edu (J.R.B)
3   Harvard Medical School, Boston, MA 02115, USA
4   Department of Biomedical Informatics, Harvard Medical School, Boston, MA 02115, USA; Nathan_Palmer@hms.harvard.edu
5   Center for Primary Care, Harvard Medical School, Boston, MA 02115, USA; Sanjay_Basu@hms.harvard.edu (S.B.); Russell_Phillips@hms.harvard.edu (R.S.P.)
6   Research and Analytics, Collective Health, San Francisco, CA 94107, USA
7   School of Public Health, Imperial College London, London SW7 2BU, UK
*   Correspondence: Sung_Choi@hsdm.harvard.edu

Abstract: Given the widespread lack of access to dental care for many vulnerable Americans, there is a growing realization that integrating dental and primary care may provide comprehensive care. We sought to model the financial impact of integrating dental care provision into a primary care practice. A microsimulation model was used to estimate changes in net revenue per practice by simulating patient visits to a primary dental practice within primary care practices, utilizing national survey and un-identified claims data from a nationwide health insurance plan. The impact of potential changes in utilization rates and payer distributions and hiring additional staff was also evaluated. When dental care services were provided in the primary care setting, annual net revenue changes per practice were −$92,053 (95% CI: −93,054, −91,052) in the first year and $104,626 (95% CI: 103,315, 105,316) in subsequent years. Net revenue per annum after the first year of integration remained positive as long as the overall utilization rates decreased by less than 25%. In settings with a high proportion of publicly insured patients, the net revenue change decreased but was still positive. Integrating primary dental and primary care providers would be financially viable, but this viability depends on demands of dental utilization and payer distributions.

Keywords: integrated care; medical–dental integration; simulation model; dental research

1. Introduction

Dentistry has traditionally remained a separate discipline from other areas of medicine in the U.S. [1], and this artificial division does not foster comprehensive and high-quality care. Evidence shows that oral health complications, such as inflammation and infections that begin in the mouth, can lead to major health complications (e.g., dental abscess) [2]. Furthermore, a growing body of research has identified a potential connection between oral health and other chronic conditions, such as diabetes and cardiovascular diseases [3–5]. The National Academy of Medicine (an American nonprofit, non-governmental organization providing expert advice on issues relating to health, medicine, and health policy) has proposed integrating oral health into primary care as a way to expand access to recommended treatments and promote better health overall [6,7]. Despite recent studies suggesting that integration of dental care may benefit patients or reduce healthcare costs [8], financing and delivery of dental care remains disconnected from other health services, even among Accountable Care Organizations (ACOs), a network of coordinated healthcare practitioners in the U.S. that shares financial and medical responsibility for providing coordinated care to patients in the hopes of improving overall population health. Integration of dental care may present an opportunity for improved accountability for total health. However, there is little financial incentive and considerable financial uncertainties for ACOs to facilitate access to these services [6,9,10].

A number of organizations have initiated efforts to adopt integrated dental–medical care. One form of these efforts is integration in a co-located setting where provision of primary dental services is within and a part of primary care or vice versa. Co-location of medical and dental services is not a new concept; Federally Qualified Health Centers across the country have offered medical and dental facilities in the same building for decades, but often, electronic health records (EHRs) lack interoperability. A more innovative co-located model would allow communication across disciplines and sharing of patient information and EHRs, which provides an opportunity for the providers to "close the loop" on care gaps for patients beyond just providing care [11,12]. This approach facilitates timely delivery of diagnostic, preventive, and treatment services to improve patient health and reduce inefficiency in care delivery, allowing easier bidirectional referrals and quicker access for medical patients with acute oral health situations (and for dental patients with potential medical issues) [3–5,13].

Currently there are co-located facilities developing in the U.S., and pilot studies are being conducted in these settings [14]. A number of integrated care projects have had promising results, including the Colorado Medical Dental Integration Project [15,16]. One of the demonstration projects, the University of California, Los Angeles (UCLA)-First 5 LA Project, showed increased access to dental care by 85%, with the majority of services in diagnostic and preventive care [17]. While these demonstration projects are effective in assessing changes in dental care access rates and identifying logistical barriers, a key gap in knowledge is the economic viability of the delivery of such services by primary care practices constrained by financial realities. In this study, we estimated the cost and revenue implications to primary care practices of embedding a dental practice to integrate primary dental and primary medical care.

2. Materials and Methods

2.1. Study Design

We estimated costs and revenues for an integrated medical and dental practice using a microsimulation model (Figure 1), an approach often used to evaluate the effects of hypothetical interventions before they are implemented in the real world [8,18]. We simulated a representative sample of 10,000 integrated practices (dental practice embedded within the primary care practice providing dental services provided by a general dentist and dental hygienist, with supporting dental assistants), per International Society for Pharmacoeconomics and Outcomes Research (ISPOR) guidelines [19]. For each of the simulated practices, we assigned a number of simulated patient visits, then for each visit, an insurance type and indicator variables for receiving certain types of procedures were assigned, matching the overall distribution of procedure utilization rates by insurance type.

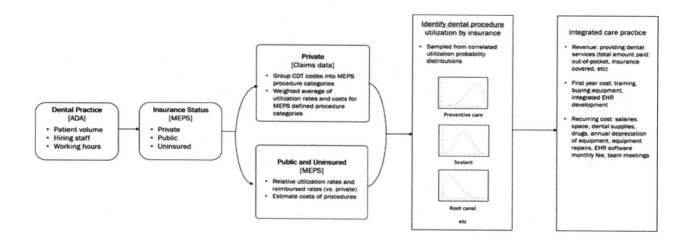

Figure 1. Simulation model flow diagram [data sources]. ADA = American Dental Association; MEPS = Medical Expenditure Panel Survey; CDT = Code on Dental Procedures and Nomenclature.

The simulation model was re-run 10,000 times while repeatedly Monte Carlo sampling from the probability distributions around the patient volume, utilization, cost, and expense data points shown in Table 1 to compute the mean and 95% credible intervals [20]. This process also accounted for the correlation among procedure utilization rates by insurance type to capture the common co-occurrence of procedures. Simulations were performed in R (v. 3.3.2, The R Foundation for Statistical Computing, Vienna, Austria). This study was reviewed by the institutional review board of the Harvard Medical School and determined to be "not-human subjects research" since the data are publicly available and de-identified.

Table 1. Input data for the dental care integration model. Data are expressed as mean (SD).

Parameters	Value	Source
Practice/patient characteristics		
Number of patient visits per dentist (including hygienist appointment) per year	3415 (347)	ADA HPI [21]
Number of patient visits per dentist (excluding hygienist appointment) per year	1831 (127)	ADA HPI [21]
Number of patient visits per hour	2.3	ADA HPI [21]
Number of hours spent on patient visits per day	6.1	ADA HP I[21]
Health insurance payer distribution of overall population (proportion with dental insurance in each group)		MEPS [22]
Private	0.66 (0.01) [0.69 (0.01)]	
Public	0.25 (0.01) [0.02 (0.01)]	
Uninsured	0.08 (0.01) [0.04 (0.01)]	

Table 1. *Cont.*

Parameters	Value	Source
Dental insurance payer distribution		MEPS [22]
Private	0.52 (0.05)	
Public	0.19 (0.03)	
Uninsured	0.29 (0.01)	
Utilization rates		
CDT procedure level utilization rate (privately insured)	Supplementary Table S1	Aetna Warehouse
Relative scales of utilization rates (public and uninsured)	Supplementary Table S1	MEPS [22]
Costs of dental procedures		
CDT procedure level costs (privately insured)	Supplementary Table S2	Aetna Warehouse
Reimbursement rates relative to private insurance	Supplementary Table S3	MEPS [22]
Expenses		
Dentist salary	152,210 (20,830)	ADA HPI [21]
Hygienist	74,070 (12,680)	Bureau of Labor Statistics [23]
Chairside assistant	37,630 (6870)	Bureau of Labor Statistics [23]
Primary care physician (hourly)	$98 (7)	MGMA [24]
Medical Assistant (hourly)	$15.1(2)	Bureau of Labor Statistics [23]
Recurring costs		
Clinical space	$1014 (290)	MGMA [24]
Dental supplies	6.4% of gross billing	ADA [25]
Drugs	0.3% of gross billing	ADA [25]
Dental lab charges	6.4% of gross billing	ADA [25]
Repairs of dental equipment	0.7% of gross billing	ADA [25]
Annual depreciation cost on dental equipment	2.2% of gross billing	ADA [25]
EHR software monthly fee	$135 (25)	Delta Dental [26]
Transition Costs (applied to the first year)		
Equipment, computers, software	$195,000 (2000)	ADA [27]
Integrated EHR development	$5000	Delta Dental [26]
Planning, coordination, informatics and workflow revision, and quality improvement during setup period	$1411 (73)	Prior pilot projects in other disciplines [28,29]

ADA = American Dental Association; HPI = Health Policy Institute; MGMA = Medical Group Management Association; EHR = electronic health records.

2.2. Model Assumption

We first estimated the patient volume that needs to be maintained at the integrated settings. On average, full-time equivalent (FTE) general dental practitioners experience 14.6 patient visits per day including dental hygienist visits [21]. An FTE primary care physician sees 19.7 patients per day on average [30]. In our model, we assumed that the minimum patient volume at the integrated settings is at least 15 patients per day, the supply of dentists remains above 61 dentists per 100,000 population with 5 primary care physicians to 1 general dental practitioner per setting. Then, we identified dental procedures that could be routinely offered by general dentists using the Code on Dental Procedures and Nomenclature (CDT Code) [31]. The final set of procedures offered in the primary care setting was determined based on the list of dental procedures covered by Adult Medicaid dental benefits in Maryland and by expert opinions from more than two general dentists to determine a conservative set of procedures (Supplementary Table S4) [32]. This final set of procedures does not include procedures that involve cost-prohibitive dental equipment for a small general dental practice, such as a Panorex machine, or are primarily billed by dentist specialists, such as orthodontic services.

2.3. Data Sources

Data sources and input data for the model are detailed in Table 1. We obtained the annual patient volume and transition costs from American Dental Association (ADA) Survey of Dental Practice [21,33]. We then subcategorized dental visits for each procedure type among patients by dental insurance type: private, public, and self-pay/uninsured based on Medical Expenditure Panel Survey (MEPS) data (for dental practices; $N = 30.5$ million) (Figure 1) [22].

We obtained the utilization rates and costs for each procedure among a privately insured population using un-identifiable member claims data from Aetna and estimated utilization rates and cost (reimbursed rates and payer distribution) among publicly insured and uninsured populations by extrapolating from MEPS (Supplementary Tables S2 and S3 and Supplementary Figure S1) [22]. Because MEPS data do not provide procedure-level utilization rates, we grouped CDT procedure codes into the procedure categories used in MEPS (Supplementary Table S4). These estimates were used to capture varying utilization and reimbursement rates by insurance status across the U.S.

2.4. Cost and Revenue Estimates from Dental–Medical Integration

We computed the cost of the embedded dental practice using procedure utilization rates and associated costs (shown in Table 1). The transition costs included the costs related to training staff and the time necessary for planning, coordination, informatics and workflow revision, and quality improvement, and start-up equipment purchase, and interoperable EHR software expenses (EHR software development cost for the first year and monthly lease fees for the subsequent years) [26]. Recurring costs included salaries for a general dental practitioner (1 full-time equivalent (FTE)), dental hygienists (1.4 FTE), and chairside assistants (1.5 FTE), and the costs associated with delivering dental services, such as dental supplies and drugs. These estimates were calculated from the fact that average general dental practitioners hire dental hygienists and chairside assistants 77.5% and 86.3% of the time, and average numbers of dental hygienists and chairside assistants per dentist among those who employ these staff are 1.8 and 1.7, respectively [34].

2.5. Primary and Secondary Outcome Metrics

The primary outcome was changes in net revenue per integrated practice per year. We computed the main outcome metric as the total reimbursements for dental services minus the total cost of service provision. Our secondary outcome metrics included (1) costs of dental service integration and (2) gross revenues for dental service integration. The primary and secondary outcomes were computed per annum for both the first and subsequent years.

2.6. Sensitivity Analyses

In an integrated setting, an increase in dental service utilization is expected due to theoretically easier access to dental care. Moreover, with recent findings on association between periodontal diseases and chronic conditions, a number of insurance companies have started offering 100% coverage for nonsurgical periodontal treatment to those with chronic conditions, such as diabetes, cardiovascular diseases, rheumatoid arthritis, and HIV/AIDS, which may increase utilization of periodontal treatment services [35–37]. The average hours per day a general dental practitioner spends in the dental office is 6.3, and 26.5% of surveyed general dentists perceived their workload to be "not busy enough" [38]. In order to estimate expected changes in net revenue from changes in utilization rates, we simulated potential increases or decreases in utilization rates in all procedure types from 50% (7 patients/day) to 120% (17 patients/day, dental practitioners spending time in the dental office for a maximum 7.6 hours per day) of baseline values.

Next, based on findings from one of the demonstration projects [17], we assessed how increases in preventive care utilization (radiographs, prophylaxis, fluoride varnish application, and sealant placement) would result in changes in net revenue. Because preventive care can be performed by hygienists, we simulated changes in net revenue from employing an additional hygienist to accommodate potential increases in preventive dental care. The number of patients a dental hygienist could accept was capped at the current average number of hygienist appointments at general dental practices nationwide [38]. We evaluated the impact of varying rates of increase in preventive care utilization on total net revenue with an additional dental hygienist.

Lastly, we simulated different payer distributions across the patient visits. In the base-case scenario, we used the national average payer distribution for medical and dental practices; 66% private, 25% public, 8 % uninsured for medical, and 52% private, 19% public, and 29% uninsured for dental practices (in dental practices, we did not include Medicare as public as dental benefits are not covered under Medicare with the exception of select Medicare Advantage plans). In this sensitivity analysis, we evaluated the impact of different patient payer distributions in certain settings. Community Health Centers (CHCs) serve a higher percentage of publicly insured or uninsured patients than the national average: 17% private, 59% public (49% Medicaid), and 24% uninsured [39]. In order to account for the fact that most patients seen by the dentist will come from the primary care practice after integration, we simulated average payer distribution at primary care practices: 45% private, 48 % public (17% Medicaid), and 7% uninsured [40]. In these scenarios, we assumed that same proportions of privately insured and Medicare patients have private dental insurance as in the base case, and calculated estimated dental insurance payer distributions for each setting.

3. Results

3.1. Base-Case Analyses

Among the fifteen procedure types that were determined to be routinely delivered by general dental practitioners, diagnostic examination and cleaning (prophylaxis) had the highest utilization rates, followed by radiographs (Supplementary Figure S2). The privately insured population visited dental practices for routine check-ups and cleanings at a higher rate than publicly insured or uninsured populations. While 62.2% (95% CI: 61.0, 63.3) of the total dental visits in a given year were for examinations in the privately insured population, publicly insured and uninsured populations visited a dental practice for examinations 57.6% (95% CI: 55.6, 59.5) and 53% (95% CI: 48.2, 58.3) of the time, respectively. However, the rate of tooth extraction was more than twice as high among publicly insured and uninsured patients, which might be due to less-frequent routine dental visits. Uninsured patients visited a dental practice for tooth extraction 21.6% (95% CI: 19.6, 23.7) of the time, whereas privately and publicly insured patients visited a dental practice for tooth extraction 5.8% (95% CI: 5.6, 6.0) and 14.4% (95% CI: 13.8, 15.0) of the time, respectively.

When dental services by a general dental practitioner were offered in the simulated integrated care setting, the primary outcome of net revenue was positive after the first year of integration. Due to transition costs and start-up expenses, the net revenue in the first year of integration was negative, -$92,053 (95% CI: −93,054, −91,052) (Table 2). After the first year, annual net revenue for the subsequent years was $104,316 (95% CI: 103,315, 105,316) per practice after the first year, assuming the same utilization rates as existing patients who completed dental visits.

Table 2. Costs and revenues from medical–dental integration, per practice per year.

	Cost, Year 1 (USD)	Cost, after Year 1 (USD)	Gross Revenue (USD)	Net Revenue, Year 1 (USD)	Net Revenue, After Year 1 (USD)
Base case	585,927 (585,335, 586,519)	389,514 (388,923, 390,104)	493,830 (492,831, 494,828)	−92,053 (−93,054, −91,052)	104,316 (103,315, 105,316)
Overall utilization (patient visit volume) change					
50%	546,758 (546,184, 547,331)	350,372 (349,799, 350,944)	247,654 (247,148, 248,160)	−299,227 (−299,929, −298,526)	−102,717 (−103,416, −102,019)
60%	554,582 (554,006, 555,158)	358,180 (357,604, 358,755)	296,759 (296,157, 297,362)	−257,842 (−258,595, −257,089)	−61,420 (−62,170, −60,669)
70%	562,408 (562,408, 561,829)	366,018 (365,439, 366,596)	346,057 (345,354, 346,760)	−216,448 (−217,256, −215,639)	−19,960 (−20,768, −19,152)
80%	570,238 (569,655, 570,821)	373,822 (373,240, 374,404)	395,141 (394,341, 395,940)	−175,034 (−175,904, −174,164)	21,318 (20,450, 22,186)
90%	578,076 (577,489, 578,663)	381,689 (381,103, 382,275)	444,617 (443,719, 445,516)	−133,575 (−134,507, −132,644)	62,928 (61,994, 63,862)
110%	593,784 (593,188, 594,381)	397,350 (396,777, 397,966)	543,252 (542,160, 544,344)	−50,490 (−51,557, −49,421)	145,880 (144,812, 146,948)
120%	601,601 (601,000, 602,202)	405,067 (404,582, 405,782)	592,374 (591,183, 593,564)	−9145 (−10,287, −8004)	187,191 (186,052, 188,330)
Preventive service utilization change with additional dental hygienist					
50% increase	673,080 (672,304, 673,857)	476,603 (475,843, 477,363)	576,377 (575,362, 577,391)	−96,703 (−97,787, −95,620)	99,774 (98,657, 100,889)
60% increase	675,706 (674,927, 676,484)	479,228 (478,469, 479,988)	592,887 (591,868, 593,907)	−82,818 (−83,897, −81,738)	113,659 (112,539, 114,778)
70% increase	678,331 (677,550, 679,112)	481,854 (481,094, 482,613)	609,399 (608,373, 610,425)	−68,932 (−70,008, −67,856)	127,545 (126,421, 128,669)
80% increase	680,955 (680,171, 681,738)	484,477 (483,717, 485,237)	625,899 (624,868, 626,931)	−55,055 (−56,127, −53,982)	141,422 (140,294, 142,550)
90% increase	683,580 (682,795, 684,366)	487,103 (486,343, 487,863)	642,413 (64,1374, 643,452)	−41,167 (−42,236, −40,097)	155,310 (154,178, 156,442)
100% increase(full capacity)	686,208 (685,420, 686,995)	489,730 (488,970, 490,491)	658,939 (657,894, 659,985)	−27,268 (−28,335, −26,201)	169,208 (168,071, 170,345)

The total gross revenue from dental practices was $493,830 (95% CI: 492,831, 494,828). The highest-revenue-generating procedure type was cleanings, with a gross revenue of $130,350 (95% CI: 130,088, 130,612), followed by diagnostic examinations and extractions, with gross annual revenues of $80,910 (95% CI: 80,747, 81,072) and $53,693 (95% CI: 53,574, 53,811), respectively (Figure 2). The least-revenue-generating procedure type was repair, such as repairing or rebasing dentures, resulting in gross annual revenue of $512 (95% CI: 508, 518).

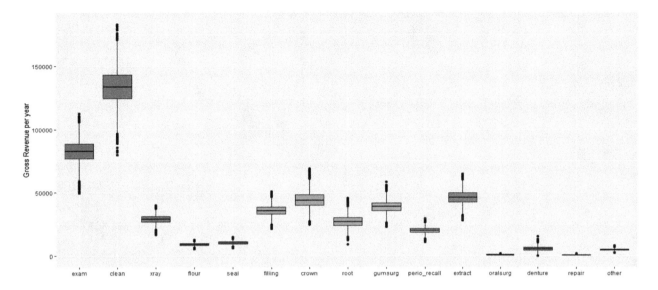

Figure 2. Gross revenue by procedure type, showing the minimum (lower whisker), maximum (upper whisker), median (center of the box), lower quartile (bottom of box), and upper quartile (top of box) values. Exam = diagnostic; clean: prophylaxis; X-ray = radiographic image; flour = fluoride; seal = sealant; root = root canal; gumsurg = periodontal scaling, root planning or gum; extract = extraction/ tooth pulled; repair = repair of bridges/dentures or relining.

3.2. Sensitivity Analyses

When overall utilization rates varied from half to twice their baseline values, net revenue per annum after the first year of integration remained positive as long as the overall utilization rates decreased by less than 25% (Table 2). Because of a greater number of adults visiting a physician annually than a dental practitioner and increased rates of enhanced dental benefits among patients with chronic conditions who are more likely to have more frequent medical visits, we expect that medical–dental integration would increase access to and utilization of dental care. When the modeled utilization rates were increased by 20%, net revenue per annum was $187,191 (95% CI: 186,052, 188,330).

Next, we evaluated the impact of hiring an additional dental hygienist to perform four types of procedures (radiographs, prophylaxis, fluoride varnish application, and sealant placement) to accommodate potential increases in preventive dental care with integration. When preventive care utilization increased by more than 53%, hiring an additional full-time dental hygienist resulted in a higher net revenue. If a full-time dental hygienist is hired and works at full capacity (performing diagnostic and preventive procedures at approximately the same rates as the average dental hygienist currently seeing patients in the U.S.), the expected net revenue was $169,208 (95% CI: 168,071, 170,345), which was a 62.2% increase from before employing the additional dental hygienist (Table 2).

When we simulated payer distributions at a CHC with a high proportion of publicly insured, the expected net revenue was $70,099 (95% CI: 69,136, 71,061), $34,217 lower than the net revenue from the base-case scenario, due primarily to lower reimbursement rates from public payers and the types of dental procedures these patients receive (Figure 3 and Supplementary Table S5). In the average primary care provider setting, the net revenue was $108,764 (95% CI: 107,744, 109,783), which was $4448 higher than the net revenue from the base-case scenario.

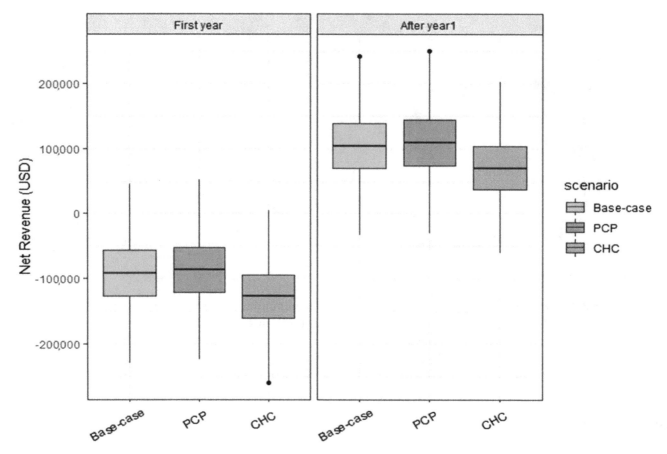

Figure 3. Impact of different payer distributions, showing the minimum (lower whisker), maximum (upper whisker), median (center of the box), lower quartile (bottom of box), and upper quartile (top of box) values. Base case = national average; PCP = primary care practice; CHC = community health center.

4. Discussion

With increased interest in the potential for integrated medical–dental care, our study evaluated the financial viability of primary integrated services—primary medicine and primary dentistry—to achieve whole-person care. We found that the net revenue changes after the first year of integration would remain positive when the integrated care could maintain at least 75% of current patient volume and the payer distribution. Serving a high proportion of patients covered by public dental insurance would result in a lower net revenue due to lower reimbursement rates. With the potential increase in utilization of basic preventive services due to integration, employing an additional hygienist to accommodate increased demand would increase the net revenue up to 62% if the hygienist worked at full capacity.

A key obstacle to successful integration of medical and dental service provision has been the substantial infrastructural investments required, such as interoperable EHRs, shared or commonly managed facilities, and a multidisciplinary workforce. While an interoperable EHR promotes well-informed care and treatment planning as well as coordination of the scheduling and billing of patient visits, it is relatively new concept and involves technical hurdles [41]. In our study, we implemented a monthly leased software option, a reasonably integrated option; however, it could be home grown with greater financial investment. For this and other reasons, the integration of medical and dental services can be a highly resource-intensive model to implement.

Our results suggest that facilities would experience negative net revenue from implementation in the first year; however, the net revenue for successful implementation would remain positive. While our study was limited to evaluating the financial viability of the integrated care, the expected benefits from this integration may extend beyond positive revenue. Integrated care facilitates timely delivery of diagnostic, preventive, and treatment services to improve patient health and reduce inefficiency in care delivery. Integrated care with dental, psychiatric, and allied health service has been also supported in other countries [42], and due to significant overlap in training between dental and medical students in many European countries, it is practically viable outside the U.S. [43]. Based on recent findings on the association between oral health status and chronic conditions [3–5] and potential cost savings from co-management of these diseases [44,45], integrated medical–dental practice could be expected to improve health outcomes of the population and result in cost savings in the overall healthcare expenditures in the U.S.

Our analysis has limitations inherent to simulation modeling based on secondary data sources. First, we simulated the utilization and cost of dental services at procedure level based on claims data from a mostly privately insured population. Although we extrapolated from nationally representative survey data to make projections about publicly insured and uninsured populations, some information loss is to be expected by grouping a number of procedure codes into different categories. An additional logical step for future research is to gain access to claims data from publicly insured populations, such as Center for Medicare and Medicaid Services (CMS) data, to identify whether incorporating procedure-level data in this population would alter the findings of our study [46]. Furthermore, we lacked sufficiently rigorous data to expand our model to incorporate regional variation in service utilization and payer distribution, such as urban vs. rural or by state. Dentist supply, dental care demand, and payer distributions vary a lot across geographic location. While our study results are based on national averages, medical–dental integration would likely yield higher revenue in one setting than the in other. In the absence of robust data about how much patient volume would change in terms of dental service need, we did not make any assumptions about the trends in dental utilization or payer distribution of the population over time. Moreover, we assumed that only a subset of dental procedures would be performed by general dental practitioners at an integrated setting under a fee-for-service scenario, and specialty services would be referred out. However, it may not be applicable to CHC where it accepts encounter-based payment, and there is a possibility that some CHCs may provide specialty services that are not covered, which would alter the financial impact of the integrated care practice. Finally, the proprietary nature of the ADA data used here is a limitation for broad usage; the potential availability of other practice cost registries or data from a strong medical–dental integrated practice may eventually lead to the wider availability of financial data for practice planning, and it remains as an area for future research.

5. Conclusions

Our findings suggest that medical–dental integration is financially viable. Given that more adults visit a physician than a dentist annually and that in some case enhanced dental benefits are being offered to patients with chronic conditions, medical–dental integration could improve patient health and reduce inefficiency in care delivery. Furthermore, it has potential value to provide comprehensive whole-person care through bidirectional referrals and sharing patient information, which would provide a critical opportunity to bridge the gap between dentistry and medicine.

Author Contributions: S.E.C.: study conception and design, statistical analysis, acquisition of data, analysis and interpretation of data, drafting of the manuscript, and critical revision of the manuscript; N.P.: acquisition of data and critical revision of the manuscript; J.R.B.: study conception and design, acquisition of data, and critical revision of the manuscript; L.S., S.B., and R.S.P.: study conception and design and critical revision of the manuscript. All authors have read and agreed to the published version of the manuscript.

References

1.   Simon, L. Overcoming Historical Separation between Oral and General Health Care: Interprofessional Collaboration for Promoting Health Equity. *AMA J. Ethics* **2016** *18*, 941–949. [CrossRef] [PubMed]

2.   Mayo Clinic. Oral Health: A Window to Your Overall Health. Available online: https://www.mayoclinic.org/
      healthy-lifestyle/adult-health/in-depth/dental/art-20047475 (accessed on 31 March 2019).
3.   Dietrich, T.; Webb, I.; Stenhouse, L.; Pattni, A.; Ready, D.; Wanyonyi, K.L.; White, S.; Gallagher, J.E. Evidence
      summary: the relationship between oral and cardiovascular disease. *Br. Dent. J.* **2017**, *222*, 381–385.
      [CrossRef] [PubMed]
4.   Kholy, K.E.; Genco, R.J.; Van Dyke, T.E. Oral infections and cardiovascular disease. *Trends Endocrinol. Metab.*
      2015, *26*, 315–321. [CrossRef] [PubMed]
5.   Preshaw, P.M.; Alba, A.L.; Herrera, D.; Jepsen, S.; Konstantinidis, A.; Makrilakis, K.; Taylor, R. Periodontitis
      and diabetes: a two-way relationship. *Diabetologia* **2012**, *55*, 21–31. [CrossRef] [PubMed]
6.   Institute of Medicine. Advancing Oral Health in America. Available online: https://www.hrsa.gov/sites/
      default/files/publichealth/clinical/oralhealth/advancingoralhealth.pdf (accessed on 1 August 2019).
7.   Institute of Medicine. Improving Access to Oral Health Care for Vulnerable and Underserved Populations.
      Available online: https://www.hrsa.gov/sites/default/files/publichealth/clinical/oralhealth/improvingaccess.
      pdf (accessed on 16 March 2019).
8.   Choi, S.E.; Sima, C.; Pandya, A. Impact of Treating Oral Disease on Preventing Vascular Diseases:
      A Model-Based Cost-effectiveness Analysis of Periodontal Treatment Among Patients With Type 2 Diabetes.
      Diabetes Care **2019**. [CrossRef] [PubMed]
9.   American Dental Association. Dental Care in Accountable Care Organizations: Insights from 5 Case Studies.
      Available online: http://www.ada.org/~{}/media/ADA/Science%20and%20Research/HPI/Files/HPIBrief_
      0615_1.ashx (accessed on 29 March 2019).
10.   American Dental Association. Dental Care Within Accountable Care Organizations: Challenges and
      Opportunities. Available online: http://www.ada.org/~{}/media/ADA/Science%20and%20Research/HPI/
      Files/HPIBrief_0316_2.pdf (accessed on 29 March 2019).
11.   Jones, J.A.; Snyder, J.J.; Gesko, D.S.; Helgeson, M.J. Integrated Medical-Dental Delivery Systems: Models in
      a Changing Environment and Their Implications for Dental Education. *J. Dent. Educ.* **2017**, *81*, eS21–eS29.
      [CrossRef] [PubMed]
12.   Centers for Medicare & Medicaid Services. EHR Incentive Programs in 2015 through 2017 Health Information
      Exchange. Available online: https://nam.edu/integration-of-oral-health-and-primary-care-communication-
      coordination-and-referral/ (accessed on 25 March 2019).
13.   Farhad, S.Z.; Amini, S.; Khalilian, A.; Barekatain, M.; Mafi, M.; Barekatain, M.; Rafei, E. The effect of chronic
      periodontitis on serum levels of tumor necrosis factor-alpha in Alzheimer disease. *Dent. Res. J.* **2014**, *11*, 549–552.
14.   McKernan, S.C.; Kuthy, R.A.; Reynolds, J.C.; Tuggle, L.; Garcia, D.T. Medical-Dental Integration in Public
      Health Settings: An Environmental Scan. Available online: http://ppc.uiowa.edu/sites/default/files/ced_
      environmental_scan.pdf (accessed on 21 October 2019).
15.   Crall, J.J.; Pourat, N.; Inkelas, M.; Lampron, C.; Scoville, R. Improving The Oral Health Care Capacity Of
      Federally Qualified Health Centers. *Health Aff.* **2016**, *35*, 2216–2223. [CrossRef] [PubMed]
16.   Colorado Medical-Dental Integration Project. One Year Highlights: Colorado Medical-Dental Integration
      Project. Available online: https://www.deltadentalcofoundation.org/wp-content/uploads/COMDI_Handout_
      web.pdf (accessed on 20 March 2019).
17.   Crall, J.J.; Illum, J.; Martinez, A.; Pourat, N. An Innovative Project Breaks Down Barriers to Oral Health Care
      for Vulnerable Young Children in Los Angeles County. *UCLA Health Policy Res* **2016**, PB2016-5. 1–8.
18.   Basu, S.; Landon, B.E.; Williams, J.W., Jr.; Bitton, A.; Song, Z.; Phillips, R.S. Behavioral Health Integration into Primary
      Care: A Microsimulation of Financial Implications for Practices. *J. Gen. Intern. Med.* **2017**, *32*, 1330–1341. [CrossRef]
      [PubMed]
19.   Briggs, A.H.; Weinstein, M.C.; Fenwick, E.A.; Karnon, J.; Sculpher, M.J.; Paltiel, A.D. Model parameter
      estimation and uncertainty analysis: A report of the ISPOR-SMDM Modeling Good Research Practices Task
      Force Working Group-6. *Med. Decis. Mak.* **2012**, *32*, 722–732. [CrossRef] [PubMed]
20.   Robert, C.P.; Casella, G. *Introducing Monte Carlo Methods with R*; Springer Verlag: New York, NY, USA, 2009.
21.   American Dental Association. Characteristics of Private Dental Practices: Selected 2017 Results from the
      Survey of Dental Practice. Available online: https://www.ada.org/en/science-research/health-policy-institute/
      data-center/dental-practice (accessed on 20 March 2019).

22. Agency for Healthcare Research and Quality. Medical Expenditure Panel Survey. Available online: https://www.meps.ahrq.gov/mepsweb/ (accessed on 20 March 2019).

23. Bureau of Labor Statistics. Occupational Outlook Handbook. Available online: https://www.bls.gov/ooh/ (accessed on 22 March 2019).

24. Medical Group Management Association. DataDive. Available online: https://www.mgma.com/data (accessed on 23 March 2019).

25. American Dental Association. Survey of Dental Practice (Annual Expenses of Operating a Private Practice). Available online: https://success.ada.org/en/practice-management/survey-of-dental-practice (accessed on 22 March 2019).

26. Delta Dental. Improving Oral Health by Integrating Medical and Dental Care—EMR/EDR. Available online: http://medicaldentalintegration.org/building-mdi-models/building-co-mdi-space/ehredr/ (accessed on 5 December 2019).

27. American Dental Association. The Real Cost of Owning a Dental Practice. Available online: http://marketplace.ada.org/blog/the-real-cost-of-owning-a-dental-practice/ (accessed on 20 March 2019).

28. Liu, C.F.; Rubenstein, L.V.; Kirchner, J.E.; Fortney, J.C.; Perkins, M.W.; Ober, S.K.; Pyne, J.M.; Chaney, E.F. Organizational cost of quality improvement for depression care. *Health Serv. Res.* **2009**, *44*, 225–244. [CrossRef] [PubMed]

29. Silk, H.; Sachs Leicher, E.; Alvarado, V.; Cote, E.; Cote, S. A multi-state initiative to implement pediatric oral health in primary care practice and clinical education. *J. Public Health Dent.* **2018**, *78*, 25–31. [CrossRef] [PubMed]

30. The Physicians Foundation. Survey of America's Physician. Available online: https://physiciansfoundation.org/wp-content/uploads/2018/09/physicians-survey-results-final-2018.pdf (accessed on 24 April 2019).

31. American Dental Association. Code on Dental Procedures and Nomenclature (CDT Code). Available online: https://www.ada.org/en/publications/cdt (accessed on 20 March 2019).

32. Maryland Department of Health. Maryland Medicaid Dental Fee Schedule and Procedure Codes. Available online: https://mmcp.health.maryland.gov/Documents/2018%20CDT%20Fee%20Schedule%20FINAL%20 (accessed on 14 December 2019).

33. American Dental Association. Income, Gross Billings, and Expenses: Selected 2017 Results from the Survey of Dental Practice. Available online: https://www.ada.org/en/science-research/health-policy-institute/dental-statistics/income-billing-and-other-dentistry-statistics (accessed on 20 March 2019).

34. American Dental Association. Employment of Dental Practice Personnel: Selected 2013 Results from the Survey of Dental Practice. Available online: https://www.ada.org/en/science-research/health-policy-institute/data-center/dental-practice (accessed on 2 April 2019).

35. Florida Blue Dental. Oral Health for Overall Health. Available online: https://www.floridabluedental.com/members/oral-health-for-overall-health/ (accessed on 12 February 2019).

36. United Concordia Dental. Smile for Health—Wellness. Available online: https://www.unitedconcordia.com/dental-insurance/employer/dental-plans/innovative-solutions-dental-plans/product-smile-for-health-wellness/ (accessed on 12 February 2019).

37. Delta Dental. SmileWay Wellness Benefits. Available online: https://www.deltadentalins.com/individuals/guidance/smileway-wellness-benefits.html (accessed on 12 February 2019).

38. American Dental Association. Supply and Profile of Dentists. Available online: https://www.ada.org/en/science-research/health-policy-institute/data-center/supply-and-profile-of-dentists (accessed on 30 March 2019).

39. National Association of Community Health Centers. Community Health Center Chartbook. Available online: http://www.nachc.org/wp-content/uploads/2017/06/Chartbook2017.pdf (accessed on 20 April 2019).

40. Gillis. K.D. *Physicians' Patient Mix—A Snapshot from the 2016 Benchmark Survey and Changes Associated with the ACA.* Available online: https://www.ama-assn.org/sites/ama-assn.org/files/corp/media-browser/public/health-policy/PRP-2017-physician-benchmark-survey-patient-mix.pdf (accessed on 22 March 2020).

41. Kalenderian, E.; Halamka, J.D.; Spallek, H. An EHR with Teeth. *Appl. Clin. Inform.* **2016**, *7*, 425–429. [CrossRef] [PubMed]

42. Tan, K.B.; Earn Lee, C. Integration of Primary Care with Hospital Services for Sustainable Universal Health Coverage in Singapore. *Health Syst. Reform* **2019**, *5*, 18–23. [CrossRef] [PubMed]

43. Martinez-Alvarez, C.; Sanz, M.; Berthold, P. Basic sciences education in the dental curriculum in Southern Europe. *Eur. J. Dent. Educ.* **2001**, *5*, 63–66. [CrossRef] [PubMed]
44. Nasseh, K.; Vujicic, M.; Glick, M. The Relationship between Periodontal Interventions and Healthcare Costs and Utilization. Evidence from an Integrated Dental, Medical, and Pharmacy Commercial Claims Database. *Health Econ.* **2017**, *26*, 519–527. [CrossRef] [PubMed]
45. Jeffcoat, M.K.; Jeffcoat, R.L.; Gladowski, P.A.; Bramson, J.B.; Blum, J.J. Impact of periodontal therapy on general health: Evidence from insurance data for five systemic conditions. *Am. J. Prev. Med.* **2014**, *47*, 166–174. [CrossRef] [PubMed]
46. Centers for Medicare & Medicaid Services. Medicaid Analytic eXtract (MAX) Chartbooks. Available online: https://www.cms.gov/Research-Statistics-Data-and-Systems/Computer-Data-and-Systems/MedicaidDataSourcesGenInfo/MAX_Chartbooks.html (accessed on 29 March 2019).

Clinical Performance of Partial and Full-Coverage Fixed Dental Restorations Fabricated from Hybrid Polymer and Ceramic CAD/CAM Materials

Nadin Al-Haj Husain [1,*][iD], Mutlu Özcan [2], Pedro Molinero-Mourelle [1][iD] and Tim Joda [3][iD]

1   Department of Reconstructive Dentistry and Gerodontology, School of Dental Medicine, University of Bern, 3010 Bern, Switzerland; pedro.molineromourelle@zmk.unibe.ch

2   Division of Dental Biomaterials, Clinic for Reconstructive Dentistry, Center for Dental and Oral Medicine, University of Zurich, 8032 Zurich, Switzerland; mutlu.ozcan@zzm.uzh.ch

3   Department of Reconstructive Dentistry, University Center for Dental Medicine Basel, University of Basel, 4058 Basel, Switzerland; tim.joda@unibas.ch

*   Correspondence: nadin.al-haj-husain@zmk.unibe.ch

Abstract: The aim of this systematic review and meta-analysis was to evaluate the clinical performance of tooth-borne partial and full-coverage fixed dental prosthesis fabricated using hybrid polymer and ceramic CAD/CAM materials regarding their biologic, technical and esthetical outcomes. PICOS search strategy was applied using MEDLINE and were searched for RCTs and case control studies by two reviewers using MeSH Terms. Bias risk was evaluated using the Cochrane collaboration tool and Newcastle–Ottawa assessment scale. A meta-analysis was conducted to calculate the mean long-term survival difference of both materials at two different periods ($\leq$24, $\geq$36 months(m)). Mean differences in biologic, technical and esthetical complications of partial vs. full crown reconstructions were analyzed using software package R ($p < 0.05$). 28 studies included in the systematic review and 25 studies in the meta-analysis. The overall survival rate was 99% (0.95–1.00, $\leq$24 m) and dropped to 95% (0.87–0.98, $\geq$36 m), while the overall success ratio was 88% (0.54–0.98; $\leq$24 m) vs. 77% (0.62–0.88; $\geq$36 m). No significance, neither for the follow-up time points, nor for biologic, technical and esthetical (88% vs. 77%; 90% vs. 74%; 96% vs. 95%) outcomes was overserved. A significance was found for the technical/clinical performance between full 93% (0.88–0.96) and partial 64% (0.34–0.86) crowns. The biologic success rate of partial crowns with 69% (0.42–0.87) was lower, but not significant compared to 91% (0.79–0.97) of full crowns. The esthetical success rate of partial crowns with 90% (0.65–0.98) was lower, but not significant compared to 99% (0.92–1.00) of full crowns.

Keywords: bonding; CAD/CAM; composite resin cement; dental; hybrid polymer; indirect; meta-analysis; systematic review

1. Introduction

Over the past two decades, metal-free computer-aided design/computer aided manufacturing (CAD/CAM) materials, including ceramics and composites, have been widely used in dentistry [1]. In the restorative clinical field, these materials have been gaining importance due to their biologic and esthetical properties resulting in favorable treatment outcomes in order to satisfy increased demands and expectations of patients and dentists [2,3].

The improvements in oral health during the last decades, have promoted less aggressive dental preparations changing the conventional indications and workflows of these restorations and adapting it for these metal-free materials [4,5]. The current state of the art of dental treatments accompanied by life changes in terms of time efficacy and patient care demands, have fostered the introduction of faster and cost-efficient digital clinical workflows using CAD/CAM technology facilitating high quality restorative treatments [6,7]. These workflows allow designing and manufacturing of chairside partial or full-contoured monolithic restorations, such as inlays, veneers, single crowns (SCs) or multi-spans fixed dental prostheses (FDPs), with esthetically favorable appearance, accurate marginal adaptation in a cost and time efficient production manner [3,8].

Digital technologies also enabled the development of high-performance materials like Lithium disilicate (LD), Lithium aluminosilicate ceramic reinforced with lithium disilicate glass–ceramic (LD-LAS), hybrid-polymer ceramic (HPC) and resin-matrix ceramics (RMC) including resin-based ceramics (RBC) and polymer infiltrated ceramic network (PICN) resins [9–11].

LD is one of the of the most commonly used chairside material due to its great clinical performance and high acceptance by patients, technicians and dentists. LD-LAS covers the same indication range as LD ceramics, while showing comparable flexural strength tests results, making it a high load-bearing material with excellent esthetic properties [12,13]. The group of hybrid materials (HPC, RMC, RBC and PICN) are of growing interest due their mechanical resistibility and high elasticity. These materials are based on a ceramic like hybrid ceramic also known as resin-matrix-ceramics, resin-based ceramics or nanoceramics, presenting promising results, as they follow esthetic trends combined with minimally invasive preparations in modern clinical workflows [11,14].

The gold standard in SCs and FDPs is still ceramic fused to metal. This "conventional" approach often presents esthetic shortcomings, requires a more aggressive tooth preparation and extended technical production time. Therefore, metal-free options have gradually become a favorite alternative compared to metal-ceramic restorations [15,16]. However, when using metal-free materials, clinicians should keep in mind the limited evidence that these materials present in terms of long-term performance, survival and complication rates and carefully evaluate the indication and processing technique in each unique clinical case [14].

The wide range of new hybrid polymer and ceramic CAD/CAM materials that are offered in the dental industry to manufacture tooth-borne restorations implies the need for an evidence-based study that evaluates the current clinical behavior of these materials. Therefore, the aim of this systematic review and meta-analysis was to analyze the clinical behavior of partial and full fixed restorations out of hybrid polymer and ceramic CAD/CAM materials. This present systematic review was performed in order to answer the PICO question defined as follows: In patients receiving tooth-borne partial or full crowns, are survival and clinical success rates of monolithic CAD/CAM restorations comparable to those of conventionally manufactured?

2. Experimental Section

2.1. Search Strategy

A preliminary search was conducted prior to the definition of the final PICO question, focusing on material choice (glass ceramic multiphase (e.g., Enamic); polymeric multiphase (e.g., Lava Ultimate)); Indication (tooth and implant-borne single-unit restoration and reconstruction design (crown vs. partial crown single unit).

The PICO question was then chosen as follows: P-population: tooth-borne partial or full crowns; I-intervention: Monolithic CAD/CAM restorations; C-control: conventionally produced/manufactured restorations (natural teeth); O-outcome: survival and clinical success (fracture, debonding, behavior); S-study designs: randomized control trials (RCT) and case–control studies.

The following MeSH terms, search terms and their combinations were used in the PubMed search: (((((((((dental crowns [MeSH]) OR (dental restoration permanent [MeSH]) OR (full crown) OR (partial crown) OR (table top))))) AND ((((computer-aided design [MeSH])) OR (computer-assisted design [MeSH]) OR ((computer-aided manufacturing [MeSH])) OR (computer-assisted manufacturing

[MeSH]) OR (cerec [MeSH]) OR (CAD/CAM) OR (rapid prototyping)))))) OR (((((ceramics [MeSH]) OR (dental porcelain [MeSH]) OR (polymers [MeSH]) OR (monolithic))))) AND (((((survival analysis [MeSH terms]) OR (survival rate [MeSH Terms]) OR (survival))))) OR (((((success) OR (failure) OR (dental restoration failure [MeSH terms]) OR (complications [MeSH terms]) OR (clinical behavior) OR (adverse event) OR (chipping) OR (debonding))))). The search strategy according to the focused PICOS question is presented in Table 1.

Table 1. Search strategy according to the focused question (PICO).

Focused Question (PICO)	In Patients Receiving Tooth-Borne Partial or Full Crowns, Are Monolithic CAD/CAM Restorations Comparable to Conventionally Manufactured Restorations in Terms of Survival and Clinical Success Rates?	
Search strategy	**Population**	Tooth-borne partial or full crowns. #1—((dental crowns [MeSH]) OR (dental restoration permanent [MeSH]) OR (full crown) OR (partial crown) OR (table top))
	Intervention	Monolithic CAD/CAM restorations. #2—((computer-aided design [MeSH])) OR (computer-assisted design [MeSH]) OR ((computer-aided manufacturing [MeSH])) OR (computer-assisted manufacturing [MeSH]) OR (cerec [MeSH]) OR (CAD/CAM) OR (rapid prototyping)) #3—((ceramics [MeSH]) OR (dental porcelain [MeSH]) OR (polymers [MeSH]) OR (monolithic))
	Comparison	Conventionally manufactured restorations. #4—((porcelain-fused to metal) OR (lost-wax technique)) #5—(dental alloys [MeSH])
	Outcome	Survival (rates) and/or clinical success. #6—((survival analysis [MeSH Terms]) OR (survival rate [MeSH Terms]) OR (survival)) #7—((success) OR (failure) OR (dental restoration failure [MeSH Terms]) OR (complications [MeSH Terms]) OR (clinical behavior) OR (adverse event) OR (chipping) OR (debonding))
	Search combination(s)	(#1) AND (#2 or #3) AND (#6 or #7)

The following terms were used in the EMBASE search: ('dental crowns'/exp OR 'dental restoration permanen'/exp OR 'full crown'/exp OR 'partial crown'/exp OR 'table top') AND (' computer-aided design' OR 'computer-assisted design' OR 'computer-aided manufacturing' OR ' computer-assisted manufacturing' OR 'cerec' OR 'CAD/CAM' OR 'rapid prototyping') OR ('ceramics' OR 'dental porcelain' OR 'polymers' OR 'monolithic') AND ('survival analysis' OR 'survival rate' OR 'survival') OR ('success' OR 'failure' OR 'dental restoration failure' OR 'complications' OR 'clinical behavior' OR 'adverse event' OR 'chipping' OR 'debonding') NOT [medline]/lim AND [embase]/lim.

The following terms were used in the Web of Science and IADR abstracts search: (((((((((dental crowns [MeSH]) OR (dental restoration permanent [MeSH]) OR (full crown) OR (partial crown) OR (table top))))) AND (((((computer-aided design [MeSH])) OR (computer-assisted design [MeSH]) OR ((computer-aided manufacturing [MeSH])) OR (computer-assisted manufacturing [MeSH]) OR (cerec [MeSH]) OR (CAD/CAM) OR (rapid prototyping))))) OR (((((ceramics [MeSH]) OR (dental porcelain [MeSH]) OR (polymers [MeSH]) OR (monolithic))))) AND (((((survival analysis [MeSH Terms]) OR (survival rate [MeSH Terms]) OR (survival))))) OR (((((success) OR (failure) OR (dental restoration failure [MeSH Terms]) OR (complications [MeSH Terms]) OR (clinical behavior) OR (adverse event) OR (chipping) OR (debonding)))).

2.2. Information Sources

A systematic electronic literature search was conducted in PubMed MEDLINE, EMBASE and Web of Science (ISI—Web of Knowledge), including Google Scholar and IADR abstracts until 16 May 2018. The search aimed for English language clinical trials and case–control studies published in the last five years, performed on human and published in dental journals. Search syntax was categorized in a population, intervention, comparison and outcome study design; each category assembled using a combination of Medical Subject Heading [MeSH Terms].

2.3. Study Selection and Eligibility Criteria

To minimize the potential for reviewer bias, two reviewers (N.A.-H.H. and T.J.) independently conducted electronic literature searches and the study selection. Both reviewers studied the retrieved titles and abstracts and disagreements were solved by discussion. Forty-eight selected studies were then obtained in full texts, and the decision of inclusion of studies was made according to preset inclusion criteria.

The following inclusion criteria were chosen for the articles included in this systematic review: (1) RCTs and case control studies; (2) Studies with observation of a follow-up period of ≥1 year; (3) Studies that considered either hybrid polymers or ceramic CAD/CAM materials.

Articles meeting one or more of the following criteria were excluded: (1) In vitro or in situ studies; (2) Studies with a follow-up period less than one year; (3) Studies testing materials other than hybrid polymers or ceramic CAD/CAM materials. For quantitative analyses (meta-analysis), studies lacking a control group or standard deviation values were excluded (Figure 1).

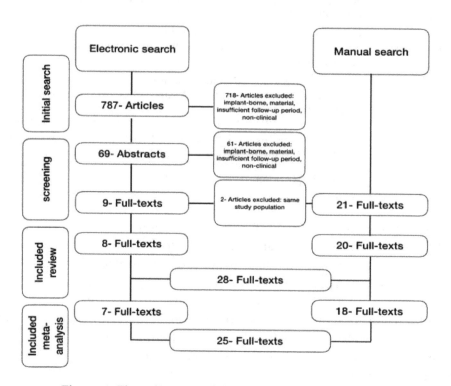

Figure 1. Flow diagram of the systematic search results.

2.4. Data Extraction and Collection

After screening the data, extracting, obtaining and screening the titles and abstracts for inclusion criteria, the selected abstracts were obtained in full texts. Titles and abstracts lacking sufficient information regarding inclusion criteria were also obtained as full texts.

Full text articles were selected in case of compliance with inclusion criteria by the two reviewers using a data extraction form. Two reviewers (N.A.-H.H. and T.J.) independently collected the following data from the included articles for further analysis: demographic information (title, authors, journal and year), study specific parameter (study type, number of treated patients, number of restorations, Ratio (restorations/patient), follow-up and drop-out), materials tested (type and commercial name, manufacturing process, luting agent, failure, survival and success rate), means and standard deviations of the clinical parameters (biologic, technical and esthetical failures).

The authors of the studies were contacted in case of unpublished data. These studies were only included if the authors provided the missing information. In order to assess the clinical performance and outcomes of the restorations, the selected studies based their evaluations on the modified United States Public Health service (USHPS) [17] criteria and the FDI World dental federation criteria [18].

For the extraction of the clinical outcomes, the relevant data of the included studies were divided into three subgroups according to their evaluated outcomes, based on the USHPS criteria and the FDI criteria: The USHPS criteria are based on an evaluation of the clinical characteristics of color, marginal adaptation, anatomic form, surface roughness, marginal staining, secondary caries and luster of restoration which is evaluated on three levels form the best to worst outcome, Alpha, Bravo and Charlie.

The FDI criteria are based on three levels that were scored into five points (Clinically very good, clinically good, clinically sufficient/satisfactory, clinically unsatisfactory, clinically poor): (A) Esthetic properties that evaluate the surface luster, the staining, color match and translucency and the esthetic anatomic form; (B) Functional properties based on the assess of fracture of material and retention, the marginal adaptation, the occlusal contour and wear, the approximal anatomic form, the radiographic examination and the patient's view; (C) Biologic properties measure the postoperative sensitivity and tooth vitality, the recurrence, the tooth integrity of caries, the periodontal response, the adjacent mucosa and the oral and general health.

2.5. Risk of Bias Assessment

The risk of bias assessment was evaluated using the Cochrane collaboration tool for randomized studies, evaluating bias risks such as sample size calculation, random sequence generation, adequate control group, materials usage following the manufacturers' instructions, tests execution by a single blinded operator, adequate statistical analysis, allocation concealment, completeness of outcome data, selective reporting and other bias. Each parameter reported by the included studies was recorded. Articles that included only one to three possible risks of bias of these items were considered at low risk for bias; four or five items, at medium risk for bias; and six to nine items, at high risk for bias.

In case of a high or unclear risk of bias the study was assigned to a judgment of risk of bias. The Newcastle–Ottawa assessment scale was applied for non-randomized studies, for the selection of the study groups, the comparability of the groups and the ascertainment of outcome or interest.

2.6. Data Analyses

The statistical analysis was performed with the software package R, Version 3.5.3 (R Core Team 2013) [19]. Both survival and success ratios were analyzed performing a meta-analysis using the logit transformation method. Results of the random effects model were reported and forest plots were drawn. Funnel plots were also produced in order to detect a possible publication bias. Overall, survival and success ratios were analyzed as well as biologic, technical and esthetical successes. The restorations instead of patients were used as the statistical unit. Studies that lacked the required information of the sample size or the follow-up time were excluded from the statistical analysis. All materials had to be pooled because of sample size considerations or missing information. The meta-analysis was done with studies reporting a follow-up time of at least 24 months.

3. Results

3.1. Study Selection

Of 795 potentially relevant studies, 48 were selected for a full-text analysis, 28 were included in the systematic review and 25 considered in the meta-analysis. Eight full text articles were selected using electronic databases and 20 further were retrieved throughout manual search. From the 25 studies included in the meta-analysis, 12 studies were randomized controlled trial, 14 prospective and 2 retrospectives (Krejci et al. 1992; Taskonak et al. 2006; Frankenberger et al. 2008; Frankenberger et al. 2009; Dukic et al. 2010; Fasbinder et al. 2010; Manhart et al. 2010; Azevedo et al. 2012; Esuivel-Opshaw et al. 2012; Murgueitio et al. 2012; Schenke et al. 2012; Taschner et al. 2012; Gehrt et al. 2013; Reich et al. 2013; Akin et al. 2014; D'all'Orologio et al. 2014; Dhima et al. 2014; Guess et al. 2014; Guess et al. 2014; Selz et al. 2014; Seydler et al. 2015; Baader et al. 2016; Botto et al. 2016; Mittal et al. 2016; Özsoy et al. 2016; Santos et al. 2016; Rauch et al. 2018) [20–46].

3.2. Study Characteristics

The characteristics of the included studies are presented in Table 2. The included articles were published between 1992 and 2018. A total of type of 28 studies including 1150 patients and 2335 reconstructions with a mean follow-up time of 4.5 years (min–max: 1–18 years) were evaluated. Materials included were composites, feldspathic ceramic, leucite reinforced glass ceramic, veneered and non-veneered lithium disilicate, veneered and monolithic zirconia and alumina. Processing techniques were stone dies incremental techniques and poured with dental stone, indirect die cast method, framework laminated with a veneering with lost-wax glaze technique, chairside and labside CAD/CAM techniques, vacuum injection mold techniques. Used luting agents were adhesive bonding systems, resin cements (Panavia, Multilink, Variolink, Tetric, Multibond) and glass ionomer luting cements (Ketac).

Table 2. Quality assessment of included studies using the Newcastle–Ottawa scale.

Study	Selection				Comparability	Outcome			Numbers of Stars (Out of 8)
	1	2	3	4	1	1	2	3	
Botto et al. 2016	–	★	–	–	★	★	★	★	5
Guess et al. 2014	★	★	★	★	★	★	★	★	8
Dhima et al. 2014	–	–	–	–	★	★	★	★	4
Dukic et al. 2010	–	–	–	–	★	★	★	★	4
Azevedo et al. 2012	★	★	★	★	★	★	★	★	8
Gehrt et al. 2013	★	★	★	★	★	★	★	★	8
Guess et al. 2014	★	★	★	★	★	★	★	★	8
Rauch et al. 2018	★	★	–	–	–	★	–	–	3
Reich et al. 2013	★	★	–	–	–	★	–	–	3
Santos et al. 2016	★	★	★	★	★	★	★	★	8
Santos et al. 2013	★	★	★	★	★	★	★	★	8
Taschner et al. 2012	★	★	★	★	★	★	★	★	8
Taskonak et al. 2006	★	★	–	★	★	★	★	–	6
Krejci et al. 1992	–	★	–	–	–	★	–	–	2

★: Each star corresponds to the subsection of quality assessment criteria.

3.3. Risks of Bias in Individual Studies

Quality and risk bias assessment of the RCTs is summarized in Figure 2 and for the case control and cohort studies reviewed in Table 1.

The Cochrane collaboration tool showed an overall low risk of bias in all the included studies. Some studies did not report enough information about the sequence generation process to allow an evaluation of either "low risk" or "high risk" (Mittal et al. 2016, Frankenberger et al. 2009). Others did not describe the allocation concealment or provide enough detail (Mittal et al. 2016, Dondi dall'Orologio et al. 2014, Ozsoy et al. 2016, Frankenberger et al. 2009). Just one study showed a high risk for the blinded outcome (Beder et al. 2016). According to the NOS scale, one study scored 2 points, two obtained 3 points, two 4 points, one 5 points, and finally seven studies obtained 8 points. These scores reflect an adequate quality of the studies included in this review.

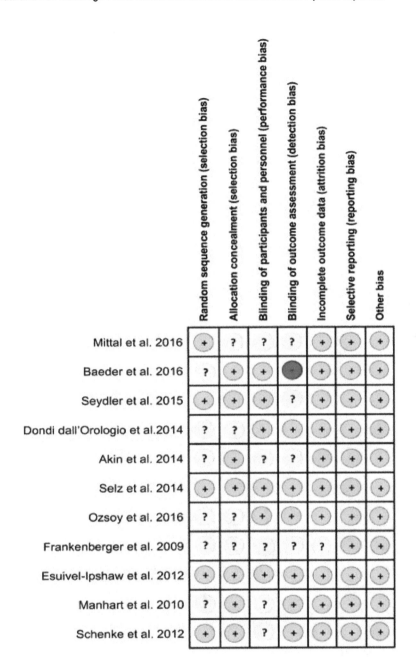

Figure 2. Summary of the Cochrane collaboration tool for assessing risk of bias for randomized controlled trials.

3.4. Meta-Analysis

Meta-analyses were performed based on 25 studies. The overall survival and success ratios of partial and full crowns were obtained using forest and funnel plots at two different time ranges: (a) ≤24 months (m); and (b) ≥36 months (m) (Table 3).

Table 3. Characteristics of included studies.

Author/ Publication Year	Journal	Study Type	Patients (N)	Restoration (n)	Ratio (n/N)	Follow-Up	Drop-Out	Material	Manufacturing Technique	Luting Agent	Failure	Survival	Success	Outcome
Mittal et al. 2016 [36]	J Clin Ped Dent	RCT	50	50	1	36 Months	0	IRC (indirect resin composite) vs. SSC (stainless steel crowns)	IRX (Composite 3-M Espe) SSC	IRC (Dual cure resin cement RelyX) SSC (luting glass ionomer cement Fuji I)	IRC (3) SSC (2)	IRC (82.9%) SSC (90.7%)	IRC (100%) SSC (95%)	Modified FDI criteria' Dental chair side treatment time and postoperative acceptability Marginal integrity IRC < SSC Time/esthetic: IRC > SSC
Botto et al. 2016 [23]	Am J Dent	Retrospective	47	93	93/47	5–18 years		13 onlays feldspathic porcelain (Vitadur Alpha), 78 onlays, 2 inlays IPS-Empress		RelyX	6 (6.5%)	87 (93.5%)	81 (93%)	Gender, age, tooth preparation, number, type, extent, location, quality and survival of the restorations, ceramic materials, luting resin cements, parafunctional habits, secondary caries and maintenance therapy, marginal adaptation, marginal discoloration, occlusal surfaces
Baader et al. 2016 [22]	J Adhes Dent	RCT	34	68	2	6.5 years	16 patients	Vita Mark II; Cerec 3D	Indirect cast	RelyX With/without enamel etching	16:11 RXU PCCs and 5 RXU+E PCCs failed. The reasons for this were fractures of restorations (3 RXU, 4 RXU+E), debonding of PCCs with no possibility of recementation (4 RXU), one endodontic treatment followed by renewal of the restoration (1 RXU) and one renewal of the PCC due to caries at another site of the tooth, necessitating a full-crown preparation (1 RXU)	RXU of 60% and for RXU+E of 82%	–	Modified USHPS postoperative hypersensitivity, anatomic form, marginal adaptation, marginal discoloration, surface texture and recurrent caries.

Table 3. *Cont.*

Author/ Publication Year	Journal	Study Type	Patients (N)	Restoration (n)	Ratio (n/N)	Follow-Up	Drop-Out	Material	Manufacturing Technique	Luting Agent	Failure	Survival	Success	Outcome
Seydler et al. 2015 [44]	J Prosthet Dent	RCT	60	60	1	2 years	0	veneered zirconia (VZ) group were made of zirconia frameworks veneered with CAD/CAM-produced lithium disilicate ceramic; monolithic lithium disilicate (MLD) ceramic	MLD crowns were milled (Cerec MC XL; Sirona Dental Systems) from a block (IPS e.max CAD; Ivoclar Vivadent AG) VZ crowns were milled from a zirconia blank (IPS e.max ZirCAD; Ivoclar Vivadent AG); the veneer structure was milled from an IPS e.max CAD lithium disilicate blank (both, Cerec MC XL; Sirona Dental Systems).	(Multilink; Ivoclar Vivadent AG	none	100		USHPS The quality of marginal fit, color and technical and biologic complications were recorded.
D'all' Orologio et al. 2014 [24]	Am J Dent	RCT	50	150		8 years	30 restoration, 10 patients	100 with the new restorative material, 50 with the composite as control, XP Bond ceram.x Duo Esthet.X		bonding system (XP Bond)	7% There were eight failures in the experimental group and four failures in the control group here were two key elements of failure: the presence of sclerotic dentin and the relationship between lesion and gingival margin.	93%		Retention, Sensitivity, Marginal Integrity, Caries, Contour
Akin et al. 2014 [20]	J Prosthodont	RCT	15	30	2	2 years	0	all-ceramic crowns	fabricated with CAD/CAM and heat-pressed (HP) techniques	Variolink II/Syntac; Ivoclar Vivadent	0	100		Porcelain fracture and partial debonding that exposed the tooth structure, secondary caries, extraction of abutment teeth and impaired esthetic quality or function were the main criteria for irreparable failure.

Table 3. *Cont.*

Author/ Publication Year	Journal	Study Type	Patients (N)	Restoration (n)	Ratio (n/N)	Follow-Up	Drop-Out	Material	Manufacturing Technique	Luting Agent	Failure	Survival	Success	Outcome
Guess et al. 2014 [32]	Int J Prosthodont	Prospective clinical study	25	86	86/25	7 years	11 patients	all-ceramic veneers with overlap (OV) and full veneer (FV) preparation designs	Leucite-reinforced glass-ceramic veneers (IPS Empress, Ivoclar Vivadent)	(Variolink II, Ivoclar Vivadent)	One OV restoration fractured (Figure 2a). cohesive ceramic fracture and crack formation within the restoration material were noted in 12 patients.	100% for FV restorations and 97.6% for OV restorations.	0.85 (CI: 0.70 to 1.00) for the FV restorations and 0.70 (CI: 0.45 to 0.95) for the OV restorations	USPHS criteria
Selz et al. 2014 [43]	Clin Oral invest	RCT	60	149	>2	5 years			In-Ceram Alumina crowns		62 Panavia, 59 Super-Bond C&B; 28 Ketac	Endodontic treatment was carried out on 7.4% of all abutment teeth and 5.4% revealed secondary caries. Unacceptable ceramic fractures were observed in 7.4%. Debonding was a rare complication (1.3%).	91.6% for Super Bond C&B, 87.4% for Ketac Cem- and 86.3% for Panavia F-bonded	82.2 Panavia, 88.7 Super-Bond C&B; 80.1 Ketac	secondary caries, clinically unacceptable fractures, root canal treatment and debonding.
Özsoy et al. 2016 [38]	JAST	RCT	60	67	>1	2 years	2 teeth	indirect composite onlays and overlays	indirect composite (Gradia, GC, Japan)	Variolink II		100	100	Anatomy, marginal adaptation, marginal discoloration, color match, surface roughness, caries
Dhima et al. 2014. CAVE: Tooth & implant-borne [25]	J Prosthet Dent	Retrospective	59	226	226/59	5 years		Ceramic single crown				95%		
Dukic et al. 2010 [26]	Oper Dent	Prospective study	51	71	71/51	3 years	0	Ind. comp	35 Ormocer, Admira, 36 Grandio	Grandio with Voco Bifix QM	0	100	No significance Ormocer/Grandio	Modified USHPS
Azevedo et al. 2012 [21]	Braz Dent J	Prospective study	25	42	42/25	1 year	0	23 etched, non-etched, 19 etched (Filtek Supreme XT; 3M ESPE)	stone dies by the incremental technique using a LED device with power density of 1000 mW/cm^2	Etched group (ETR)—selective enamel phosphoric-acid etching + RelyX Unicem clicker; 2. Non-etched group (NER)—RelyX Unicem	0	100		More than 99% of the scores were considered clinically excellent (Alpha 1) or good (Alpha 2). Only 3 scores (0.9%) were classified as clinically sufficient (Bravo): 2 from ETR group (MS = 1, Figure 3; SE = 1) and 1 from NER group

Table 3. *Cont.*

Author/ Publication Year	Journal	Study Type	Patients (N)	Restoration (n)	Ratio (n/N)	Follow-Up	Drop-Out	Material	Manufacturing Technique	Luting Agent	Failure	Survival	Success	Outcome
Fasbinder et al. 2010 [28]	J Am Dent Assoc	Prospective study	43	62	62/43	2 years	1.6%	lithium disilicate (IPS e.max CAD, Ivoclar Vivadent, Amherst, N.Y.) all-ceramic crowns.	chairside computer-aided design/computer-aided manufacturing (CAD/CAM) system (CEREC 3, Sirona Dental Systems, Charlotte, N.C.) e.max CAD Crystall./Glaze paste (Ivoclar Vivadent) with shade tints	Multilink Automix, Ivoclar Vivadent OR: experimental self-adhesive, dual-curing cement (EC) developed by Ivoclar Vivadent.	0	100		Modified USPHS
Frankenberger et al. 2008 [29]	J Adhes Dent	Controlled clinical trial	34	96	96/34	12 years	40%	Leucite-reinforced glass ceramic IPS Empress	according to the manufacturer's instructions	4 cements: Dual Cement (n = 9), Variolink Low (n = 32), Variolink Ultra (n = 6) and Tetric (n = 49) (all Ivoclar Vivadent).	16% (15/96) without dropout	58 86%		luted with dual-cured resin composites revealed significantly fewer bulk fractures Surface roughness (loss of gloss), color match (improving with time), marginal integrity (distinct deterioration with marginal fractures in two cases with charlie scores after 12 years), tooth integrity (enamel cracks, one case rated Delta), inlay integrity (continuous deterioration over time, predominantly chipping of the ceramic, two charlie and two delta scores) and hypersensitivity

Table 3. *Cont.*

Author/ Publication Year	Journal	Study Type	Patients (N)	Restoration (n)	Ratio (n/N)	Follow-Up	Drop-Out	Material	Manufacturing Technique	Luting Agent	Failure	Survival	Success	Outcome
Frankenberger et al. 2009 [30]	Dent Mater	RCT	39	98	98/39	4 years	3%	Cergogold glass ceramic inlays	One dental ceramist produced all inlays according to the manufacturer's instructions and recommendations within 2 weeks after impression taking.	Multibond and Definite Ormocer resin composite Definite Multibond/Definite (n = 45) Syntac/Variolink Ultra (n = 53)	21 restorations had to be replaced due to inlay fracture (n = 11), tooth fracture (n = 4), hypersensitivities (n = 3) or marginal gap formation (n = 3).	77 survival rate 89.9%,	significantly changed over time: color match, marginal integrity, tooth integrity, inlay integrity, sensitivity, hypersensitivity and X-ray control Color match was inferior for Variolink, but only at the 2-year recall (Mann–Whitney U-test, p < 0.05), marginal integrity was inferior for Variolink, but only at the 0.5 and 1-year recall (Mann–Whitney U-test, p < 0.05) and proximal contacts were inferior in the definite group, but only at baseline	criteria marginal integrity, tooth integrity and inlay integrity
Gehrt et al. 2013 [31]	Clin Oral invest	prospective study	41	104	104/41	9 years	4 patients, 10 crowns	lithium-disilicate crowns	frameworks were laminated by a prototype of a veneering material combined with an experimental glaze. lost-wax technique	adhesively luted (69.2%) or inserted with glass–ionomer cement (30.8%). adhesively luted (IPS Ceramic etchant/Monobond S/dual-cured Variolink II, Ivoclar Vivadent) and 32 (30.8%) crowns were inserted with glass–ionomer cement (Vivaglass, Ivoclar Vivadent)	4 (4.3%)	97.4% after 5 years and 94.8% after 8 years	There were five rated technical complications (5.3%). Three crowns (3.3%) suffered from minor chipping of the veneering material. Major chippings did not occur. There were four biologic complications (4.3%). Two anterior crowns (2.1%) had to be treated endodontically 94.7 months after insertion.	Biologic complications such as loss of vitality joined by declined endodontic condition, endodontic disease and occurrence of caries & Technical complications such as loss of retention, minor chipping

Table 3. *Cont.*

Author/ Publication Year	Journal	Study Type	Patients (N)	Restoration (n)	Ratio (n/N)	Follow-Up	Drop-Out	Material	Manufacturing Technique	Luting Agent	Failure	Survival	Success	Outcome
Guess et al. 2014 [32]	Int J Prosthodont	Prospective Study	25	80	80/25	7 years	42 restorations	40 lithium disilicate pressed PCRs (IPS e.max-Press, Ivoclar Vivadent) and 40 leucite-reinforced glass–ceramic CAD/CAM PCRs (ProCAD, Ivoclar Vivadent).	computer-aided design/computer-assisted manufacture (CAD/CAM) ProCAD, Ivoclar Vivadent; Cerec 3 InLab, Sirona	hybrid composite resin material (Tetric/Syntac Classic, Ivoclar Vivadent)	1 restoration	100% for pressed PCRs and 97% for CAD/CAM PCR	No secondary caries, endodontic complications or postoperative complaints were ob- served. Minimal cohesive ceramic fractures (Figure 2a,b) were noted in 5 patients, but all affected restorations remained in situ 0.84 (CI: 0.70–0.98) for the pressed PCRs and 0.58 for the CAD/CAM PCRs (CI: 0.38–0.78).	modified United States Public Health Service (USPHS)
Murgueitio et al. 2012 [37]	J Prosthodont	Prospective study	99	210	210/99	3 years	?	leucite-reinforced IPS Empress Onlays and Partial Veneer Crowns	the manufacturer's instructions using the vacuum injection mold technique for leucite-reinforced ceramic material (IPS Empress).	Variolink II, Ivoclar Vivadent	The mode of failure was classified and evaluated as (1) adhesive, (2) cohesive, (3) combined failure, (4) decementation, (5) tooth sensitivity and (6) pulpal necrosis 33%	96.66%	Increased material thickness produced less probability of failures. Vital teeth were less likely to fail than nonvital teeth. Second molars were five times more susceptible to failure than first molars. Tooth sensitivity postcementation and the type of opposing dentition were not statistically significant in this study.	USPHS

Table 3. *Cont.*

Author/ Publication Year	Journal	Study Type	Patients (N)	Restoration (n)	Ratio (n/N)	Follow- Up	Drop- Out	Material	Manufacturing Technique	Luting Agent	Failure	Survival	Success	Outcome
Esuivel-Ipshaw et al. 2012 [27]	J Prosthodont	RCT	32	37	37/32	3 years	1 restoration	(1) metal-ceramic crown (MC) made from a Pd-Au-Ag-Sn-In alloy (Argedent 62) and a glass-ceramic veneer (IPS d.SIGN veneer); (2) non-veneered (glazed) lithium disilicate glass-ceramic crown (LDC) (IPS e.max Press core and e.max Ceram Glaze); and (3) veneered lithia disilicate glass-ceramic crown (LDC/V) with glass-ceramic veneer (IPS Empress 2 core and IPS Eris).		Variolink II, Ivoclar Vivadent	0?	100?	Statistically significant differences in surface texture ($p = 0.0013$) and crown wear ($p = 0.0078$) were found at year 3 between the metal-ceramic crowns and the lithium-disilicate-based crowns.	tissue health, marginal integrity, secondary caries, proximal contact, anatomic contour, occlusion, surface texture, cracks/chips (fractures), color match, tooth sensitivity and wear (of crowns and opposing enamel). Numeric rankings ranged from 1 to 4, with 4 being excellent and 1 indicating a need for immediate replacement. between years 2 and 3, gradual roughening of the occlusal surface occurred in some of the ceramic-ceramic crowns, possibly caused by dissolution and wear of the glaze.
Manhart et al. 2010 [35]	Quintessence Int	RCT	89	155	155/89	3 years	Artglass inlays (35%) and Charisma inlays (21%)	Resin composite	The inlays were postcured in a light oven (Uni-XS, Heraeus Kulzer)	adhesive system Solid Bond (Heraeus Kulzer)	five Artglass and 10 Charisma inlays failed mainly because of postoperative symptoms, bulk fracture and loss of marginal integrity	5 Artglass and ten Charisma inlays had to be (3 years)	Small Charisma inlays exhibited a statistically significant better performance for the "integrity of the restoration" parameter ($p = 0.022$).	Modified USPHS
Rauch et al. 2018 [39]	Clin Oral invest	Prospective	34	41	41/34	10 years	15 restorations	monolithic lithium disilicate crowns	chairside CAD/CAM technique.	Multilink Sprint, Ivoclar Vivadent	5 five failures occurred due to one crown fracture, an abutment fracture, one endodontic problem, a root fracture and a replacement of one crown caused by a carious	24/29	Due to the small amount of technical complications and failures, the clinical performance of monolithic lithium disilicate crowns was completely satisfying.	Modified USHPS

Table 3. *Cont.*

Author/ Publication Year	Journal	Study Type	Patients (N)	Restoration (n)	Ratio (n/N)	Follow- Up	Drop- Out	Material	Manufacturing Technique	Luting Agent	Failure	Survival	Success	Outcome
Reich et al. 2013 [40]	Clin Oral invest	Prospective clinical trial	34	41	41/34	4 years	12 restoration	lithium disilicate crowns	chairside CAD/CAM technique (Cerec)	Multilink Sprint (Ivoclar-Vivadent)	1 failure 96.3% after 4 years according to Kaplan–Meier	28	The complication-free rate comprising all events after 4 years was 83%, whereas the rate dropped down to 71% after 4.3 years	Modified USHPS
Santos et al. 2016 [41]	Clin Oral invest	Prospective clinical trial	35	86	86/35	5 year	17.91% restoration	sintered Duceram (Dentsply Degussa) and pressable IPS Empress (Ivoclar Vivadent).	poured with dental stone type IV (Durone, Dentsply).	Variolink II, Ivoclar Vivadent	8 failures Four IPS restorations were fractured, two restorations presented secondary caries (one from IPS and one from Duceram) and two restorations showed unacceptable defects at the restoration margin and needed replacement (one restoration from each ceramic system).	56	87% significant differences in relation to marginal discoloration, marginal integrity and surface texture between the baseline and five-year recall for both systems	Modified USHPS
Schenke et al. 2012 [42]	Clin Oral invest	RCT	29	58	58/29	2 years	0	ceramic blocks (Vita 3D Master CEREC Mark II, CAD/CAM designed and machined with the CEREC III system (Sirona CEREC III Software Version 3.0 (600/800), Sirona, Bensheim, Germany)	an indirect method on a die cast	RelyX Unicem with/without enamel etching	4 failures	54	Statistically significant changes were observed for marginal adaptation (MA) and marginal discoloration (MD) between BL and 2 years, but not between the two groups (RXU, RXU+E). Percentage of alfa values at BL for MA (RXU, 97% and RXU+E, 100%) and for MD (RXU, 97% and RXU+E, 97%) decreased to RXU, 14% and RXU+E, 28% for MA and to RXU, 50% and RXU+E, 59% for MD after 24 months.	Modified USHPS

Table 3. *Cont.*

Author/ Publication Year	Journal	Study Type	Patients (N)	Restoration (n)	Ratio (n/N)	Follow-Up	Drop-Out	Material	Manufacturing Technique	Luting Agent	Failure	Survival	Success	Outcome
Taschner et al. 2012 [45]	Dent Mater	Prospective controlled clinical study	30	83	83/30	2 years	0	IPS-Empress	at a commercial dental laboratory according to manufacturer's instructions	Group 1: 43 inlays/onlays were luted with RX; group 2: 40 inlays/onlays were luted with Syntac/Variolink II low viscosity (SV, Ivoclar Vivadent).	1	82/83 restorations	Indirect restorations luted with RX showed lower tooth and marginal integrity compared to the multistep approach.	Surface roughness, Color match, Anatomic form, Marginal integrity, Integrity tooth, Integrity inlay, Proximal contact, Changes in sensitivity, Radiographic check, Subjective satisfaction
Taskonak et al. 2006 [46]	Dent Mater	Prospective clinical trial	15	40	40/15	2 years		lithia-disilicate-based all-ceramic (Empress II) FDP/Crowns (20 FDPs/ 20 crowns)			10 (50%) catastrophic failures of FPDs occurred			marginal adaptation, color match, secondary caries and visible fractures in the restorations
Krejci et al. 1992 [34]	Quintessence Int	Prospective clinical trial	10	10	1	1.5 years	0	IPS/Empress Inlays	According to manufacturer's instruction	Dual curing composite, Dual cement, Vivadent, Inc.	0	100	1 hypersensitivity, Discoloration at the marginal	Modified USHPS
Azevdo et al. 2012 [21]	Braz Dent J	Prospective clinical trial	25	42	42/25	1 year	0	Indirect resin composite	The composite resin restorations were built over plaster casts using the incremental technique with a LED device for light-curing the increments	1. Etched group (ETR)—selective enamel phosphoric-acid etching + RelyX Unicem clicker; 2. Non-etched group (NER)—RelyX Unicem RelyX	0	100	More than 99% of the scores were considered clinically excellent (Alpha 1) or good (Alpha 2) (Figure 2). Only 3 scores (0.9%) were classified as clinically sufficient (Bravo): 2 from ETR group (MS = 1, Figure 3; SE = 1) and 1 from NER group (SE).	Modified USHPS

3.5. Survival Ratios

As for the survival ratios it could be observed that at the time frame up to 24 m the estimated survival is 99%, while after at least 36 m it dropped to 95%. Forest and funnel plots ≤24 m revealed homogeneous results (heterogeneity $I^2 = 47\%$, $p = 1.00$) and low suspicion for a publication bias, while forest and funnel plots ≥36 m demonstrated heterogeneous results (heterogeneity $I^2 = 93\%$, $p < 0.01$) and a slight suspicion of a publication bias (Figures 3–7).

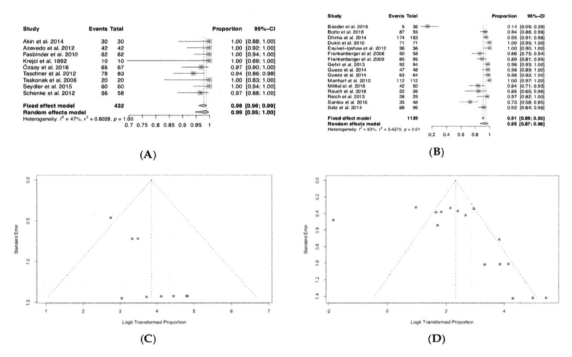

Figure 3. Survival ratios of all included specimens. (**A**) Forest plot ≤24 months; (**B**) forest plot ≥36 months; (**C**) funnel plot ≤24 months; (**D**) funnel plot ≥36 months.

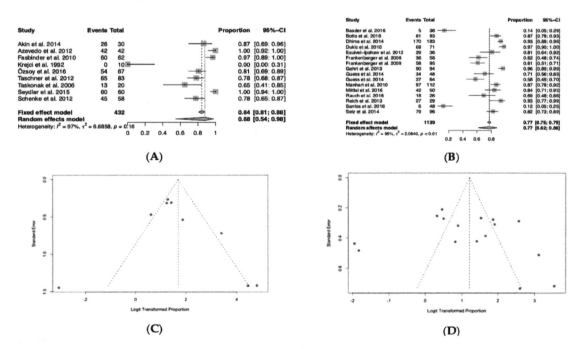

Figure 4. Success ratios of all biologic, technical and esthetical aspects. (**A**) Forest plot ≤24 months; (**B**) forest plot ≥36 months; (**C**) funnel plot ≤24 months; (**D**) funnel plot ≥36 months.

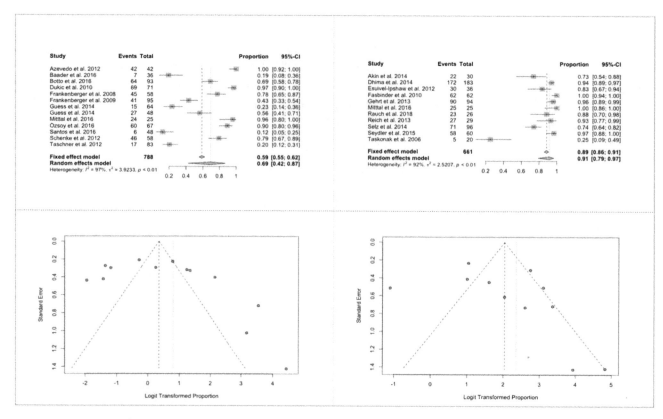

Figure 5. Success ratios of all biologic aspects. (**A**) Forest plot for partial and (**B**) full crowns; (**C**) funnel plot for partial and (**D**) full crowns.

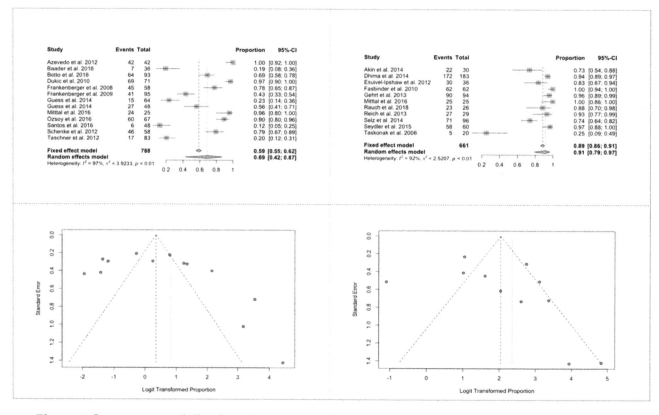

Figure 6. Success ratios of all technical aspects. (**A**) Forest plot for partial and (**B**) full crowns; (**C**) funnel plot for partial and (**D**) full crowns.

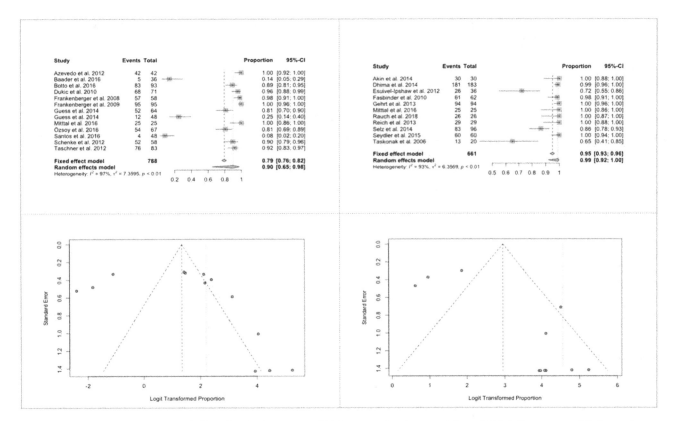

Figure 7. Success ratios of all esthetical aspects. (**A**) Forest plot for partial and (**B**) full crowns; (**C**) funnel plot for partial and (**D**) full crowns.

3.6. Success Ratios of All Biologic, Technical and Esthetical Aspects

The estimated success ratio at ≤24 m was 88% (95% COI: 0.54–0.98), while after at least 36 m it dropped to 77% (95% COI: 0.62–0.88). Forest plot ≤24 m revealed not strongly homogeneous results (heterogeneity $I^2 = 97\%$, $p = 0.16$). However, heterogeneity is not statistically significant. Funnel plot ≤24 m showed very small and extremely large values. Forest plot ≥36 m demonstrated highly heterogeneous results ($I^2 = 95\%$, $p < 0.01$). The plot illustrates the studies with the remarkably noticeable results. The wide range and heterogeneity of included material types (composites, feldspathic ceramic, leucite reinforced glass ceramic, veneered and non-veneered lithium disilicate, veneered and monolithic zirconia and alumina), processing techniques and luting agents did not allow any further statistical analysis as regards to an analysis for the material type only.

3.7. Success Ratios of All Biologic Criteria

The estimated success ratio at ≤24 m was 88% (95% COI: 0.58–0.97), while after at least 36 m it dropped to 75% (95% COI: 0.56–0.88). Results of the forest Plot <24 m presented very heterogeneous results ($I^2 = 96\%$, $p < 0.01$). The funnel Plot <24 m showed, apart from the before mentioned two studies the distribution of published results, a slight skew in favor of high success rates, indicating a possible publication bias.

For forest plot >36 m (I^2 of 97%, $p < 0.01$) these study results were also very heterogeneous, and a large dispersion could be observed. In general, the results of the funnel Plot >36 m presented great variability among the published studies.

3.8. Success Ratios of All Technical Criteria

After 2 years the estimated success ratio was 90% (95% COI: 0.74–0.97), while after 3 years it dropped to 74% (95% COI: 0.50–0.89). Forest plot <24 m presented (I^2 of 93%, $p < 0.01$) heterogenous results and after 3 years (I^2 of 97%, $p < 0.01$). The funnel plot after 2 years showed a tendency towards overproportioned high success rates studies.

3.9. Success Ratios of All Esthetical Criteria

The success ratios are very high at 24 m 96% (95% COI: 0.87–0.99) and dropped very slightly after 36 m 95% (95% COI: 0.78–0.99). Forest plot <24 m presented (I^2 of 86%, $p = 0.08$) statistically insignificant heterogenous results and after 3 years (I^2 of 97%, $p < 0.01$) heterogenous results, because of 3 studies showing only 8%–25% success rates, while all other included studies presented ≥72%. Funnel plot did not show any bias during the first 2 years, while the 3 mentioned studies presented very low success rates, many others shower too high success rates. The overall results did not show any bias.

The biologic success rates of full crowns were much higher than those of partial crowns. Forest plot of partial (I^2 of 97%, $p < 0.01$) and full (I^2 of 92%, $p < 0.01$) crowns showed very heterogeneous studies, while funnel plots exhibited a possibility of publication bias for partial and low possibility of bias for full crowns, even though there was a slight hint of too high success rates.

The technical success rates of full crowns were much higher and significantly different ($p < 0.05$) compared to partial crowns. Forest plot showed heterogeneous results for partial crowns (I^2 of 98%, $p < 0.01$) and homogeneous results for full crowns (I^2 of 66%, $p = 0.63$). Funnel plot for partial crowns showed a rather unlikely publication bias, the variation is very high, for full crowns the results were all in the expected range, with an asymmetric distribution. Higher success rates were often demonstrated as statistically expected. A publication bias seems to be possible.

The esthetical success of partial crowns was also higher compared to full crowns, but not as high as it was for biologic and technical success rates. Forest plot of partial crowns (I^2 of 97%, $p < 0.01$) revealed heterogeneous results with three studies showing low success rates, the funnel plot exhibited at both sides a high prevalence of studies in the upper and lower end of the graph with more studies presenting high results. The forest plot of full crowns (I^2 of 93%, $p < 0.01$) showed also heterogeneous results, because of the two studies Esquivel-Ipshaw et al. and Taskonak et al. reporting low results. The funnel plot showed many results with high success rates and three with low results. Because of the sample size it was not possible to conclude if a bias was possible or not.

4. Discussion

This systematic review including meta-analysis was conducted to evaluate the clinical short- and long-term survival rates and biologic, technical and esthetical success ratios of partial and full crowns using hybrid polymer and ceramic CAD/CAM materials.

Some data were reported on CAD/CAM processing methods regarding survival and clinical survival rates. However, to best of author's knowledge, no similar systematic review based on hybrid polymer and ceramic materials on survival and complications rates has been published yet. Since these materials have been developed recently, their indications and clinical applicability are still being studied. In the present review, the existence of a great variety and heterogeneity of hybrid polymer and ceramic materials and their indications has been observed.

The meta-analysis of this study was performed for mean long-term survival rates and for biologic, technical and esthetic complication ratios for partial vs. full crown reconstructions at two different follow-up periods. Due to the variety of the CAD/CAM materials, their differing compositions and the lack of homogeneity, the variable "material" could not be included in the meta-analysis. This finding was also observed in the systematic review by Alves de Carvalho et al. [47]. investigating clinical survival rates in single restorations using CAD/CAM technologies with a minimum follow-up of three years, describing a great variety of studies analyzing different materials. Their results are in agreement with the present systematic review related to the heterogeneity caused by the variety of the materials assessed [47]. The review of Rodrigues et al. included studies on CAD/CAM materials for single crown, multiple- unit or partial ceramic crown with a 24 to 84-month follow-up based on the longevity and failures rates, suggesting that the longevity of CAD/CAM restorations is lower compared to the conventionally fabricated restorations [48], as they presented a 1.84 higher failure rate during a follow-up period of 24 to 84 months. However, the results of the present systematic review showed that when partial and full crown reconstructions made of hybrid polymer and ceramic CAD/CAM materials were analyzed, the overall survival rate was 99% (0.95–1.00) up to 24 months and dropped to 95% (0.87–0.98) at ≥36 months.

These results were assessed based on the restoration type, given higher success rates for the overall clinical performance in full crown reconstructions compared to partial crowns. Similar data were found for survival rates of full crowns, estimated 5-year survival rate for leucite or lithium-disilicate reinforced glass ceramic (96.6%) and sintered alumina and zirconia (96%) were similar [16]. For partial restorations, our results are also in agreement with the literature, Sampaio FBWR et al. found estimated survival rates for CAD/CAM of 97% after five years [49].

Current trends for material selection in tooth-supported single restorations showed that, both clinicians and patients are favoring esthetic and nonmetallic restorations. However, for full crowns, literature is still supporting the porcelain-fused-to-metal crowns as the gold standard, with results of 5-year survival rates exceeding 95% [16,50]. Furthermore, in terms of longevity, the literature showed that full and partial CAD/CAM ceramic crowns have lower long-term survival compared to the ones produced through conventional techniques [48]. Analyzing the results of other studies of full ceramic crowns, the literature provided data on leucite or disilicate reinforced ceramics survival rates of 96.6% and 95%, respectively [16], these results are comparable to those found in this review.

The other large CAD/CAM processed material group was zirconia, showing a 5-year survival of 91.2% (82.8–95.6%) [16]. Digital developments, new materials and advanced processing techniques enabled the minimal invasive approach in dentistry throughout partial restorations. Partial crowns have been widely used for years, as composite resins were a less predictable treatment option for direct restorations. Among other factors, the longevity of partial restorations depended on the restorative material, the patient and the experience of the clinician. Previous reviews show survival rates of 92% and 95% at five years and 91% at 10 years, (Morimoto et al.) or in a more recent study the survival rate data for inlays was 90.89% and 93.50% in a follow-up period of one to five years [51].

Gold alloys have served as gold standard for partial crowns for years [52]. However, the increasing price of gold and the high esthetic demands of patients have caused advancement of materials such as hybrid polymer and ceramic CAD/CAM materials. The current evidence of gold restorations is limited, suggesting a survival rate of 95.4% observed in a retrospective, clinical study studying 1314 gold restorations; whereas inlays had a failure rate of 4.7% after more than 20 years [53]. Another study evaluated 391 posterior gold inlays during a mean follow-up period of 11.6 years and observed 82.9% of success rate and a 6.4% failure rate [52].

The development, evolution and improvement of composite resins, high strength ceramics and adhesive techniques have allowed the development of hybrid materials to compensate the deficiencies and limitations of gold alloys. In this regard, a systematic review evaluating 5811 restorations showed a survival rate of feldspathic porcelain and glass–ceramics for five-year follow-up of 95% and at the 10-year follow-up of 2154 restorations, a survival rate of was 91% [54].

In addition to ceramics and gold alloys composite resin materials have been increasingly used due to improvements in the composition and thereby related mechanical properties. Previous reviews on resins were inconclusive whether longevity and survival rates of resins are higher compared to ceramics [55]. However, a recent review on CAD/CAM materials for full and partial crowns that included resin-matrix ceramic showed an estimated survival rate after five years of 82.5% [47,49].

Survival rates are a reliable indicator to assess clinical performance. However, after placement and during exposure to the oral cavity restorations can present complications compromising their longevity, survival and clinical success. The clinical performance based on the overall success ratio of biologic, technical and esthetical aspects was 88% (0.54–0.98; ≤24 m) vs. 77% (0.62–0.88; ≥36 m) for the different follow-up periods. The meta-analysis could not find any significance regarding both follow-up time (≤24 m or ≥36 m) and their biologic, technical and esthetical (88% vs. 77%; 90% vs. 74%; 96% vs. 95%) outcome. However, it presented a significant difference in the technical clinical performance between full 93% (0.88–0.96) and partial 64% (0.34–0.86) crowns, in favor of full crown reconstructions ($p < 0.05$). Biologic and esthetical success rates of full crowns (91% (0.79–0.97) vs. 99% (0.92–1.00)) were comparable to those of partial crowns (69% (0.42–0.87) vs. 90% (0.65–0.98)). This meta-analysis suggests that in case of possible technical failure a full crown reconstruction should be preferred compared to a partial crown.

Restoration failures are considered as such when they need repair or replacement, the general assessment of these failures can also be considered in terms of success rates. The success rates, assessed by biologic, technical and esthetical aspects showed a decrease in success from 24 to 36 months. Compared to previous reviews the present data were higher compared to ceramic, zirconia and CAD/CAM single crown reconstructions reported in previous studies [16,48,56].

This study assessed the failures as either biologic, technical and esthetic complications, although during the analysis of the included studies, the lack of homogeneity of the results did not allow for its specific analysis resulting in an overall complications analysis. Considering tooth-supported restorations complications, the success ratio of biologic complications decreased in case of caries occurrence, loss of pulp vitality, endodontic treatment, tooth fracture and hypersensitivity. The present study showed a biologic success rate of 88% at the follow-up period ≤24 m and 75% at ≥36 m. The most frequent biologic complication reported in the literature was caries and loss of pulp vitality. Comparing full and partial restorations higher biologic complications rates (21% more) were observed in partial reconstructions. Considering the characteristics of partial restorations, in terms of indications and dental preparation, full crowns could hide biologic complications. Therefore, caries can be diagnosed more easily in partial crowns compared to full crowns and could explain the results obtained in this study. The biologic complications for full crowns were lower in metal-ceramic restorations than in full ceramic reconstructions [16,57].

Technical complications include ceramic fracture, cracks, core failure, chipping, problems with microleakage and the loss of retention. Ceramic chipping has been described as the most common technical complication, finding similar ranges for metal ceramics and fully ceramic crowns with no statistic differences between materials. However, the overall technical complication rates in the present study were higher compared to conventional and other CAD/CAM materials [16,57].

Missing clinical workflows and lacking experience with these newly developed materials could have an influence in the complications derived from bonding techniques and microleakage, factors such as polymerization of resin cement, degradation of adhesive, enzymatic degradation of bonding of these materials composition could explain the higher failure rates compared to conventional groups or metal-ceramic restorations regarding biologic and technical complication rates [51].

The technical complications in partial restorations are increasing during the follow-up assessment and between groups showing less complications for full coverage restorations. Considering the design and the manufacturing process, the complications could have been due to defects of the thickness and the roughness of the final preparations milled by CAD/CAM chairside units. Some partial crowns are designed and milled using chairside devices, lacking a verification of material thickness throughout the technician. Technical complications may also result in esthetical problems, such as discoloration or wear of glace. The results of the review for esthetic were higher at 36 months and however lower compared to the other studies. Considering the posterior localization of the restorations, it is possible that the results are due to the fact that materials are biomimetic, and patients do notice esthetical failures less than in the anterior sites.

Given these data, the results for the CAD/CAM crowns of hybrid polymer and ceramics are comparable regarding the 5-year success rates performance with other materials.

A tendency for lower failure rate for glass-matrix ceramics and polycrystalline ceramics compared to leucite and feldspathic ceramic could be observed. The high survival rate of glass-matrix ceramics—followed by resin-matrix ceramics and polycrystalline ceramics—should, however, be considered with caution due to shorter follow-up periods of the latter materials.

Dual curing agents are preferred for ceramic and resin-matrix ceramic inlays in order to compensate for the light transmission throughout the restoration and to allow complete polymerization even at the bottom of the cavity, where the access of LED curing light is limited [58]. Despite the wide diversity of included materials, most studies used chemically polymerized or LED polymerized dual curing agents. In studies where chemical and dual curing cements were compared, the dual curing systems achieved better results and presented lower failure rates compared to only chemical luting agents.

According to the findings of this systematic review, a great heterogeneity of the methodological data between studies with lack of properly comparisons (control and study groups), no homogeneous restoration material type groups and a short follow-up examination was observed. More homogeneous studies with the more comparable materials, manufacturing techniques and CAD/CAM software system with a control groups in a split-mouth randomized controlled study design should be conducted.

The density of published high survival rates is statistically slightly conspicuously high. In the lower section, there is the study by Baader et al. 2016, which stands out regarding the low survival ratios. However, further small studies, which published a low outcome are lacking.

5. Conclusions

Summary for success rates and different follow-up times including all biologic, technical and esthetical parameters could be listed as follows:

- All success rates decreased after 36 or more months compared to 24 months;
- The esthetic success rates were greatest, followed by the almost identical rate of technical and biologic success rates;
- There were no significant differences at the 95% level between the two follow-up times nor between the biologic, technical and esthetic aspects;
- Both the biologic, technical and esthetic success rates were higher for full crowns than for partial crowns;
- The technical success rate of full crowns was statistically significantly higher than that of partial crowns;
- The esthetic success rates are greater than the biologic or technical ones, but neither for the full crowns nor for the partial crowns these comparisons were of significance.

Author Contributions: Conceptualization, N.A.-H.H., M.Ö. and T.J.; methodology, N.A.-H.H., M.Ö. and T.J.; software, N.A.-H.H., M.Ö., P.M.-M. and T.J.; validation, N.A.-H.H., M.Ö., P.M.-M. and T.J.; formal analysis, N.A.-H.H., M.Ö., P.M.-M. and T.J.; investigation, N.A.-H.H., M.Ö. and T.J.; resources, N.A.-H.H., M.Ö. and T.J.; data curation, N.A.-H.H., M.Ö. and T.J.; writing—original draft preparation, N.A.-H.H., M.Ö., P.M.-M. and T.J.; writing—review and editing, N.A.-H.H., M.Ö., P.M.-M. and T.J.; visualization, N.A.-H.H., M.Ö., P.M.-M. and T.J.; supervision, N.A.-H.H., M.Ö., P.M.-M. and T.J.; project administration, N.A.-H.H., M.Ö., P.M.-M. and T.J.; funding acquisition, none. All authors have read and agreed to the published version of the manuscript.

References

1. Ruse, N.D.; Sadoun, M.J. Resin-composite blocks for dental CAD/CAM applications. *J. Dent. Res.* **2014**, *93*, 1232–1234. [CrossRef] [PubMed]
2. Mainjot, A.K.; Dupont, N.M.; Oudkerk, J.C.; Dewael, T.Y.; Sadoun, M.J. From artisanal to CAD-CAM blocks: State of the art of indirect composites. *J. Dent. Res.* **2016**, *95*, 487–495. [CrossRef] [PubMed]
3. Spitznagel, F.A.; Boldt, J.; Gierthmuehlen, P.C. CAD/CAM Ceramic Restorative Materials for Natural Teeth. *J. Dent. Res.* **2018**, *97*, 1082–1091. [CrossRef] [PubMed]

4.   Abt, E.; Carr, A.B.; Worthington, H.V. Interventions for replacing missing teeth: Partially absent dentition. *Cochrane Database Syst. Rev.* **2012**, *15*, CD003814. [CrossRef]

5.   Schneider, C.; Zemp, E.; Zitzmann, N.U. Oral health improvements in Switzerland over 20 years. *Eur. J. Oral Sci.* **2017**, *125*, 55–62. [CrossRef]

6.   Joda, T.; Brägger, U. Digital vs. conventional implant prosthetic work-flows: A cost/time analysis. *Clin. Oral Implants Res.* **2015**, *26*, 1430–1435. [CrossRef]

7.   Berrendero, S.; Salido, M.P.; Ferreiroa, A.; Valverde, A.; Pradíes, G. Comparative study of all-ceramic crowns obtained from conventional and digital impressions: Clinical findings. *Clin. Oral Investig.* **2019**, *23*, 1745–1751. [CrossRef]

8.   Tsirogiannis, P.; Reissmann, D.R.; Heydecke, G. Evaluation of the marginal fit of single-unit, complete-coverage ceramic restorations fabricated after digital and conventional impressions: A systematic review and meta-analysis. *J. Prosthet. Dent.* **2016**, *116*, 328–335. [CrossRef]

9.   Coldea, A.; Swain, M.V.; Thiel, N. Mechanical properties of polymer- infiltrated ceramic-network materials. *Dent. Mater.* **2013**, *29*, 419–426. [CrossRef]

10. Mörmann, W.H.; Stawarczyk, B.; Ender, A.; Sener, B.; Attin, T.; Mehl, A. Wear characteristics of current aesthetic dental restorative CAD/CAM materials: Two-body wear, gloss retention, roughness and martens hardness. *J. Mech. Behav. Biomed. Mater.* **2013**, *20*, 113–125. [CrossRef]

11. Gracis, S.; Thompson, V.P.; Ferencz, J.L.; Silva, N.R.; Bonfante, E.A. A new classification system for all-ceramic and ceramic-like restorative materials. *Int. J. Prosthodont.* **2015**, *28*, 227–235. [CrossRef] [PubMed]

12. Belli, R.; Petschelt, A.; Hofner, B.; Hajtó, J.; Scherrer, S.S.; Lohbauer, U. Fracture rates and lifetime Estimations of CAD/CAM All-ceramic Restorations. *J. Dent. Res.* **2016**, *95*, 67–73. [CrossRef] [PubMed]

13. Homsy, F.R.; Özcan, M.; Khoury, M.; Majzoub, Z.A.K. Comparison of fit accuracy of pressed lithium disilicate inlays fabricated from wax or resin patterns with conventional and CAD-CAM technologies. *J. Prosthet. Dent.* **2018**, *120*, 530–536. [CrossRef] [PubMed]

14. Aslan, Y.U.; Coskun, E.; Ozkan, Y.; Dard, M. Clinical evaluation of three types of CAD/CAM inlay/onlay materials after 1-Year clinical follow up. *Eur. J. Prosthodont. Restor. Dent.* **2019**, *27*, 131–140.

15. Zarone, F.; Russo, S.; Sorrentino, R. From porcelain-fused-to-metal to zirconia: Clinical and experimental considerations. *Dent. Mater.* **2011**, *27*, 83–96. [CrossRef]

16. Sailer, I.; Makarov, N.A.; Thoma, D.S.; Zwahlen, M.; Pjetursson, B.E. All-ceramic or metal-ceramic tooth-supported fixed dental prostheses (FDPs)? A systematic review of the survival and complication rates. Part I: Single crowns (SCs). *Dent. Mater.* **2015**, *31*, 603–623. [CrossRef]

17. Ryge, G.; Snyder, M. Evaluating the clinical quality of restorations. *J. Am. Dent. Assoc.* **1973**, *87*, 369–377. [CrossRef]

18. Hickel, R.; Peschke, A.; Tyas, M.; Mjör, I.; Bayne, S.; Peters, M.; Hiller, K.A.; Randall, R.; Vanherle, G.; Heintze, S.D. FDI World Dental Federation—Clinical criteria for the evaluation of direct and indirect restorations. Update and clinical examples. *J. Adhes. Dent.* **2010**, *12*, 259–272. [CrossRef]

19. R Foundation for Statistical Computing, Vienna, Austria. Available online: http://www.R-project.org (accessed on 27 June 2020).

20. Akin, A.; Toksavul, S.; Toman, M. Clinical Marginal and Internal Adaptation of Maxillary Anterior Single Ceramic Crowns and 2-year Randomized Controlled Clinical Trial. *J. Prosthodont.* **2015**, *24*, 345–350. [CrossRef]

21. Azevedo, C.G.S.; De Goes, M.F.; Ambrosano, G.M.B.; Chan, D.C.N. 1-year Clinical Study of Indirect Resin Composite REstorations Luted with a Self-Adhesive Resin Cement: Effect of Enamel Etching. *Braz. Dent. J.* **2012**, *23*, 97–103. [CrossRef]

22. Baader, K.; Hiller, K.A.; Buchalla, W.; Schmalz, G.; Federlin, M. Self-adhesive Luting of Partial Ceramic Crowns: Selective Enamel Etching Leads to Higher Survival after 6.5 Years in Vivo. *J. Adhes. Dent.* **2016**, *18*, 69–79. [PubMed]

23. Botto, E.B.; Baró, R.; Borgia Botto, J.L. Clinical performance of bonded ceramic inlays/onlays: A 5- to 18-year retrospective longitudinal study. *Am. J. Dent.* **2016**, *29*, 187–192.

24. D'all'Orologio, G.D.; Lorenzi, R. Restorations in abrasion/erosion cervical lesions: 8-year results of a triple blind randomized controlled trial. *Am. J. Dent.* **2014**, *27*, 245–250.

25. Dhima, M.; Paulusova, V.; Carr, A.B.; Rieck, K.L.; Lihse, C.; Salinas, T.J. Practice-based clinical evaluation of ceramic single crowns after at least five years. *J. Prosthet. Dent.* **2014**, *3*, 124–130. [CrossRef]

26. Dukic, W.; Dukic, O.L.; Milardovic, S.; Delija, B. Clinical evaluation of indirect composite restorations at baseline and months after placement. *Oper. Dent.* **2010**, *35*, 156–164. [CrossRef]

27. Esuivel-Opshaw, J.; Rose, W.; Oliveira, E.; Yang, M.; Clark, A.E.; Anusavice, K. Randomized, controlled clinical trial of bilayer ceramic and metal-ceramic crown performance. *J. Prosthodont.* **2012**, *22*, 166–173. [CrossRef]

28. Fasbinder, D.J.; Dennison, J.B.; Heys, D.; Neiva, G. A Clinical Evaluation of Chairside Lithium Disilicate CAD/CAM Crowns: A two-year report. *J. Am. Dent. Assoc.* **2010**, *141*, 10S–14S. [CrossRef]

29. Frankenberger, R.; Taschner, M.; Garcia-Godoy, F.; Petschelt, A.; Krämer, N. Leucite-reinforced glass ceramic inlays and onlays after 12 years. *J. Adhes. Dent.* **2008**, *10*, 393–398.

30. Frankenberger, R.; Reinelt, C.; Petschelt, A.; Krämer, N. Operator vs. material influence on clinical outcome of bonded ceramic inlays. *Dent. Mater.* **2009**, *25*, 960–968. [CrossRef]

31. Gehrt, M.; Wolfart, S.; Rafai, N.; Reich, S.; Edelhoff, D. Clinical results of lithium-disilicate crowns after up to 9 years of service. *Clin. Oral Investig.* **2013**, *17*, 275–284. [CrossRef]

32. Guess, P.C.; Selz, C.F.; Voulgarakis, A.; Stampf, S.; Stappert, C.F. Prospective clinical study of press-ceramic overlap and full veneer restorations: 7-year result. *Int. J. Prosthodont.* **2014**, *27*, 355–358. [CrossRef] [PubMed]

33. Guess, P.C.; Selz, C.F.; Steinhart, Y.N.; Stampf, S.; Strub, J.R. Prospective clinical split-mouth study of pressed and CAD/CAM all-ceramic partial-coverage restorations: 7-year results. *Int. J. Prosthodont.* **2013**, *26*, 21–26. [CrossRef] [PubMed]

34. Krejci, I.; Krejci, D.; Lutz, F. Clinical evaluation of a new pressed glass ceramic inlay material over 1.5 years. *Oper. Dent.* **1992**, *23*, 181–186.

35. Manhart, J.; Chen, H.Y.; Mehl, A.; Hickel, R. Clinical study of indirect composite resin inlays in posterior stress-bearing preparations placed by dental students: Results after 6 months and 1, 2, and 3 years. *Quintessence Int.* **2010**, *41*, 399–410.

36. Mittal, H.C.; Goyal, A.; Gauba, K.; Kapur, A. Clinical Performance of Indirect Composite Onlays as Esthetic Alternative to Stainless Steel Crowns for Rehabilitation of a Large Crarious Primary Molar. *J. Clin. Pediatr. Dent.* **2016**, *40*, 345–352. [CrossRef]

37. Murgueitio, R.; Bernal, G. Three-Year Clinical Follow-Up of Posterior Teeth Restored with Leucite-Reinforced IPS Empress ONlays and Partial Veneer Crowns. *J. Proshtodont.* **2012**, *21*, 340–345. [CrossRef]

38. Özsoy, A.; Kuşdemir, M.; Öztürk-Bozkurt, F.; Toz Akalın, T.; Özcan, M. Clinical performance of indirect composite onlays and overlays: 2-year follow up. *J. Adhes. Sci. Technol.* **2016**, *30*, 1808–1818.

39. Rauch, A.; Reich, S.; Dalchau, L.; Schierz, O. Clinical survival of chair-side generated monolithic lithium disilicate crowns: 10-year results. *Clin. Oral Investig.* **2018**, *22*, 1763–1769. [CrossRef]

40. Reich, S.; Schierz, O. Chair-side generated posterior lithium disilicate crowns after 4 years. *Clin. Oral Investig.* **2013**, *17*, 1765–1772. [CrossRef]

41. Santos, M.J.; Freitas, M.C.; Azeedo, L.M.; Santos, G.C., Jr.; Navarro, M.F.; Francisschone, C.E.; Mondelli, R.F. Clinical evaluation of ceramic inlays and onlays fabricated with two systems: 12-year follow-up. *Clin. Oral Investig.* **2016**, *20*, 1683–1690. [CrossRef]

42. Schenke, F.; Federlin, M.; Hiller, K.A.; Moder, D.; Schmalz, G. Controlled, prospective, randomized, clinical evaluation of partial ceramic crowns inserted with RelyX Unicem with or without selective enamel etching. Results after 2 years. *Clin. Oral Investig.* **2012**, *16*, 451–461. [CrossRef] [PubMed]

43. Selz, C.F.; Strub, J.R.; Cach, K.; Guess, P.C. Long-term performance of posterior InCeram Alumina crowns cemented with different luting agents: A prospective, randomized clinical split-mouth study over 5 years. *Clin. Oral Investig.* **2014**, *18*, 1695–1703. [CrossRef] [PubMed]

44. Seydler, B.; Schmitter, M. Clinical Performance of two different CAD/CAM-fabricated ceramic crowns: 2-Year results. *J. Prosthet. Dent.* **2015**, *114*, 212–216. [CrossRef] [PubMed]

45. Taschner, M.; Krämer, N.; Lohbauer, U.; Pelka, M.; Breschi, L.; Petschelt, A.; Frankenberger, R. Leucite-reinforced glass ceramic inlays luted with self-adhesive resin cement: A 2-year in vivo study. *Dent. Mater.* **2012**, *28*, 535–540. [CrossRef] [PubMed]

46. Taskonak, B.; Sertgöz, A. Two-year clinical evaluation of lithia-disilicate-based all-ceramic crowns and fixed partial dentures. *Dent. Mater.* **2006**, *22*, 1008–1113. [CrossRef]

47. Alves de Carvalho, I.F.; Santos Marques, T.M.; Araujo, F.M.; Azevedo, L.F.; Donato, H.; Correia, A. Clinical Performance of CAD/CAM Tooth-Supported Ceramic Restorations: A systematic Review. *Int. J. Periodontics. Restorative. Dent.* **2018**, *38*, e68–e78. [CrossRef]

48. Rodrigues, S.B.; Franken, P.; Celeste, R.K.; Leitune, V.C.B.; Collares, F.M. CAD/CAM or conventional ceramic materials restorations longevity: A systematic review and meta-analysis. *J. Prosthodont. Res.* **2019**, *63*, 389–395. [CrossRef]

49. Sampaio, F.B.W.R.; Özcan, M.; Gimenez, T.C.; Moreira, M.S.N.A.; Tedesco, T.K.; Morimoto, S. Effects of manufacturing methods on the survival rate of ceramic and indirect composite resotorations: A systematic review and meta-analysis. *J. Esthet. Restor. Dent.* **2019**, *31*, 561–571. [CrossRef]

50. Rekow, E.D.; Silva, N.R.; Coelho, P.G.; Zhang, Y.; Guess, P.; Thompson, V.P. Performance of dental ceramics: Challenges for improvement. *J. Dent. Res.* **2011**, *90*, 937–952. [CrossRef]

51. Vagropoulou, G.I.; Klifopoulou, G.L.; Vlahou, S.G.; Hirayama, H.; Michalakis, K. Complications and survival rates of inlays and onlays vs complete coverage restorations: A systematic review and analysis of studies. *J. Oral Rehabil.* **2018**, *5*, 903–920. [CrossRef]

52. Mulic, A.; Svendsen, G.; Kopperud, S.E. A retrospective clinical study on the longevity of posterior class II cast gold inlays/onlays. *J. Dent.* **2018**, *70*, 46–50. [CrossRef] [PubMed]

53. Donovan, T.; Simonsen, R.J.; Guertin, G.; Tucker, R.V. Retrospective clinical evaluation of 1314 cast gold restorations in service from 1 to 52 years. *J. Esthet. Restor. Dent.* **2014**, *16*, 194–204. [CrossRef] [PubMed]

54. Morimoto, S.; Rebello de Sampaio, F.B.; Braga, M.M.; Sesma, N.; Özcan, M. Survival Rate of Resin and Ceramic Inlays, Onlays and Overlays: A systematic Review and Meta-analysis. *J. Dent. Res.* **2016**, *95*, 985–994. [CrossRef] [PubMed]

55. Grivas, E.; Roudsari, R.V.; Satterthwaite, J.D. Composite inlays: A systematic review. *Eur. J. Prosthodont. Restor. Dent.* **2014**, *22*, 117–124.

56. Angeletaki, F.; Gkogkos, A.; Papazoglou, E.; Kloukos, D. Direct versus indirect inlay/onlay composite restorations in posterior teeth. A systematic review and meta-analysis. *J. Dent.* **2016**, *53*, 12–21. [CrossRef]

57. Poggio, C.E.; Ercoli, C.; Rispoli, L.; Maiorana, C.; Esposito, M. Metal-free materials for fixed prosthodontic restorations. *Cochrane Database Syst. Rev.* **2017**, *20*, 12CD009606. [CrossRef]

58. Hofmann, N.; Papsthart, G.; Hugo, B.; Klaiber, B. Comparison of photo-activation versus chemical or dual-curing of resin-based luting cements regarding flexural strength, modulus and surface hardness. *J. Oral Rehabil.* **2001**, *28*, 1022–1028. [CrossRef]

Recent Trends and Future Direction of Dental Research in the Digital Era

Tim Joda [1,*], Michael M. Bornstein [2], Ronald E. Jung [3], Marco Ferrari [4], Tuomas Waltimo [2] and Nicola U. Zitzmann [1]

[1] Department of Reconstructive Dentistry, University Center for Dental Medicine Basel, University of Basel, 4058 Basel, Switzerland; n.zitzmann@unibas.ch

[2] Department of Oral Health & Medicine, University Center for Dental Medicine Basel, University of Basel, 4058 Basel, Switzerland; michael.bornstein@unibas.ch (M.M.B.); tuomas.waltimo@unibas.ch (T.W.)

[3] Department of Reconstructive Dentistry, Center for Dental Medicine Basel, University of Zurich, 8032 Zurich, Switzerland; ronald.jung@zzm.uzh.ch

[4] Department of Prosthodontics & Dental Material, University School of Dental Medicine, University of Siena, 53100 Siena, Italy; ferrarm@gmail.com

* Correspondence: tim.joda@unibas.ch

Abstract: The digital transformation in dental medicine, based on electronic health data information, is recognized as one of the major game-changers of the 21st century to tackle present and upcoming challenges in dental and oral healthcare. This opinion letter focuses on the estimated top five trends and innovations of this new digital era, with potential to decisively influence the direction of dental research: (1) rapid prototyping (RP), (2) augmented and virtual reality (AR/VR), (3) artificial intelligence (AI) and machine learning (ML), (4) personalized (dental) medicine, and (5) tele-healthcare. Digital dentistry requires managing expectations pragmatically and ensuring transparency for all stakeholders: patients, healthcare providers, university and research institutions, the medtech industry, insurance, public media, and state policy. It should not be claimed or implied that digital smart data technologies will replace humans providing dental expertise and the capacity for patient empathy. The dental team that controls digital applications remains the key and will continue to play the central role in treating patients. In this context, the latest trend word is created: augmented intelligence, e.g., the meaningful combination of digital applications paired with human qualities and abilities in order to achieve improved dental and oral healthcare, ensuring quality of life.

Keywords: digital transformation; rapid prototyping; augmented and virtual reality (AR/VR); artificial intelligence (AI); machine learning (ML); personalized dental medicine; tele-health; patient-centered outcomes

1. Introduction

Digital transformation is the ubiquitous catchword in a variety of business sectors, and (dental) medicine is no exception [1]. Continuous progress in information technology (IT) has made it possible to overcome the limitations and hurdles that existed in clinical and technological workflows just a few years ago [2]. In addition, social and cultural behaviors of civilized society in industrial countries have changed and fostered the trend of digitalization: urbanism, centralization, and mobility, permanent accessibility via smartphones and tablets combined with the internet of things (IoT), as well as convenience-driven markets striving for efficiency [3].

The implementation of digital tools and applications reveals novel options facing today's chief problems in healthcare, such as a demographic development of an aging population with an increased prevalence of chronic diseases and increased treatment costs over an individual's lifespan [4]. In dental medicine, several digital workflows for production processing have already been integrated into treatment protocols, especially in the rapidly growing branch of computer-aided design/computer-aided manufacturing (CAD/CAM) and rapid prototyping (RP) [5].

New possibilities have opened up for automated processing in radiological imaging using artificial intelligence (AI) and machine learning (ML). Moreover, augmented and virtual reality (AR/VR) is the technological basis for the superimposition of diverse imaging files creating virtual dental patients and non-invasive simulations comparing different outcomes prior to any clinical intervention. Increased IT-power has fostered these promising technologies, whose possible uses can only be assessed in the future [6]. Not all digital options are currently exhausted, and their (valuable) advantages are not completely understood. Basic science, clinical trials, and subsequently derived knowledge for innovative therapy protocols need to be re-directed towards patient-centered outcomes, enabling the linkage of oral and general health instead of merely industry-oriented investigations [7].

To sum up, unseen opportunities will arise due to digital transformation in oral healthcare and dental research. Therefore, this opinion letter highlights the estimated top five healthcare trends and innovations of the dawning digital era that might influence the direction of dental research and their stakeholders in the near future.

2. Top Five Healthcare Trends and Innovations

2.1. Rapid Prototyping (RP)

RP is a technique to quickly and automatically construct three-dimensional (3D) models of a final product or a part of a whole using 3D-printers. The additive manufacturing process allows inexpensive production of complex 3D-geometries from various materials and minimal material wastage [8]. However, while the future looks very promising from a technical and scientific point of view, it is not clear how RP and its products will be regulated. This uncertainty is problematic for the producing industry, healthcare provider, and patients as well.

In dentistry, one of the main difficulties today is the choice of materials. Commercially available materials commonly used for RP are currently permitted for short to medium-term intraoral retention only and are, therefore, limited to temporary restorations and not yet intended for definitive dental reconstructions. RP offers great potential in dental technology for mass production of dental models, but also for the fabrication of implant surgical guides [9]. For those indications, prolonged intraoral retention is not required. From an economic point of view, a great advantage is the production in large quantities at the same time in a reproducible and standardized way. Another important area of application is the use of 3D-printed models in dental education based on CBCT or μCT. An initial study, however, has revealed that 3D-printed dental models can show changes in dimensional accuracy over periods of 4 weeks and longer. In this context, further investigations comparing different 3D-printers and material combinations are compellingly necessary for clarification [10].

In the near future, those material-related barriers and limitations will probably be broken down. Many research groups are focusing on the development of printable materials for dental reconstructions, such as zirconium dioxide (ZrO_2) [11]. This different mode of fabrication of ZrO_2 structures could allow us to realize totally innovative geometries with hollow bodies that might be used, for example, for time-dependent low-dose release of anti-inflammatory agents in implant dentistry [12]. A completely revolutionary aspect would be the synthesis of biomaterials to artificially create lost tooth structures using RP technology [13]. Instead of using a preformed dental tooth databank, a patient-specific digital dental dataset could be acquired at the time of growth completion and used for future dental reconstructions. Furthermore, the entire tooth can be duplicated to serve as an individualized implant. RP will most likely offer low-cost production and highly customized solutions in various fields of dental medicine that can be tailored to suit the specific needs of each patient.

2.2. Augmented and Virtual Reality (AR/VR)

AR is an interactive technology enhancing a real-world environment by computer-animated perceptual information. In other words, AR expands the real world with virtual content. In most cases, it is the superimposition of additional digital information on live images or videos. VR, in contrast, uses only artificial computerized scenarios without connection to reality [14]. Depending on the technique, every conceivable way of sensation can be used, mainly visual, auditory, and haptic, independently or in any combination [15]. Today, there is a rapidly increasing number of applications for AR/VR technologies in dental medicine as a whole, as well as many intriguing developments for both patients and healthcare providers [16–18].

AR/VR software allows users to superimpose virtually created visualizations onto recordings of the patient in natural motion. Any 3D-model, for instance, a prosthetic design of a possible reconstruction, can be augmented into the individual patient situation to simulate diverse, prospective outcomes in advance without invasive work steps [19]. These digital models can then be viewed in real-time and facilitate communication not only with the patient to demystify the complex treatment steps but also between dental professionals to make the treatment more predictable and efficient. In the future, the possibilities will continue to grow and help facilitate the dental routine. An interesting indication is the augmentation of CBCT-based virtual implant planning directly into the oral cavity or while using intraoral scanners (IOS), projection, and display of the optically detected area with AR glasses.

Another promising area of interest is the sector of dental education, transferring theoretical knowledge and practical exercises to offer interactive teaching with 24/7-access and objective evaluation. AR/VR-based motor skill training for tooth preparation especially facilitates efficient and autonomous learning for dental students. Initial studies have shown that AR/VR technologies stimulate more senses to learn meritoriously [20]. Moreover, in postgraduate education, challenging and complex clinical protocols can be trained in a complete virtual environment without risk or harm for real patients; additionally, specialists can continuously maintain their skills while training with AR/VR-simulations. Within a few years, AR/VR will have the potential to revolutionize dental education radically [21,22].

2.3. Artificial Intelligence (AI) and Machine Learning (ML)

AI (including ML) has already invaded and established itself in our daily lives, although in more subtle means, such as virtual assistants named "Siri" or "Alexa". The basis for AI is the increasing power of computers to think like and complete tasks currently performed by humans with greater speed, accuracy, and lower resource utilization [23,24]. Therefore, AI technology is perfect for work that requires the analysis and evaluation of large amounts of data. Repetitive activities are boring and tiring for humans in the long-run with increased risk of error, while AI-based applications do not show signs of fatigue. In contrast to humans, the artificial learning process results in constant better performance with increasing workload. Additionally, computers are not biased compared to humans, who come with innate biases and may judge things prematurely and differently from each other [25,26].

The most valuable indication for the use of AI and ML in dentistry is the entire field of diagnostic imaging in dento-maxillofacial radiology [27,28]. Currently, applications and research in AI purposes in dental radiology focus on automated localization of cephalometric landmarks, diagnosis of osteoporosis, classification/segmentation of maxillofacial cysts and/or tumors, and identification of periodontitis/periapical disease. Computer software analyzing radiographs has to be trained on huge datasets ("big data") to recognize meaningful patterns. The diagnostic performance of AI models varies among different algorithms used, is also dependent on the observers labeling the datasets, and it is still necessary to verify the generalizability and reliability of these models by using adequate, representative images. AI software must be able to understand new information presented by images as well as written text or spoken language with proper context. Finally, the software must be able to make intelligent decisions regarding this new information, and then, learn from mistakes to improve the decision-making for future processing [29].

A beneficial AI system should realize all of this in about the same time that a human being can perform the given task. Up to now, applications of AI on a broad scale were not technically feasible or cost-effective, so the reality of AI has not yet matched the possibilities in routine dental applications [30], although the technical progress is exponential, and very soon, a large number of AI models will be developed for automated diagnostics of 3D-imaging identifying pathologies, prediction of disease risk, to propose potential therapeutic options, and to evaluate prognosis.

2.4. Personalized (Dental) Medicine

Electronic health records (eHR) with standardized diagnostics and generally accepted data formats are the mandatory door opener to personalized medicine and predictive models investigating a broader population. The structured assessment and systematic collection of patient information is an effective instrument in health economics [31]. Health data can be obtained from routine dental healthcare and clinical trials, as well as from diverse new sources, as IoT in general, and specifically, data on the social determinants of health [3].

The linkage of individual patient data gathered from various sources enables the diagnosis of rare diseases and completely novel strategies for research [32]. Examining large population-based patient cohorts could detect unidentified correlations of diseases and create prognostic models for new treatment concepts. The linkage of patient-level information to population-based citizen cohorts and biobanks provides the required reference of diagnostic and screening cutoffs that could identify new biomarkers through personalized health research [33].

eHR has great power for a change of research both ways. On the other side, the digitized transparent patient could be stigmatized and categorized by insurance companies, provoking adverse effects that have not yet been determined socially [3,6]. Therefore, linked biomedical data supporting register-based research pose several risks and methodological challenges for clinical research: appropriate security settings and the development of algorithms for statistical calculations, including interpretation of collected health data [34,35]. A generally accepted code of conduct has to be defined and established for the ethical and meaningful use of register-based patient data.

Overall, personalized medicine holds the key to unlocking a new frontier in dental research. Genomic sequencing, combined with the developments in medical imaging and regenerative technology, has redefined personalized medicine using novel molecular tools to perform patient-specific precision healthcare [36,37]. It has the potential to revolutionize healthcare using genomics information for individual biomarker identification [38]. The vision is an interdisciplinary approach to dental patient sample analysis, in which dentists, physicians, and nurses can collaborate to understand the inter-connectivity of disease in a cost-effective way [39].

2.5. Tele-Healthcare

Tele-healthcare enables a convenient way for patients to increase self-care while potentially reducing office visits and travel time [40]. Considering the growing number of the elderly population with reduced mobility and/or nursing home-stay, special-care patients, as well as people living in rural areas, these patient groups would benefit significantly from tele-dentistry [41,42]. Measures to be taken in case of dental trauma can be effectively communicated by telephone counselors and can be frequently used during out-of-office hours [43]. In general, it facilitates easier access to care and also represents a cost-reduced option for patients, as instead of expensive treatments, tele-dentistry shifts towards prevention practices and allows patients to consult with otherwise unavailable dental professionals, for example, using a live consult via video-streaming [44,45]. Nevertheless, it must be emphasized that tele-dentistry can never replace a real dentist; rather, it must be understood as an additional tool [30].

Today, tele-dentistry is only in an early start-up phase [46]. Early studies have mainly focused on specific and rare diseases that might require surgery, but there are findings that suggest that a teleradiology system in general dental practice could be helpful for the differential diagnosis of common lesions and may result in a reduction of unnecessary costs [47]. There is a fundamental need to regulate the expanding field of tele-healthcare, with guidelines to secure clinical quality standards. The legislation must be clearly defined and clarified for routine implementation of a national-wide tele-dentistry platform. The technical requirements must be met and security standards for sensitive patient information guaranteed, with well-defined regulatory affairs.

3. Conclusions

The future direction of dental research should foster the linkage of oral and general health in order to focus on personalized medicine considering patient-centered outcomes. In this context, dental research must have an impact as a deliverable to society, not just research to churn out scientific publications but to truly change protocols applied in the clinic. Moreover, here, digitization with AI/ML and AR/VR represents the most promising tools for innovative research today. Furthermore, research in a digital era will also be more and more assessed in terms of "impact" as a deliverable good. Impact assessment is still very much debated by scientists, healthcare policy-makers, and politicians. Additionally, general public health societies are increasingly dependent on solid data sets, gaining knowledge to enable innovations and result in recommendations, guidelines, and healthcare policies of utmost importance. These are supposed to generate economic and social benefits on every and each level from an individual to a population. Scientists in dental medicine have also to be aware that funding might be increasingly dependent on the possibility to demonstrate an impact on a large scale. Thus, the use of impact assessments in the future will most likely serve the following two tasks: (1) demonstrating the value of research, and (2) increasing the value of research through a more effective way of financing research in order to have a societal impact [48,49].

For digital dentistry, this requires managing expectations pragmatically and ensuring transparency for all stakeholders: patients, healthcare providers, university and other research institutions, the medtech industry, insurance, public media, and state policy. It should not be claimed or implied that digital smart data technologies will replace humans who possess dental expertise and the capacity for patient empathy. Therefore, the dental team controlling the power of the digital toolbox is the key and will continue to play a central role in the patient's journey to receive the best possible individual treatment, and to provide emotional support. The collection, storage, and analysis of digitized biomedical patient data pose several challenges. In addition to technical aspects for the handling of huge amounts of data, considering internationally defined standards, an ethical and meaningful policy must ensure the protection of patient data for safety optimal impact.

Nowadays, the mixed term "augmented intelligence" is perhaps somewhat prematurely introduced in social media. However, the benefits of digital applications will complement human qualities and abilities in order to achieve improved and cost-efficient healthcare for patients. Augmented intelligence based on big data will help to reduce the incidence of misdiagnosis and offers more useful insights—quickly, accurately, and easily. This is all achievable without losing the human touch, improving the quality of life.

Author Contributions: Conceptualization, T.J.; Methodology, T.J. and N.U.Z.; Writing—Original Draft Preparation, T.J. and N.U.Z.; Writing—Review and Editing, M.M.B., R.E.J., M.F., and T.W.; Supervision, T.J.; Project Administration, T.J. All authors have read and agreed to the published version of the manuscript.

References

1. Gopal, G.; Suter-Crazzolara, C.; Toldo, L. Digital transformation in healthcare—Architectures of present and future information technologies. *Clin. Chem. Lab. Med.* **2019**, *57*, 328–335. [CrossRef] [PubMed]

2. Weber, G.M.; Mandl, K.D.; Kohane, I.S. Finding the missing link for big biomedical data. *J. Am. Med. Assoc.* **2014**, *311*, 2479–2480. [CrossRef] [PubMed]

3. Joda, T.; Waltimo, T.; Pauli-Magnus, C.; Probst-Hensch, N.; Zitzmann, N.U. Population-based linkage of big data in dental research. *Int. J. Environ. Res. Public Health* **2018**, *15*, 2357. [CrossRef] [PubMed]

4. Glick, M. Taking a byte out of big data. *J. Am. Dent. Assoc.* **2015**, *146*, 793–794. [CrossRef]

5. Miyazaki, T.; Hotta, Y. CAD/CAM systems available for the fabrication of crown and bridge restorations. *Aust. Dent. J.* **2011**, *56* (Suppl. 1), 97–106. [CrossRef]

6. Jones, K.H.; Laurie, G.; Stevens, L.; Dobbs, C.; Ford, D.V.; Lea, N. The other side of the coin: Harm due to the non-use of health-related data. *Int. J. Med. Inform.* **2017**, *97*, 43–51. [CrossRef]

7. Joda, T.; Waltimo, T.; Probst-Hensch, N.; Pauli-Magnus, C.; Zitzmann, N.U. Health data in dentistry: An attempt to master the digital challenge. *Public Health Genom.* **2019**, *22*, 1–7. [CrossRef]

8. Joda, T.; Ferrari, M.; Gallucci, G.O.; Wittenben, J.-G.; Bragger, U. Digital technology in fixed implant prosthodontics. *Periodontology 2000* **2017**, *73*, 178–192. [CrossRef]

9. Dawood, A.; Marti Marti, B.; Sauret-Jackson, V.; Darwood, A. 3D printing in dentistry. *Br. Dent. J.* **2015**, *219*, 521–529. [CrossRef]

10. Lech, G.; Nordström, E. Dimensional Stability of 3D Printed Dental Models. Master's Thesis, Malmö University Electronic Publishing, Malmö, Sweden, 2018.

11. Galantea, R.; Figueiredo-Pinaa, C.G.; Serro, A.P. Additive manufacturing of ceramics for dental applications: A review. *Dent. Mater.* **2019**, *35*, 825–846. [CrossRef]

12. Zocca, A.; Colombo, P.; Gomes, C.M.; Gunster, J. Additive manufacturing of ceramics: Issues, potentialities, and opportunities. *J. Am. Ceram. Soc.* **2015**, *98*, 1983–2001. [CrossRef]

13. Bose, S.; Ke, D.; Sahasrabudhe, H.; Bandyopadhyay, A. Additive manufacturing of biomaterials. *Prog. Mater. Sci.* **2018**, *93*, 45–111. [CrossRef] [PubMed]

14. Sutherland, J.; Belec, J.; Sheikh, A.; Chepelev, L.; Althobaity, W.; Chow, B.J.W.; Mitsouras, D.; Christensen, A.; Rybicki, F.J.; La Russa, D.J. Applying modern virtual and augmented reality technologies to medical images and models. *J. Digit. Imaging* **2019**, *32*, 38–53. [CrossRef] [PubMed]

15. Pensieri, C.; Pennacchini, M. Overview: Virtual reality in medicine. *J. Virtual Worlds Res.* **2014**, *7*, 1–34. [CrossRef]

16. Kwon, H.B.; Park, Y.S.; Han, J.S. Augmented reality in dentistry: A current perspective. *Acta Odontol. Scand.* **2018**, *76*, 497–503. [CrossRef]

17. Joda, T.; Gallucci, G.O.; Wismeijer, D.; Zitzmann, N.U. Augmented and virtual reality in dental medicine: A systematic review. *Comput. Biol. Med.* **2019**, *108*, 93–100. [CrossRef]

18. Farronato, M.; Maspero, C.; Lanteri, V.; Fama, A.; Ferrati, F.; Pettenuzzo, A.; Farronato, D. Current state of the art in the use of augmented reality in dentistry: A systematic review of the literature. *BMC Oral Health* **2019**, *19*, 135. [CrossRef]

19. Joda, T.; Gallucci, G.O. The virtual patient in dental medicine. *Clin. Oral Implant. Res.* **2015**, *26*, 725–726. [CrossRef]

20. Lee, S.H. Research and development of haptic simulator for dental education using virtual reality and user motion. *Int. J. Adv. Smart Conv.* **2018**, *7*, 114–120.

21. Ayoub, A.; Pulijala, Y. The application of virtual reality and augmented reality in Oral & Maxillofacial Surgery. *BMC Oral Health* **2019**, *19*, 238.

22. Durham, M.; Engel, B.; Ferrill, T.; Halford, J.; Singh, T.P.; Gladwell, M. Digitally augmented learning in implant dentistry. *Oral Maxillofac. Surg. Clin. N. Am.* **2019**, *31*, 387–398. [CrossRef] [PubMed]

23. Currie, G. Intelligent imaging: Anatomy of machine learning and deep learning. *J. Nucl. Med. Technol.* **2019**, *47*, 273–281. [CrossRef] [PubMed]

24. Park, W.J.; Park, J.B. History and application of artificial neural networks in dentistry. *Eur. J. Dent.* **2018**, *12*, 594–601. [CrossRef] [PubMed]

25. Chen, Y.W.; Stanley, K.; Att, W. Artificial intelligence in dentistry: Current applications and future perspectives. *Quintessence Int.* **2020**, *51*, 248–257. [PubMed]

26. Kulkarni, S.; Seneviratne, N.; Baig, M.S.; Khan, A.H.A. Artificial intelligence in medicine: Where are we now? *Acad. Radiol.* **2020**, *27*, 62–70. [CrossRef] [PubMed]

27. Tuzoff, D.V.; Tuzova, L.N.; Bornstein, M.M.; Krasnov, A.S.; Kharchenko, M.A.; Nikolenko, S.I.; Sveshnikov, M.M.; Bednenko, G.B. Tooth detection and numbering in panoramic radiographs using convolutional neural networks. *Dentomaxillofac. Radiol.* **2019**, *48*, 20180051. [CrossRef]

28. Hung, K.; Montalvao, C.; Tanaka, R.; Kawai, T.; Bornstein, M.M. The use and performance of artificial intelligence applications in dental and maxillofacial radiology: A systematic review. *Dentomaxillofac. Radiol.* **2020**, *49*, 20190107. [CrossRef]

29. Leite, A.F.; Vasconcelos, K.F.; Willems, H.; Jacobs, R. Radiomics and machine learning in oral healthcare. *Proteom. Clin. Appl.* **2020**, e1900040, [Epub ahead of print]. [CrossRef]

30. Goldhahn, J.; Rampton-Branco-Weiss, V.; Spinas, G.A. Could artificial intelligence make doctors obsolete? *BMJ* **2018**, *363*, k4563. [CrossRef] [PubMed]

31. Tokede, O.; White, J.; Stark, P.C.; Vaderhobli, R.; Walji, M.F.; Ramoni, R.; Schoonheim-Klein, M.; Kimmes, N.; Tavares, A.; Kalenderian, E. Assessing use of a standardized dental diagnostic terminology in an electronic health record. *J. Dent. Educ.* **2013**, *77*, 24–36. [PubMed]

32. Harron, K.L.; Doidge, J.C.; Knight, H.E.; Gilbert, R.E.; Goldstein, H.; Cromwell, D.A.; van der Meulen, J.H. A guide to evaluating linkage quality for the analysis of linked data. *Int. J. Epidemiol.* **2017**, *46*, 1699–1710. [CrossRef] [PubMed]

33. Manolopoulos, V.G.; Dechairo, B.; Huriez, A.; Kühn, A.; Llerena, A.; van Schaik, R.H.; Yeo, K.T.; Ragia, G.; Siest, G. Pharmacogenomics and personalized medicine in clinical practice. *Pharmacogenomics* **2011**, *12*, 597–610. [CrossRef] [PubMed]

34. Aldridge, R.W.; Shaji, K.; Hayward, A.C.; Abubakar, I. Accuracy of probabilistic linkage using the enhanced matching system for public health and epidemiological studies. *PLoS ONE* **2015**, *10*, e0136179. [CrossRef] [PubMed]

35. Jorm, L. Routinely collected data as a strategic resource for research: Priorities for methods and workforce. *Public Health Res. Pract.* **2015**, *25*, e2541540. [CrossRef]

36. Garcia, I.; Kuska, R.; Somerman, M.J. Expanding the foundation for personalized medicine: Implications and challenges for dentistry. *J. Dent. Res.* **2013**, *92*, 3–10. [CrossRef]

37. Marrazzo, P.; Paduano, F.; Palmieri, F.; Marrelli, M.; Tatullo, M. Highly efficient in vitro reparative behavior of dental pulp stem cells cultured with standardized platelet lysate. *Stem Cells Int.* **2016**, *2016*, 7230987. [CrossRef]

38. Emmert-Streib, F. Personalized medicine: Has it started yet? A reconstruction of the early history. *Front. Genet.* **2013**, *3*, 313. [CrossRef]

39. Di Sanzo, M.; Borro, M.; La Russa, R.; Cipolloni, L.; Santurro, A.; Scopetti, M.; Simmaco, M.; Frati, P. Clinical applications of personalized medicine: A new paradigm and challenge. *Curr. Pharm. Biotechnol.* **2017**, *18*, 194–203. [CrossRef]

40. Wang, S.; Parsons, M.; Stone-McLean, J.; Rogers, P.; Boyd, S.; Hoover, K.; Meruvis-Pastor, O.; Gong, M.; Smith, A. Augmented reality as a telemedicine platform for remote procedural training. *Sensors* **2017**, *17*, 2294. [CrossRef]

41. Jampani, N.D.; Nutalapati, R.; Dontula, B.S.; Boyapati, R. Applications of teledentistry: A literature review and update. *J. Int. Soc. Prev. Community Dent.* **2011**, *1*, 37–44.

42. Estai, M.; Kruger, E.; Tennant, M.; Bunt, S.; Kanagasingam, Y. Challenges in the uptake of telemedicine in dentistry. *Rural. Remote. Health* **2016**, *16*, 3915. [PubMed]

43. Lienert, N.; Zitzmann, N.U.; Filippi, A.; Weiger, R.; Krastl, G. Teledental consultations related to trauma in a Swiss telemedical center: A retrospective survey. *Dent. Traumatol.* **2010**, *26*, 223–227. [CrossRef] [PubMed]

44. Daniel, S.J.; Kumar, S. Teledentistry: A key component in access to care. *J. Evid. Based Dent. Pract.* **2014**, *14*, 201–208. [CrossRef] [PubMed]

45. Irving, M.; Stewart, R.; Spallek, H.; Blinkhom, A. Using teledentistry in clinical practice as an enabler to improve access to clinical care: A qualitative systematic review. *J. Telemed. Telecare* **2018**, *24*, 129–146. [CrossRef] [PubMed]

46. Wang, G.; Xiang, W.; Pickering, M. A cross-platform solution for light field based 3D telemedicine. *Comput. Methods Programs Biomed.* **2016**, *125*, 103–116. [CrossRef]

47. Estai, M.; Bunt, S.; Kanagasingam, Y.; Tennant, M. Cost savings from a teledentistry model for school dental screening: An Australian health system perspective. *Aust. Health Rev.* **2018**, *42*, 482–490. [CrossRef]

48. Greenhalgh, T.; Raftery, J.; Hanney, S.; Glover, M. Research impact: A narrative review. *BMC Med.* **2016**, *14*, 78. [CrossRef]

49. Newson, R.; King, L.; Rychetnik, L.; Milat, A.; Bauman, A. Looking both ways: A review of methods for assessing research impacts on policy and the policy utilisation of research. *Health Res. Policy Syst.* **2018**, *16*, 54. [CrossRef]

10

Efficacy of Plasma-Polymerized Allylamine Coating of Zirconia after Five Years

Nadja Rohr [1,2,*]⦿, Katja Fricke [3]⦿, Claudia Bergemann [2]⦿, J Barbara Nebe [2]⦿ and Jens Fischer [1]

[1] Biomaterials and Technology, Department of Reconstructive Dentistry, University Center for Dental Medicine, University of Basel, 4058 Basel, Switzerland; jens.fischer@unibas.ch

[2] Department of Cell Biology, Rostock University Medical Center, 18057 Rostock, Germany; claudia.bergemann@med.uni-rostock.de (C.B.); barbara.nebe@med.uni-rostock.de (J.B.N.)

[3] Leibniz Institute for Plasma Science and Technology e.V. (INP), 17489 Greifswald, Germany; k.fricke@inp-greifswald.de

* Correspondence: nadja.rohr@unibas.ch

Abstract: Plasma-polymerized allylamine (PPAAm) coatings of titanium enhance the cell behavior of osteoblasts. The purpose of the present study was to evaluate a PPAAm nanolayer on zirconia after a storage period of 5 years. Zirconia specimens were directly coated with PPAAm (ZA0) or stored in aseptic packages at room temperature for 5 years (ZA5). Uncoated zirconia specimens (Zmt) and the micro-structured endosseous surface of a zirconia implant (Z14) served as controls. The elemental compositions of the PPAAm coatings were characterized and the viability, spreading and gene expression of human osteoblastic cells (MG-63) were assessed. The presence of amino groups in the PPAAm layer was significantly decreased after 5 years due to oxidation processes. Cell viability after 24 h was significantly higher on uncoated specimens (Zmt) than on all other surfaces. Cell spreading after 20 min was significantly higher for Zmt = ZA0 > ZA5 > Z14, while, after 24 h, spreading also varied significantly between Zmt > ZA0 > ZA5 > Z14. The expression of the mRNA differentiation markers collagen I and osteocalcin was upregulated on untreated surfaces Z14 and Zmt when compared to the PPAAm specimens. Due to the high biocompatibility of zirconia itself, a PPAAm coating may not additionally improve cell behavior.

Keywords: zirconia implant; human osteoblasts; cell viability; cell spreading; gene expression; plasma-polymerized allylamine; X-ray photoelectron spectroscopy

1. Introduction

To replace missing teeth, dental implants made of titanium are a valuable treatment option. However, in recent years, titanium implants have been critically discussed regarding the release of titanium particles and biologic complications [1]. There are some indications that Ti ions released from the implant surface upregulate the expression of chemokines and cytokines in human osteoclasts and osteoblasts. Consequently, osteoclastogenesis is induced, which may contribute to the pathomechanism of aseptic loosening [2,3]. Dental implants made of zirconia can be considered promising alternatives to titanium implants [4–6]. Clinical data are available, reporting survival rates of 95.4% after 3 years [4] and 98.4% after 5 years in situ [5].

Permanent osseointegration, indicated by the formation of a direct bone–implant contact, is the most important requirement for the clinical success of an implant [7]. The endosseous part of the implant is shaped as screw to achieve a certain primary stability after insertion. Additionally, most implant surfaces are micro-structured, which is reported to enhance osseointegration [8]. For zirconia implants, different approaches are undertaken to structure the endosseous surface such as sandblasting, acid-etching, laser structuring, additive sintering or injection molding [9–11]. The currently available surfaces providing long-term clinical data for zirconia implants are sandblasted followed by acid etching [4,12] and, optionally, heat treated [5].

Another approach is the creation of a biologically active implant surface by applying an additional functional layer, which has been done for titanium surfaces [13,14]. Nitrogen-rich surface chemistry is known to promote cellular attachment because it contains polar groups [15]. The most common plasma precursors used to generate amine functionalities on biomaterials are allylamine [16–18], ethylendiamine [19], cyclopropylamine [20,21] as well as mixtures of hydrocarbon-containing gases and molecular nitrogen [22]. Due to the presence of positively charged carriers such as NH_2 groups on the surface coating [23,24], the net negative charged eukaryotic cells are attracted. For instance, plasma-polymerized allylamine (PPAAm) coatings have been applied on titanium [25–30], titanium alloy (Ti6Al4V) [22], porous calcium phosphate [31] and yttria-stabilized zirconia (Y-TZP) [32] to improve their hydrophilic properties by generating positively charged amine groups. The resulting zeta potential changed from negative into positive values, e.g., untreated titanium: −82.3 mV and PPAAm-coated Ti: +8.6 mV (pH 7.4) [33]. On all tested materials, the cell spreading of human osteoblastic cells MG-63 was accelerated by the PPAAm coating. PPAAm-coated titanium plates have also been inserted in the muscular neck tissue of rats, revealing lower macrophage-related reactions in the mid (14 d) and late (56 d) phases of the study than uncoated titanium specimens [29]. However, the PPAAm coating is susceptible to aging. Within 7 days after coating, 70% of the primary amino groups of the PPAAm layer were already converted into amides. Zeta potential remained positive and even increased with prolonged storage of 200 d from 13.9 ± 1.2 mV to 26.3 ± 0.5 mV (pH 6.0), probably due to the increased density of imines, nitriles and acid amides [30]. Nevertheless, the cell spreading of human osteoblasts on PPAAm-coated titanium alloys that were stored over 360 d was accelerated compared to uncoated specimens [30]. To evaluate the differentiation behavior of osteoblastic cells, gene expression of differentiation markers such as alkaline phosphatase (ALP), collagen type 1 (COL) or osteocalcin (OCN) are measured. COL and ALP are considered early differentiation markers in the osteoblast lineage, while the transcription of OCN is enhanced in a later differentiation stage. The purpose of the present study is to test whether a PPAAm coating on zirconia is stable up to 5 years, which is the common shelf life of ready-for-sale implants. The reaction of human osteoblasts to the PPAAm coating on zirconia has therefore been assessed by evaluating cell viability, spreading, cell morphology and gene expression.

2. Materials and Methods

Zirconia discs with a diameter of 13 mm and a height of 2 mm were produced. The discs were machine overdimensioned in the green state, sintered and isostatically hot pressed in order to get disc-shaped specimens. The zirconia was composed of 93.0 wt% ZrO_2, 5.0 wt% Y_2O_3, 0.1 wt% Al_2O_3, 1.9 wt% HfO_2; its grain size was 0.3 μm (MZ111, CeramTec, Plochingen, Germany). Four different surfaces were produced according to Table 1: ZA0: as-sintered zirconia, heat treated for 1 h at 1250 °C, PPAAm coating, ZA5: as-sintered zirconia, heat treated for 1 h at 1250 °C, PPAAm coating, aged 5 years in sealed package, Zmt: as-sintered zirconia, heat treated for 1 h at 1250 °C, Z14: sandblasted Al_2O_3 105 μm, etched for 1 h in hydrofluoric acid 38–40%, heat treated for 1 h at 1250 °C. Z14 is the endosseous surface of a clinically tested implant [5] (cer.face 14, Vita, Bad Säckingen, Germany) and served as the clinically relevant control. Z14 displayed the following roughness parameters: arithmetical mean (Ra) = 1.47 ± 0.0.6 μm, maximum height of profile (Rz) = 10.85 ± 0.67 μm [34]. Specimens were heat treated at 1250 °C for 1 h to achieve a higher tetragonal phase of zirconia and consequently increase its resistance to aging. The surface of Zmt (Ra = 0.33 ± 0.0.2 μm, Rz = 2.71 ± 0.24 μm [34]) served as a substrate for the specimens treated with PPAAm (ZA0 and ZA5). Those specimens were coated with a thin (approximately 40 nm) PPAAm layer using a low-pressure plasma reactor (V55G, Plasma Finish, Germany) according to the following two-step procedure: (1) activation of the substrates by a continuous wave oxygen/argon plasma (500 W, 50 Pa, 1000-sccm O2/5 sccm Ar) for 60 s and (2) deposition of PPAAm by microwave-excited (2.45 GHz) pulsed plasma (500 W, 50 Pa, 50 sccm Ar) for 480 s (effective treatment time). Prior to flushing the reactor with allylamine, the precursor was carefully purified of air by evacuating and purging with N_2. Substrates were treated in a downstream position 9 cm from the microwave coupling window. ZA0 and ZA5 were then immediately stored in aseptic packaging until use. Specimens of ZA5 were stored in aseptic packaging at room temperature for a period of 5 years. Prior to all experiments, Z14 and Zmt specimens were cleaned in an ultrasonic bath, 70% ethanol for 5 min, distilled water for 5 min, sterilized in a heating chamber at 200 °C for 2 h (FED-240, Binder, Tuttlingen, Germany) and stored in sterile petri dishes that were wrapped with aluminum foil for at least 2 weeks. The specimen surfaces were then characterized in terms of their elemental composition and visualized using scanning electron microscopy (SEM).

Table 1. Pretreatment of zirconia surfaces of the respective groups.

Group	Surface Pretreatment
ZA0	heat treated for 1 h at 1250 °C, plasma-polymerized allylamine coating September 2018
ZA5	heat treated for 1 h at 1250 °C, plasma-polymerized allylamine coating August 2013
Zmt	heat treated for 1 h at 1250 °C
Z14	sandblasted Al_2O_3 105 µm, etched 1 h hydrofluoric acid 38–40%, heat treated for 1 h at 1250 °C

2.1. Specimen Characterization

2.1.1. Elemental Composition (XPS)

The elemental surface composition was analyzed by high-resolution scanning XPS. The spectra were acquired using an Axis Supra delay-line detector (DLD) electron spectrometer (Kratos Analytical, Manchester, UK) equipped with a monochromatic Al K_α source (1486.6 eV). The analysis area was approximately 250 µm in diameter during the acquisition, obtained by using the medium magnification lens mode (field of view 2) and by selecting the slot mode. The core level spectra of each element, which were identified in the survey spectra, were collected at a pass energy of 80 eV by applying an emission current of 10 mA and a high voltage of 15 kV. Charge neutralization was implemented by a low-energy electron injected into the magnetic field of the lens from a filament located directly atop the sample. For each sample, spectra were recorded on three different spots and randomly distributed. Data processing was carried out using CasaXPS software, version 2.3.22PR1.0 (Casa Software Ltd., Teighnmouth, UK). Due to sample charging, the binding energy scale was corrected for all samples by setting the carbon C1s binding energy to 285.0 eV. Concentrations are provided in atomic percent (at%). The labeling of primary amino groups was performed with 4-trifluoromethyl-benzaldehyde (TFBA, Alfa Aesar, Haverhill, MA, USA) at 40 °C in a saturated gas phase for 2 h. The density of the amino groups, the ratio of NH_2 to carbon atoms (NH_2/C), was determined from the fluorine elemental fraction.

2.1.2. SEM Imaging

The specimens' surfaces were gold-sputtered and visualized with a scanning electron microscope (SEM) using mixed secondary electrons (SE) and backscattered electrons (BSE) modes at 15 kV (ESEM XL30, Philips, Eindhoven, the Netherlands).

2.2. Cell Behavior

2.2.1. Cell Cultivation

The human osteoblastic cell line MG-63 (American Type Culture Collection ATCC, CRL1427) was cultivated in Dulbecco's modified Eagle medium (DMEM + GlutaMAX-l + 4.5 g/L DGlucose + Pyruvate; gibco, Thermo Fisher Scientific, Waltham, MA, USA) with the addition of 10% fetal calf serum (FCS superior standardized S0615 0879F, Biochrom, Berlin, Germany) and 1% antibiotic (gentamicin, ratiopharm, Ulm, Germany) to 70–80% confluency up to passages 8–21 [35] at 37 °C in a humidified atmosphere with 5% CO_2. Cells were detached with 0.05% trypsin/0.02% ethylenediaminetetraacetate (EDTA, PAA Laboratories GmbH) for 5 min at 37 °C. After stopping trypsinization by the addition of a complete cell culture medium, an aliquot of 100 μL was put into 10 mL of CASY ton buffer solution (Roche Innovatis, Reutlingen, Germany) and the cell number was measured in the counter CASY Model DT (Schärfe System, Reutlingen, Germany). Specimens were seeded with the appropriate cell number and incubated in 24-well plates (Greiner Bio-One, Frickenhausen, Germany) for the respective time intervals. All cell experiments were performed independently three times using different cell passages.

2.2.2. Cell Viability

The mitochondrial dehydrogenase activity of MG-63 cells on the respective specimens was measured by 3-(4,5-dimethylthiazol-2-yl)-2,5-diphenyltetrazolium bromide (MTS) assay to determine cell viability. A drop of 120 μL cell culture medium containing 5×10^4 MG-63 cells was carefully placed on each specimen (n = 2 per group) and incubated for 20 min to ensure cell attachment on the specimens. Afterwards, 1 mL of cell culture medium was added per well and the specimens were incubated for 24 h at 37 °C. Specimens were transferred to a new 24-well plate with MTS solution (CellTiter 96 ONE-Solution Cell Proliferation Assay, Promega, Madison, WI, USA) and culture medium (1:5) was added to each specimen. Blanks containing a specimen of each group with culture medium but without cells and a control group with cells growing on polystyrene were additionally tested. After 80 min, supernatants were transferred to a 96-well plate (for each specimen 3×80 μL were analyzed). The optical density (OD) was recorded at 490 nm with a micro-plate reader (Anthos, Mikrosysteme, Krefeld, Germany). Relative cell viability was calculated using the following equation:

$$\text{Relative cell viability} = (\text{OD}_{\text{specimen}} - \text{OD}_{\text{blank specimen}})/(\text{OD}_{\text{control}} - \text{OD}_{\text{blank control}})$$

2.2.3. Cell Spreading

Cell spreading was assessed on all surfaces after 20 min and 24 h, respectively. In total, 10^6 cells were suspended in 250 μL diluent C and their cell membranes were stained with PKH-26, a lipophilic membrane dye (PKH-26 general cell linker kit, Sigma-Aldrich, Steinheim, Germany) for 5 min at 37 °C using a dilution of 2 μL PKH-26 + 248 μL diluent C. After stopping the staining reaction using FCS, cells were washed with Dulbecco's phosphate buffered saline (PBS), resuspended in cell culture medium and 3×10^4 cells were seeded per specimen. After 20 min or 24 h, cells were rinsed twice with Dulbecco's phosphate buffered saline (PBS) (Sigma-Aldrich), fixed with 4% paraformaldehyde for 10 min at room temperature (RT), rinsed with PBS and embedded with mounting medium (Fluoroshield with DAPI, Sigma-Aldrich) and a cover slip. Cells were examined with a water immersion objective (C Apochromat 40×, 1.2 W, Carl Zeiss, Oberkochen, Germany) at a wavelength of 546 nm using a confocal laser scanning microscope (LSM780, Carl Zeiss, Oberkochen, Germany; ZEN 2011 software black version, Carl Zeiss, Oberkochen, Germany). The mean spreading area in μm² of 40 cells per specimen was then calculated using image processing software (ImageJ, v2.0.0, National Institutes of Health, Bethesda, Maryland, USA).

2.2.4. Cell Morphology

The morphology of 4×10^4 cells on the respective specimens after 20 min and 24 h was visualized using SEM. Cells on the specimens were rinsed with PBS after the respective time intervals, fixed with 2.5% glutaraldehyde (Merck KGaA, Darmstadt, Germany) for 30 min at 4 °C, rinsed with PBS, dehydrated with ethanol (30%, 50%, 70%, 90%, abs.), dried in a desiccator with silica gel and gold-sputtered.

2.2.5. Gene Expression

On each specimen, 3×10^4 cells were seeded (n = 2 per group) and cultivated for 24 h or 3 d, respectively. Total RNA was purified using the NucleoSpin RNA kit (Machery-Nagel, Düren, Germany) after the cell lysate of the 2 specimens per group was pooled. The RNA concentration for each group was measured using NanoDrop 1000 (Peqlab/VWR, Erlangen, Germany).

After isolating total RNA, first-strand cDNA was synthesized from at least 400 ng total RNA by reverse transcription with SuperScript II (Life Technologies, Darmstadt, Germany) using 2.5-µM random hexamers (Life Technologies) (MiniCycler, MJ Research/Biozym Diagnostik, Hess, Germany). cDNA of each group, resulting from the reverse transcription, was diluted with RNase free H_2O 1:2.5. Twelve-µL Mastermix. composed of 10-µL TaqMan Universal PCR Master Mix (Life Technologies), 1-µL RNase free H_2O and 1-µL Assays-on-Demand gene expression assay mix (Life Technologies) for the detection of either alkaline phosphatase (ALP, #Hs00758162_m1ALPL), collagen type 1 (COL I, #Hs00164004_m1COLA1) or osteocalcin (OCN, #Hs01587813_g1BGLAP) and for glyceraldehyde 3-phosphate dehydrogenase as an endogenous control (GAPDH, #Hs99999905_m1GAPDH, housekeeping gene) was analyzed with 8 µL of cDNA.

Quantitative real-time PCR assays were performed with a 3×20-µL reaction mix per group, marked and monitored with the ABI PRISM 7500 sequence detection system (Applied Biosystems, Darmstadt, Germany). Relative mRNA expression for each marker protein was calculated based on the comparative $\Delta\Delta CT$-method, normalized to GAPDH as an endogenous control and calibrated to the control cells grown on polystyrene after 24 h.

2.3. Statistical Analysis

Data are presented as the mean and its standard deviation. Values were analyzed for normal distribution using the Shapiro–Wilk test. For normally distributed data, one-way ANOVA was applied followed by a post-hoc Fisher least significant difference (LSD) test to determine differences between groups. Values of gene expression were analyzed with Student's t-test. The level of significance was set to $\alpha = 0.05$.

3. Results

3.1. Specimen Characterization

The elemental surface compositions of the coated samples, ZA0 and ZA5, determined with XPS, are listed in Table 2. The PPAAm coating on ZA0 is mainly composed of carbon and nitrogen, which were the constituents of the precursor used for the plasma polymerization (except for hydrogen, which cannot be analyzed by XPS), as well as a marginal fraction of oxygen that originates from post-oxidation processes. For the aged PPAAm coating (ZA5), a remarkably higher portion of oxygen was determined compared to ZA0 and, furthermore, traces of zirconium, silicon, fluorine and chloride at a total amount of <1 at% were detected. The amino group density of NH_2/C was found to be 3.4% for the as-deposited PPAAm coating (ZA0) and 0.3% for the 5-year aged layer (ZA5).

Table 2. Elemental composition of plasma-polymerized allylamine (PPAAm)-coated zirconia surfaces (ZA0) and aged surfaces (ZA5) determined with XPS.

	C (at.%)	N (at.%)	O (at.%)	N/C (%)	O/C (%)	NH₂/C (%)
ZA0	74.5 ± 2.1	22.9 ± 2.3	2.6 ± 0.3	30.7 ± 3.8	3.5 ± 0.3	3.4 ± 0.1
ZA5	73.9 ± 0.8	13.9 ± 0.8	11.4 ± 0.3	18.8 ± 1.3	15.4 ± 0.1	0.3 ± 0.1

The high-resolution XPS C1s spectra of ZA0 and ZA5 are shown in Figure 1. The PPAAm C1s peak of ZA0 can be fitted with three components: one at 285.0 eV, characteristic for C–H or/and C–C aliphatic bonds, another at 285.9 eV assigned to C–NH, and a third component at 286.8 eV, which corresponds to C–O, C–O–C, C = N or nitriles. In contrast, the highly resolved C1s spectrum of ZA5 shows drastic changes in the shape of the C1s peak with two further components at 287.9 eV and 289.0 eV attributed to C = O and O–C = O, respectively.

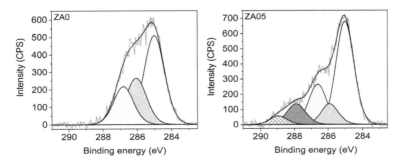

Figure 1. XPS C1s high resolution spectra of PPAAm after preparation (ZA0) and aging in a sealed aseptic packing at ambient conditions for 5 years (ZA5).

SEM images of specimens are displayed in Figure 2. No differences between the surfaces of Zmt, ZA0 and ZA5 could be observed in SEM images. Granules can be observed on all surfaces. Z14 displayed a rougher surface with micro-rough lacunae due to sandblasting with Al_2O_3 particles (105 μm) and hydrofluoric acid etching.

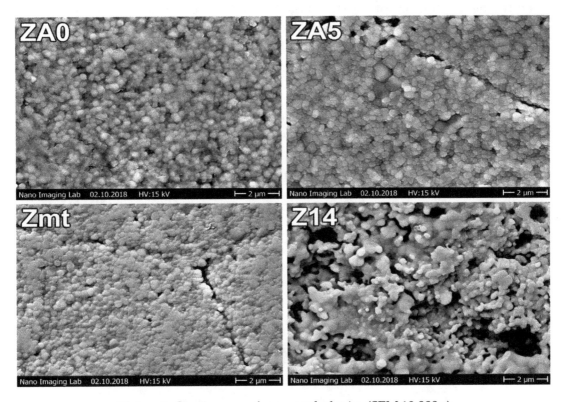

Figure 2. Specimen surface morphologies (SEM 10,000×).

3.2. Cell Behavior

Cell viability after 24 h was significantly higher for Zmt than for all other specimens ($p < 0.001$) (Figure 3a). Cell spreading after 20 min was significantly highest for Zmt = ZA0 > ZA5 > Z14, while, after 24 h, spreading was also significantly different between Zmt > ZA0 > ZA5 > Z14 ($p < 0.001$) (Figure 3b), possibly influenced by the increased roughness of Z14.

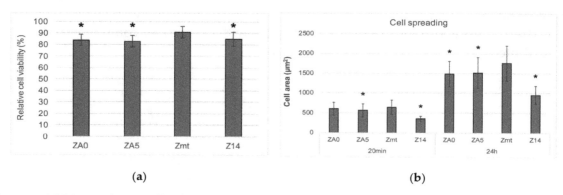

(a)   (b)

Figure 3. (**a**) Mean relative cell viability and standard deviation after 24 h in% normalized to the control cells grown on well bottoms. Statistically significant differences in specimens compared to uncoated zirconia specimens (Zmt), determined with a post-hoc Fisher LSD test, are indicated with * ($p < 0.001$). (**b**) Human osteoblastic cell (MG-63) area after 20 min and 24 h on differently treated zirconia specimens. Statistically significant differences in specimens compared to the control Zmt of the respective group of either 20 min or 24 h, determined with a post-hoc Fisher LSD test, are indicated with * ($p < 0.001$), n = 40 cells per group × 3 independent experiments, mean ± standard deviations.

The cell morphology visible in SEM images in Figure 4a was in accordance with the spreading determined with LSM. After 20 min, cells start to change from spherical into planar shapes; this process proceeds even further on the smooth surfaces of ZA0, ZA5 and Zmt compared to Z14. After 24 h, cells appear to be spread further on Zmt than on all other surfaces. Exposed nucleoli can be observed in the center of the cells on surfaces ZA0, ZA5 and Zmt. Due to the higher roughness on Z14, cells are less spread, but they are extended into the microstructures, where they anchor their filopodia (Figure 4b).

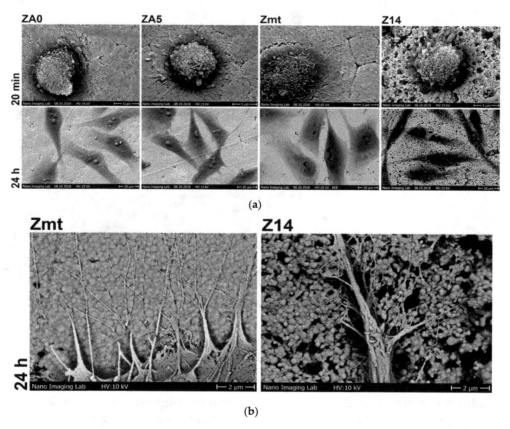

Figure 4. (**a**) MG-63 cells on differently treated zirconia surfaces. First row: spreading after 20 min (SEM, 5000×, bar 5 μm); second row: spreading after 24 h (SEM, 1000×, bar 20 μm). (**b**) MG-63 cell filopodia formation and interaction with the substrates Zmt and the micro-structured endosseous surface of a zirconia implant (Z14) (SEM, 10,000×, bar 2 μm).

The gene expression of early osteogenic marker ALP and late markers COL and OCN is displayed in Figure 5. The relative mRNA of ALP was significantly reduced on all specimens after 3 d when compared to the control cells grown on well bottoms for 24 h; COL remained stable and OCN was significantly increased for all specimens except ZA5. Significant differences when compared to Zmt at the respective time intervals are displayed in Figure 5 ($p < 0.05$).

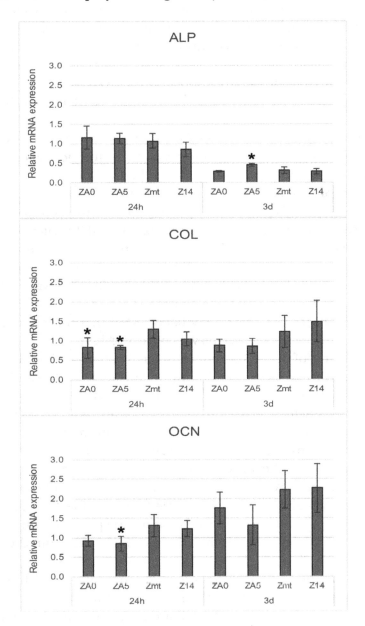

Figure 5. Relative mRNA expression of alkaline phosphatase (ALP), collagen type 1 (COL) and osteocalcin (OCN) in MG-63 cells on zirconia surfaces ZA0, ZA5, Zmt and Z14. The relative mRNA expression is normalized to the control cells grown on well bottoms after 24 h (=1.0), statistically significant differences in Zmt after 24 h or 3 d, respectively, determined with Student's t-test, are indicated with * ($p < 0.05$).

4. Discussion

The purpose of the present study was to determine whether a PPAAm coating on zirconia is stable for up to 5 years and still able to improve the osteoblast reactions compared to previously reported results on titanium [25–29], porous calcium phosphate [31] and Y-TZP [32]. Surprisingly, the control surface of the as-sintered and heat-treated zirconia (Zmt) was the substrate that accelerated initial cell behavior. In contrast to previous findings for Y-TZP [32], in this study, a coating with PPAAm on the

Zmt surface did not have an additional positive effect on the cells and even reduced their viability and spreading capability. The five-year aging of the PPAAm surfaces resulted in the oxidation of the coating, which, however, did not affect cell behavior differently than for freshly coated specimens, as also previously reported for titanium [30].

PPAAm films on ZA0 exhibited a N/C value of almost 32%—close to the theoretical N/C value of 33% for the precursor allylamine—which indicates the presence of nitrogen-containing functional groups at the surface. Additionally, XPS analysis revealed no further elements originating from the zirconia substrate (i.e., Al, Hf, Y, Zr), which confirms the homogeneous coverage of the substrate with a nanometer-thin PPAAm film. Amine-bearing plasma polymer coatings are susceptible to oxidation when stored under ambient conditions [30]. Hence, for PPAAm-coated specimen ZA5, stored for 5 years, the uptake of the oxygen content and a considerable depletion of the amino group density were determined by XPS.

The SEM images of the specimens revealed a surface structure with rounded granules sized around 100 nm. Due to the sandblasting and etching with hydrofluoric acid of Z14, niches were formed and surface roughness consequently increased. Since the thickness of the PPAAm layer is around 40 nm, the surface textures of ZA0 and ZA5 are comparable to the control Zmt.

Cell viability was significantly highest for Zmt than for all other surfaces. It has been previously seen that viability on smooth surfaces is increased compared to micro-structured surfaces [34]. The presence of the PPAAm layer also reduced cell viability when compared to the control without a coating. However, the viability of cells on the PPAAm-coated surfaces was comparable to Z14 and was above 80%; consequently, no toxic effect was initiated by the PPAAm coating when considering ISO standard 10993-5, which indicates no toxic effects for cell viability > 75%. The biocompatibility of a PPAAm coating on titanium has previously been tested in a rat model and no increased local inflammation compared to uncoated specimens was observed [29].

The initial cell spreading of MG-63 osteoblasts has been identified as the main factor that is highly accelerated by the PPAAm coating on titanium surfaces [27,30,31]. However, spreading on zirconia could not be improved when the coating was applied in the present study and was even lower than on uncoated specimens after 20 min as well as after 24 h. In contrast to the present study using 10% FCS, previously, no serum was added to the cell culture medium when cells were seeded on the PPAAm-coated specimens. Serum proteins improve initial cell adhesion and the spreading of osteoblasts on zirconia [36] and the addition of fetal calf serum to the culture medium may have masked the potential effects of PPAAm. That spreading was generally higher on smooth than on micro-roughened surfaces has been previously observed for osteoblasts on zirconia [37,38], as well as on titanium [39]. Adequate spreading is a crucial factor for the proliferation of adherent cells because maximum extracellular matrix contact with the whole cell body is aspired to maintain osteoblastic function [40,41].

The cell morphology visible in SEM images was in accordance with the measured cell areas in LSM images. On Z14 surfaces, cells anchored their filopodia on the micro-roughened surface and spread into the depths of the niches; hence, the cell area appeared smaller than for cells on all other surfaces, as previously seen for primary human osteoblasts (HOB) [38].

For the gene expression of RNA markers, the downregulation of ALP after 3 d, stable COL and upregulated OCN in MG-63 cells, as observed, can be considered typical reactions in osteoblast maturation. COL and ALP are early differentiation markers in the osteoblast lineage; hence, mRNA expression of these markers is increased in preosteoblasts and declines during osteoblast maturation [42]. mRNA expression of COL was significantly increased for cells on Zmt when compared to PPAAm-coated specimens after 24 h. OCN is first expressed at very low levels and, later in osteoblast maturation, transcription is enhanced [43]. In the present study, after 3 d, this was noticeable for ZA0 but further progressed for Zmt and Z14. In general, gene expression on Zmt and Z14 was comparable. Another study compared the gene expression of the same markers of human primary osteoblasts on machined as well as on sandblasted, etched and heat-treated zirconia [38]. ALP and COL mRNA expression of primary human osteoblasts on both zirconia surfaces was downregulated after 3 d. OCN was further upregulated for cells on the machined surface than on the sandblasted, etched and heat-treated surface after 3 d [38]. These gene expression results support the finding of the present study that smoother zirconia surfaces are favorable for initial cell behavior. Contrary to previous findings on titanium, calcium phosphate and Y-TZP, a coating of zirconia with PPAAm in the presence of serum in the culture medium does not improve cell behavior further. Five-year aging of PPAAm-coated zirconia resulted in the oxidation of the layer, but did not affect cell behavior differently than for freshly coated zirconia.

5. Conclusions

Within the limitations of this study, it can be concluded that zirconia coated with PPAAm does not additionally improve osteoblast behavior in cell culture experiments due to the high biocompatibility of zirconia.

Author Contributions: Conceptualization, N.R. and J.F.; methodology, N.R., J.B.N. and K.F.; formal analysis, N.R. and J.F. investigation, N.R., C.B. and K.F.; writing—original draft preparation, N.R. and K.F.; writing—review and editing N.R., K.F., C.B., J.B.N. and J.F. All authors have read and agreed to the published version of the manuscript.

Acknowledgments: The authors would like to thank Fredy Schmidli, Martina Grüning, Petra Müller and Petra Seidel for the laboratory support.

References

1. Mombelli, A.; Hashim, D.; Cionca, N. What is the impact of titanium particles and biocorrosion on implant survival and complications? A critical review. *Clin. Oral Implant. Res.* **2018**, *29*, 37–53. [CrossRef] [PubMed]
2. Cadosch, D.; Gautschi, O.P.; Chan, E.; Filgueira, L.; Simmen, H.-P. Titanium induced production of chemokines CCL17/TARC and CCL22/MDC in human osteoclasts and osteoblasts. *J. Biomed. Mater. Res. Part A* **2009**, *9999*, 475–483. [CrossRef] [PubMed]
3. Cadosch, D.; Al-Mushaiqri, M.S.; Gautschi, O.P.; Meagher, J.; Simmen, H.-P.; Filgueira, L. Biocorrosion and uptake of titanium by human osteoclasts. *J. Biomed. Mater. Res. Part A* **2010**, *95*, 1004–1010. [CrossRef]
4. Bormann, K.H.; Gellrich, N.-C.; Kniha, H.; Schild, S.; Weingart, D.; Gahlert, M. A prospective clinical study to evaluate the performance of zirconium dioxide dental implants in single-tooth edentulous area: 3-year follow-up. *BMC Oral Health* **2018**, *18*, 181. [CrossRef] [PubMed]
5. Balmer, M.; Spies, B.C.; Kohal, R.-J.; Hämmerle, C.H.; Vach, K.; Jung, R.E. Zirconia implants restored with single crowns or fixed dental prostheses: 5-year results of a prospective cohort investigation. *Clin. Oral Implant. Res.* **2020**, *31*, 452–462. [CrossRef] [PubMed]
6. Adánez, M.H.; Nishihara, H.; Att, W. A systematic review and meta-analysis on the clinical outcome of zirconia implant–restoration complex. *J. Prosthodont. Res.* **2018**, *62*, 397–406. [CrossRef] [PubMed]
7. Binon, P.P. Implants and components: Entering the new millennium. *Int. J. Oral Maxillofac. Implant.* **2000**, *15*, 76–94.
8. Wennerberg, A.; Albrektsson, T. Effects of titanium surface topography on bone integration: A systematic review. *Clin. Oral Implant. Res.* **2009**, *20*, 172–184. [CrossRef]
9. Fischer, J.; Schott, A.; Martin, S. Surface micro-structuring of zirconia dental implants. *Clin. Oral Implant. Res.* **2015**, *27*, 162–166. [CrossRef]
10. Pieralli, S.; Kohal, R.-J.; Hernandez, E.L.; Doerken, S.; Spies, B.C. Osseointegration of zirconia dental implants in animal investigations: A systematic review and meta-analysis. *Dent. Mater.* **2017**, *34*, 171–182. [CrossRef]
11. Nishihara, H.; Adanez, M.H.; Att, W. Current status of zirconia implants in dentistry: Preclinical tests. *J. Prosthodont. Res.* **2019**, *63*, 1–14. [CrossRef] [PubMed]
12. Kniha, K.; Schlegel, K.; Kniha, H.; Modabber, A.; Hölzle, F. Evaluation of peri-implant bone levels and soft tissue dimensions around zirconia implants—A three-year follow-up study. *Int. J. Oral Maxillofac. Surg.* **2018**, *47*, 492–498. [CrossRef] [PubMed]
13. Morra, M. Biomolecular modification of implant surfaces. *Expert Rev. Med Devices* **2007**, *4*, 361–372. [CrossRef] [PubMed]
14. Narayanan, R.; Seshadri, S.K.; Kwon, T.Y.; Kim, K.H. Calcium phosphate-based coatings on titanium and its alloys. *J. Biomed. Mater. Res. Part B Appl. Biomater.* **2008**, *85*, 279–299. [CrossRef] [PubMed]

15. Faucheux, N.; Tzoneva, R.; Nagel, M.D.; Groth, T. The dependence of fibrillar adhesions in human fibroblasts on substratum chemistry. *Biomaterials* **2006**, *27*, 234–245. [CrossRef]

16. Aziz, G.; De Geyter, N.; Morent, R. Incorporation of Primary Amines via Plasma Technology on Biomaterials. In *Advances in Bioengineering*; Serra, P.A., Ed.; InTech: London, UK, 2015. [CrossRef]

17. Liu, X.; Feng, Q.; Bachhuka, A.; Vasilev, K. Surface Modification by Allylamine Plasma Polymerization Promotes Osteogenic Differentiation of Human Adipose-Derived Stem Cells. *ACS Appl. Mater. Interfaces* **2014**, *6*, 9733–9741. [CrossRef]

18. Gallino, E.; Massey, S.; Tatoulian, M.; Mantovani, D. Plasma polymerized allylamine films deposited on 316L stainless steel for cardiovascular stent coatings. *Surf. Coatings Technol.* **2010**, *205*, 2461–2468. [CrossRef]

19. Crespin, M.; Moreau, N.; Masereel, B.; Feron, O.; Gallez, B.; Vander Borght, T.; Michiels, C.; Lucas, S. Surface properties and cell adhesion onto allylamine-plasma and amine-plasma coated glass coverslips. *J. Mater. Sci. Mater. Electron.* **2011**, *22*, 671–682. [CrossRef]

20. Testrich, H.; Rebl, H.; Finke, B.; Hempel, F.; Nebe, B.; Meichsner, J. Aging effects of plasma polymerized ethylenediamine (PPEDA) thin films on cell-adhesive implant coatings. *Mater. Sci. Eng. C* **2013**, *33*, 3875–3880. [CrossRef]

21. Manakhov, A.; Landová, M.; Medalová, J.; Michlíček, M.; Polčák, J.; Nečas, D.; Zajíčková, L. Cyclopropylamine plasma polymers for increased cell adhesion and growth. *Plasma Process. Polym.* **2016**, *14*, 1600123. [CrossRef]

22. Chan, K.V.; Asadian, M.; Onyshchenko, I.; Declercq, H.; Morent, R.; De Geyter, N. Biocompatibility of Cyclopropylamine-Based Plasma Polymers Deposited at Sub-Atmospheric Pressure on Poly (ε-caprolactone) Nanofiber Meshes. *Nanomaterials* **2019**, *9*, 1215. [CrossRef] [PubMed]

23. Buddhadasa, M.; Lerouge, S.; Girard-Lauriault, P.-L. Plasma polymer films to regulate fibrinogen adsorption: Effect of pressure and competition with human serum albumin. *Plasma Process. Polym.* **2018**, *15*, 1800040. [CrossRef]

24. Schweikl, H.; Müller, R.; Englert, C.; Hiller, K.-A.; Kujat, R.; Nerlich, M.; Schmalz, G.; Müller, R. Proliferation of osteoblasts and fibroblasts on model surfaces of varying roughness and surface chemistry. *J. Mater. Sci. Mater. Electron.* **2007**, *18*, 1895–1905. [CrossRef] [PubMed]

25. Nebe, J.B.; Finke, B.; Lüthen, F.; Bergemann, C.; Schröder, K.; Rychly, J.; Liefeith, K.; Ohl, A. Improved initial osteoblast functions on amino-functionalized titanium surfaces. *Biomol. Eng.* **2007**, *24*, 447–454. [CrossRef]

26. Finke, B.; Luethen, F.; Schroeder, K.; Mueller, P.D.; Bergemann, C.; Frant, M.; Ohl, A.; Nebe, J.B. The effect of positively charged plasma polymerization on initial osteoblastic focal adhesion on titanium surfaces. *Biomaterials* **2007**, *28*, 4521–4534. [CrossRef]

27. Rebl, H.; Finke, B.; Lange, R.; Weltmann, K.-D.; Nebe, J.B. Impact of plasma chemistry versus titanium surface topography on osteoblast orientation. *Acta Biomater.* **2012**, *8*, 3840–3851. [CrossRef]

28. Staehlke, S.; Rebl, H.; Finke, B.; Mueller, P.; Gruening, M.; Nebe, J.B. Enhanced calcium ion mobilization in osteoblasts on amino group containing plasma polymer nanolayer. *Cell Biosci.* **2018**, *8*, 22. [CrossRef]

29. Hoene, A.; Walschus, U.; Patrzyk, M.; Finke, B.; Lucke, S.; Nebe, B.; Schroeder, K.; Ohl, A.; Schlosser, M. In vivo investigation of the inflammatory response against allylamine plasma polymer coated titanium implants in a rat model. *Acta Biomater.* **2010**, *6*, 676–683. [CrossRef]

30. Finke, B.; Rebl, H.; Hempel, F.; Schäfer, J.; Liefeith, K.; Weltmann, K.-D.; Nebe, J.B. Aging of Plasma-Polymerized Allylamine Nanofilms and the Maintenance of Their Cell Adhesion Capacity. *Langmuir* **2014**, *30*, 13914–13924. [CrossRef]

31. Rebl, H.; Finke, B.; Schmidt, J.; Mohamad, H.S.; Ihrke, R.; Helm, C.A.; Nebe, J.B. Accelerated cell-surface interlocking on plasma polymer-modified porous ceramics. *Mater. Sci. Eng. C* **2016**, *69*, 1116–1124. [CrossRef]

32. Nebe, J.B.; Rebl, H.; Schlosser, M.; Staehlke, S.; Gruening, M.; Weltmann, K.-D.; Walschus, U.; Finke, B. Plasma Polymerized Allylamine—The Unique Cell-Attractive Nanolayer for Dental Implant Materials. *Polymers* **2019**, *11*, 1004. [CrossRef]

33. Moerke, C.; Mueller, P.; Nebe, J.B. Sensing of micropillars by osteoblasts involves complex intracellular signaling. *J. Mater. Sci. Mater. Med.* **2017**, *28*, 171. [CrossRef]

34. Rohr, N.; Zeller, B.; Matthisson, L.; Fischer, J. Surface structuring of zirconia to increase fibroblast viability. *Dent. Mater.* **2020**, *36*, 779–786. [CrossRef]

35. Staehlke, S.; Rebl, H.; Nebe, B. Phenotypic stability of the human MG-63 osteoblastic cell line at different passages: MG-63 cells: Receptors, cell cycle, signaling. *Cell Boil. Int.* **2018**, *43*, 22–32. [CrossRef]

36. Luo, F.; Hong, G.; Matsui, H.; Endo, K.; Wan, Q.; Sasaki, K. Initial osteoblast adhesion and subsequent differentiation on zirconia surfaces are regulated by integrins and heparin-sensitive molecule. *Int. J. Nanomed.* **2018**, *13*, 7657–7667. [CrossRef]

37. Rohr, N.; Nebe, J.B.; Schmidli, F.; Müller, P.; Weber, M.; Fischer, H.; Fischer, J. Influence of bioactive glass-coating of zirconia implant surfaces on human osteoblast behavior in vitro. *Dent. Mater.* **2019**, *35*, 862–870. [CrossRef]

38. Bergemann, C.; Duske, K.; Nebe, J.B.; Schöne, A.; Bulnheim, U.; Seitz, H.; Fischer, J. Microstructured zirconia surfaces modulate osteogenic marker genes in human primary osteoblasts. *J. Mater. Sci. Mater. Med.* **2015**, *26*, 26. [CrossRef]

39. Hempel, U.; Hefti, T.; Dieter, P.; Schlottig, F. Response of human bone marrow stromal cells, MG-63, and SaOS-2 to titanium-based dental implant surfaces with different topography and surface energy. *Clin. Oral Implant. Res.* **2011**, *24*, 174–182. [CrossRef]

40. Lüthen, F.; Lange, R.; Becker, P.; Rychly, J.; Beck, U.; Nebe, J.B. The influence of surface roughness of titanium on β1- and β3-integrin adhesion and the organization of fibronectin in human osteoblastic cells. *Biomaterials* **2005**, *26*, 2423–2440. [CrossRef]

41. Hidalgo-Bastida, L.A.; Cartmell, S. Mesenchymal Stem Cells, Osteoblasts and Extracellular Matrix Proteins: Enhancing Cell Adhesion and Differentiation for Bone Tissue Engineering. *Tissue Eng. Part B Rev.* **2010**, *16*, 405–412. [CrossRef]

42. Schünemann, F.H.; Galárraga-Vinueza, M.E.; Magini, R.; Fredel, M.; Silva, F.; De Souza, J.C.M.; Zhang, Y.; Henriques, B. Zirconia surface modifications for implant dentistry. *Mater. Sci. Eng. C* **2019**, *98*, 1294–1305. [CrossRef]

43. Billiard, J.; Moran, R.A.; Whitley, M.Z.; Chatterjee-Kishore, M.; Gillis, K.; Brown, E.L.; Komm, B.; Bodine, P. Transcriptional profiling of human osteoblast differentiation. *J. Cell. Biochem.* **2003**, *89*, 389–400. [CrossRef]

11

Big Data and Digitalization in Dentistry: A Systematic Review of the Ethical Issues

Maddalena Favaretto [1,*], **David Shaw** [1], **Eva De Clercq** [1], **Tim Joda** [2] and **Bernice Simone Elger** [1]

[1] Institute for Biomedical Ethics, University of Basel, 4056 Basel, Switzerland; david.shaw@unibas.ch (D.S.); eva.declercq@unibas.ch (E.D.C.); b.elger@unibas.ch (B.S.E.)

[2] Department of Reconstructive Dentistry, University Center for Dental Medicine Basel, 4058 Basel, Switzerland; tim.joda@unibas.ch

[*] Correspondence: maddalena.favaretto@unibas.ch

Abstract: Big Data and Internet and Communication Technologies (ICT) are being increasingly implemented in the healthcare sector. Similarly, research in the field of dental medicine is exploring the potential beneficial uses of digital data both for dental practice and in research. As digitalization is raising numerous novel and unpredictable ethical challenges in the biomedical context, our purpose in this study is to map the debate on the currently discussed ethical issues in digital dentistry through a systematic review of the literature. Four databases (Web of Science, Pub Med, Scopus, and Cinahl) were systematically searched. The study results highlight how most of the issues discussed by the retrieved literature are in line with the ethical challenges that digital technologies are introducing in healthcare such as privacy, anonymity, security, and informed consent. In addition, image forgery aimed at scientific misconduct and insurance fraud was frequently reported, together with issues of online professionalism and commercial interests sought through digital means.

Keywords: Big Data; digital dentistry; oral health; ethical issues

---

1. Introduction

The sophistication and increased use of Internet and Communication Technologies (ICT), the rise of Big Data and algorithmic analysis, and the origin of the Internet of Things (IOT) are a plethora of interconnected phenomena that is currently having an enormous impact on today's society and that is affecting almost all spheres of our lives. In recent years, we have seen an exponential growth in the generation, storage, and collection of computational data and the digital revolution is transforming an increasing number of sectors in our society [1,2].

In the biomedical context, for instance, digital technologies are finding numerous novel applications to improve healthcare, cut costs for hospitals, and maximize treatment effectiveness for patients. Examples of such implementations include the development of electronic health records (EHRs) and smarter hospitals for increased workflow [3], personalized medicine and linkage of health data [4], clinical decision support for novel treatment concepts [5], and deep learning and Artificial Intelligence (AI) for diagnostic analysis [6]. In addition, the implementation of mobile technologies into the medical sector is fundamentally altering the ways in which healthcare is perceived, delivered, and consumed. Thanks to the ubiquity of smartphones and wearable technologies, mobile health (mHealth) applications are currently being explored by healthcare providers and companies for remote measurement of health and provision of healthcare services [7].

Dentistry, as a branch of medicine, has not remained unaffected by the digital revolution. The trend in digitalization has led to an increased production of computer-generated data in a growing number of dental disciplines and fields—for example, oral and maxillofacial pathology and surgery, prosthodontics and implant dentistry, and oral public health [8–10]. For this reason, research in the field of dental medicine is currently focusing on exploring the numerous potential beneficial applications of digital and computer-generated data both for dental practice and in research. Population-based linkage of patient-level information could expand new approaches for research such as assisting with the identification of unknown correlations of oral diseases with suspected and new contributing factors and furthering the creation of new treatment concepts [11]. AI applications could help enhance the analysis of the relationship between prevention and treatment techniques in the field of oral health [12]. Digital imaging could promote accurate tracking of the distribution and prevalence of oral diseases to improve healthcare service provisions [13]. Finally, the creation of the digital or virtual dental patient, through the application of sophisticated dental imaging techniques (such as 3D con-beam computed tomography (CBCT) and 3D printed models) could be used for precise pre-operative clinical assessment and simulation of treatment planning in dental practice [9,14]. As these technologies are still at the early phases of implementation, technical issues and disadvantages might also emerge. For instance, data collection for the implementation of Big Data applications and AI must be done systematically according to harmonized and inter-linkable data standards, otherwise issues of data managing and garbage data accumulation might arise [15]. AI for diagnostic purposes is still in the very early phases, where its accuracy is being assessed, and although they are revealing themselves to be valuable for image-based diagnoses, analysis of diverse and massive EHR data still remains challenging [16]. Finally, with regards to the simulation of a 3D virtual dental patient, dataset superimposition techniques are still experimental and none of the currently available imaging techniques are sufficient to capture the complete dataset needed to create the 3D output in a single-step procedure [9].

In the past few years, alongside the ambitious promises of digital technologies in healthcare, the research community has also highlighted many of the potential ethical issues that Big Data and ICT are raising for both patients and other members of society. In the biomedical context, data technologies have been claimed to exacerbate issues of informed consent for both patients and research participants [17,18], and to create new issues regarding privacy, confidentiality [19–21], data security and data protection [22], and patient anonymization [23] and discrimination [24–26]. In addition, recent research has also emphasized additional pressing challenges that could emerge from the inattentive use of increasingly sophisticated digital technologies, such as issues of accuracy and accountability in the use of diagnostic algorithms [27] and the exacerbation of healthcare inequalities [25].

As dentistry is also undergoing the digital path, similar ethical issues might emerge from the application of ICT and Big Data technologies. To the best of our knowledge, there is currently no systematic evaluation of the different ethical issues raised by Big Data and ICT in the field of dentistry, as most of the literature on the topic generally focuses on non-dental medicine and healthcare [28]. As timely ethical evaluation is a consistent part of appropriate health technology assessment [29] and because recent literature has focused on the ethical issues concerning health-related Big Data [28], it is of the utmost importance to map the occurrence of the ethical issues related to the application of heterogeneous digital technologies in dental medicine and to investigate if specific ethical issues for dental Big Data are emerging.

We thus performed a systematic review of the literature. The study has the following aims: (1) mapping the identified ethical issues related to the digitalization of dental medicine and the applications of Big Data and ICT in oral healthcare; (2) investigating the suggested solutions proposed by the literature; and (3) understanding if some applications and practices in digital dentistry could also help overcome some ethical issues.

2. Materials and Methods

We performed a systematic literature review by searching four databases: PubMed, Web of Science, Scopus, and Cinahl. The following search terms were used: "big data", "digital data", "data linkage", "electronic health record *", "EHR", "digital *", "artificial intelligence", "data analytics", "information technology", "dentist *", "dental *", "oral health", "orthodont *", "ethic *", and "moral *". No restriction was placed on the type of methodology used in the paper (qualititative, qualitative, mixed methods, or theoretical). No time restriction was used. In order to enhance reproducibility of the study, we only included original research articles from peer-reviewed journals; therefore, grey literature, books (monographs and edited volumes), conference proceedings, dissertations, and posters were omitted. English was selected as it is the designated language of the highest number of peer-reviewed academic journals. The search was performed on 24 of January 2020 (see Table 1).

Table 1. Search terms.

No.	Match Search Terms	Pub Med	Web of Science	Scopus	Cinahl
1	("big data" OR "digital data" OR "data linkage" OR "electronic health record*" OR "EHR" OR "digital*" OR "artificial intelligence" OR "data analytics" OR "information technology")	251,004	4,682,526	1,750,766	67,116
2	("dentist*" OR "dental *" OR "oral health" OR "orthodont*")	827,547	1,409,796	613,348	158,231
3	("ethic *" OR "moral*")	334,537	582,299	528,738	98,246
4	1 AND 2 AND 3	190	186	71	63

We followed the protocol from the Preferred Reporting Item for Systematic Reviews and Meta-Analyses (PRISMA) method [30], which resulted in 510 papers. We scanned the results for duplicates (125) and 385 papers remained. In this phase, we included all articles that focused on digitalization of dentistry or on one specific digital technology in the field of dentistry and that mentioned, enumerated, discussed, or described one or more ethical challenge related to digitalization. Papers that only described a technology from a technical point of view, that did not focus on dentistry or focused generally on medical practice, or that did not relate to the ethical challenges of digitalization were excluded. Additional papers (27) were excluded because they were book sections, posters, conference proceedings, or not in English. In total, 356 papers were excluded.

We subsequently scanned the references of the remaining 29 articles to identify additional relevant studies. We added five papers through this process. The final sample included 34 articles. During the next phase, the first author read the full texts in their length. After thorough evaluation, eight articles were excluded for the following reasons: (1) they did not discuss or mention any ethical issue related to the technology discussed in the study; and (2) they did not refer to any digital implementation in dentistry (see Figure 1).

The subsequent phase of the study involved the analysis of the remaining 26 articles. Regarding data analysis, we carried out a narrative synthesis of included publications [31]. Therefore, we extracted the following information relevant to the aim of the present study and to the research question from the papers: year and country of publication; methodology; type of technology or digital application discussed; field of application of the article; ethical issues that emerge from the use of the technology; technical issues that might exacerbate the ethical issues discussed; suggested potential solutions to the issue(s); and ethical issues that the technology could help overcome.

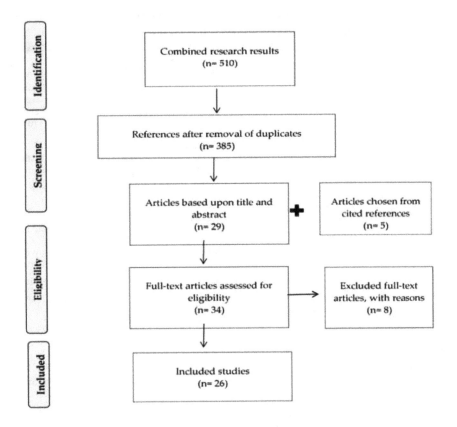

Figure 1. Preferred Reporting Item for Systematic Reviews and Meta-Analyses (PRISMA) flowchart.

3. Results

Among the 26 papers included in our analysis, 22 were theoretical papers that critically discussed the impact of digitalization in the field of dentistry or that discussed a specific technology highlighting its promises and some of its ethical challenges. Among the remaining papers, three applied empirical methods and one was a feasibility study. The majority of papers (n = 20) were published after 2010, five were published between 2008 and 2010, and one of them was from 1996. Half of the articles (n = 13) were from the United States, five came from the United Kingdom, and four from India. The remaining ones came from Belgium, Brazil, Germany, and South Africa. Regarding the type of technological application they discussed, almost one-third of the papers (n = 8) analyzed digital photography, radiology and computed imaging; six papers discussed the impact of digital communication and social media in dentistry; three articles focused on electronic health records (EHRs) and patient records; another three discussed the promises and challenges of mobile health and teledentistry; and an additional three records focused on data linkage and personalized medicine. In addition, two papers broadly discussed the challenges and promises of ICT and digital implementations in dentistry, while one paper focused on search engine optimizations in dental practices. Finally, concerning the field of application of the different papers, 10 articles discussed the ethical issues of digitalization regarding dental practice, nine discussed digitalization and digital application for dentistry without a specific focus, five focused on education and dental school, and two discussed applications in research (see Table 2).

Table 2. Retrieved papers. EHR, electronic health record; mHealth, mobile health; CBCT, con-beam computed tomography; ICT, internet and communication technologies.

Author, Year, Country	Design	Participants	Technology Discussed	Field of Application	Ethical Issues
Boden (2008), USA	Theoretical		Digital transfer of patient records	Dental practice	Justice and autonomy- high charges for the patient prevent beneficial use of records for future patient treatment
Calberson et al. (2008), Belgium	Theoretical		Digital radiography	General	Fraudulent use of radiographs
Cederberg and Valenza (2012), USA	Theoretical		EHR (in dental schools)	Dental school	Justice, patient privacy and security, shift in doctor patient relationship, misconduct from students
Chambers (2012), USA	Theoretical		Digital Communication	Dental practice	Shift in doctor patient relationship, patient privacy and security, professionalism
Cvrker (2018), USA	Theoretical		mHealth	General	Patient access, data ownership, patient privacy and security, bystanders
da Costa et al. (2012), Brazil	Theoretical		Teleorthodontics	General	Patient privacy and security
Day et al. (2018), UK	Feasibility Study	Birth cohort in the United Kingdom	Data linkage	Research	Anonymization, data ownership
Eng et al. (2012), USA	Theoretical		Personalized dentistry	General	Discrimination, confidentiality
Gross et al. (2019), Germany	Theoretical		Digitalization in dentistry	General	Shift in doctor patient relationship, data literacy, responsibility and accountability for AI, digital footprint
Indu et al. (2015), India	Empirical	A sample of postgraduate students and teaching faculties of oral pathology in India	Digital photography	General	Anonymity and security
Jampani et al (2011), India	Theoretical		Teledentistry	General	Confidentiality, patient privacy and security, consent
Kapoor (2015), India	Empirical		Digital photography and radiology	General	Fraudulent use of radiographs/photographs, scientific misconduct
Khelemsky (2011), USA	Theoretical		CBCT	Dental practice	Harm to patient, consent
Knott (2013), UK	Theoretical		ICT	Dental practice	Anonymity, data security, patient privacy
Luther (2010), UK	Theoretical		Digital forensics	Research	Fraudulent use of images, scientific misconduct,
Neville and Waylen (2015), UK	Theoretical		Social Media	Dental practice	Shift in doctor patient relationship, patient Confidentiality, privacy, anonymity
Oakley and Spallek (2012), USA	Theoretical		Social Media	Dental School	Shift in doctor patient relationship, patient privacy and confidentiality, miscommunication, boundary violation
Peltier and Curley (2013), USA	Theoretical		Social Media	Dental practice	Dishonest/unlawful advertising, patient confidentiality
Rao et al. (2010), India	Empirical	A sample of randomly selected clinicians in India	Digital photography	General	Fraudulent use of photographs, scientific misconduct
Spallek er al. (2015), USA	Theoretical		Social Media	Dental School	Shift in doctor patient relationship, patient privacy and confidentiality, miscommunication, boundary violation
Stieber et al. (2015), USA	Theoretical		Electronic media and digital photography	Dental School	Patient privacy and confidentiality, autonomy and consent
Swirsky at al. (2018), USA	Theoretical		Search engine optimization	Dental practice	Beneficence, autonomy, consent, conflict of interest and undue influence

Table 2. *Cont.*

Author, Year, Country	Design	Participants	Technology Discussed	Field of Application	Ethical Issues
Sykes et al (2017), South Africa	Theoretical		Social Media	Dental practice	Patient privacy, anonymity, confidentiality and consent, professionalism, shift in patient doctor relationship, misleading advertisement
Szekely et al. (1996), USA	Theoretical		EHR	Dental practice	Patient privacy and confidentiality, security
Wenworth (2010), USA	Theoretical		Digital Radiography	Dental practice	Patient privacy and confidentiality, misleading advertisement
Zijlstra-Shaw and Stokes (2018), UK	Theoretical		Big Data analytics (in dental education)	Dental school	Consent and data ownership

3.1. Implementation of Digital Technologies in Dentistry

Two papers generally discussed the ethical implications that ICT and digitalization are introducing in dentistry [32,33]. According to Gross et al. [32], digitalization of dentistry is influencing the patient doctor relationship as the integration of digital technologies could distract attention away from the patient during the visit. Issues of data literacy can arise for both the dentist—who will need to constantly be updated on the latest technologies—and the patient—who will need to understand how new technologies work, possibly disfavoring people with poor computer literacy such as the elderly. The application of AI for diagnostic purposes could create issues of responsibility and accountability. A shift might occur towards overtreatment of the patient owing to increased demand for the use of digitized systems. In addition, the constant use, refurbishment, and replacement of increasingly new technology leaves a remarkable digital footprint and aggravates digital pollution. Finally, digital technologies create issues of data security, data falsification, and privacy issues regarding identifiable patient information [33].

3.2. Big Data and Data Analytics

Nine papers discussed the increased employment of Big Data and data analytics in dentistry related to different applications such as data linkage [34], data analytics in dental schools [35], personalized medicine [36], EHRs [37–39], and mHealth and teledentistry [40–42].

3.2.1. Electronic Health Records (EHRs)

Three papers focused on the implementation of EHRs both in private practices and in dental education [37–39]. Ethical issues that arise from this technology are data security, as sensitive patient information could be more easily accessed by unauthorized third parties, resulting in a breach of patient privacy and confidentiality [38,43].

In addition, Cederberg and Valenza [38] argue that the use of digital records might compromise the doctor patient relationship in the future, as easy access to all relevant information through digital means and forced focus on the computer screen could accustom students to becoming more detached from patients.

Suggested solutions for privacy and security issues related to EHR are as follows: (a) the implementation of a three-zone confidentiality model of medical information for databases both linked (networked) and non-linked (network), where different levels of access and security are put in place for different areas—from a more secured inner area that holds the highest sensitive information about the patients (e.g., HIV status and psychiatric care) to an outer, less secured area containing generally publicly available information [37].

3.2.2. mHealth and Teledentistry

Ethical concerns related to mHealth and teledentisry—that is, the use of information technologies and telecommunications to provide remotely dental care, education and raise oral health awareness— were raised by three articles [40–42]. As for other Big Data technologies, issues of data security and patient anonymity [40,41] and confidentiality [42] were the most mentioned, as networked transfer through unsecure means could enable unwarranted third parties to obtain easier access to sensitive patient data.

mHealth might also have an impact on consent both for the patient who might not have been appropriately informed about all of the risks that teledentistry implies [42] and for non-consenting bystanders, whose data might be collected by the device the patient is using [41].

Furthermore, Cvkrel [41] argued that first, mHealth creates additional vulnerability as smartphones gather additional data that are usually not collected by healthcare practitioners (e.g., fitness data, sleep patterns), and, as it is an object of everyday use, it might be easily accessible to unauthorized people. Second, easy access through the smartphone to raw data including data related to dental care could be counterproductive and harmful for patients who might self-adjust the prescription given by the practitioner.

Among the suggested solutions are the following: (a) the establishment of secured networking communication such as the development of state-of-the-art firewalls and antiviruses to mitigate security concerns in telecommunications [40]; (b) the formulation of high quality consent processes that appropriately make the user aware of the risks and all relative factors [41]; and (c) the implementation of information and education about the specific issues that such technology raises for dentists who want to employ teledentistry in their practice.

3.2.3. Personalized Medicine and Data Linkage

In the context of data linkage in dental practices, personalized medicine, and dental schools, the analyzed articles reported how consent issues might arise concerning data usage when the student or the patient cannot be completely informed about the ways in which the collected data is used [35]. Data anonymization [34] and patient confidentiality [36] were again both mentioned as issues of data linkage. Finally, Eng et al. [36] highlighted how discrimination based on higher risk for specific diseases might appear from the linkage of different databases in personalized medicine.

In order to overcome these issues, Eng et al. [36] suggested to develop protective measures at both at a legal and a clinical level to ensure patient data confidentiality and security.

3.3. Digital Communication and Social Media in Dentistry

Seven papers discussed the impact that the employment of digital communication and social media could have upon dental practices and the dentist–patient relationship [44–50].

According to the retrieved studies, one of the main issues is the possibility that commercial values might creep into the management of private practices' websites and official social media pages [44]. For instance, digital media broadcasts might deliver a distorted image of the practice, resulting in misleading or dishonest advertisement of state-of-the-art dental technologies or dental practices, thus exercising an undue influence on patients [47,49]. In addition, Swirsky [50] also raised a concern regarding unethical search engine optimization, an aggressive marketing technique aimed at making your own website appear before others in popular search engines. This practice creates conflict of interest between the dental profession and the patient/public.

Furthermore, the introduction of digital communication in dental practices has heavy effects on the dentist–patient relationship. Neville and Waylen [45] indicate how the use of social media pages is blurring the personal and professional divide. Via social media, patients might have access to information about their dental providers that could compromise the doctor–patient relationship and create issues of trust between the two parties. For instance, shared posts and messages of doctors might be misinterpreted by the users (patients) and be considered unprofessional. Likewise, privacy issues might occur in the case where a dentist visits the personal social media page of their patient and uncovers information that the patient did not want to share with them [46,48]. In addition, doctor–patient confidentiality could be breached by dentists both willingly and inadvertently, if information about a patient is disclosed online, such as identifiable patient photographs or sensitive treatment details [47,49].

Suggested practices to avoid such issues are the development of adequate social media policies for the use of social media in dental practices and increased education for dental practitioners regarding online professionalism in social media—such as awareness of the ethical issues and of the rules of conduct to be used while using social media [48,49].

3.4. Digital Photography and Radiography

The technology discussed by eight of the collected papers was digital photography and digital radiography [51–58]. Among them, four articles [51,53,55,56] highlighted that image modification, made easier by digitalization of both dental photography and radiography, could result in misconduct in science and fraudulent use of modified pictures. Practitioners could be tempted to modify radiographs to deceive insurance companies [51] and researchers might do the same to falsify the results of their research [55].

Three papers correlated the ethical issues of digital imagery to digital sharing and storage of images [52,57,58]. For instance, issues of security of data and patient privacy and confidentiality might arise owing to inattentive storage of images (if digital photographs are stored for too long on an SD-card or if images are shared via electronic means such as using emails and smartphones or networking apps as Whatsapp) [52]. In addition, Stieber et al. [57] indicate how even patient autonomy and consent might be breached if the images are used in an unauthorized manner, such as posting them on a public forum.

Finally, one paper that discussed the ethical issues of digital dental imaging focused on a particular diagnostic technology: cone beam computed tomography (CBCT) [54]. Highlighted issues related to this particular technology are related to its routine use potentially causing harm to patients, especially children and adolescents, owing to the excessive exposure to radiation and consent if patients are not appropriately informed about the health risks they are exposed to when undergoing this diagnostic exam.

Some papers also highlighted some potential solutions. Regarding image modification, the application of state-of-the-art anti-forgery techniques was suggested [51], as well as the development of appropriate guidelines to set an acceptable standard for image modification in dentistry [53]. As for image sharing issues, Stieber et al. [57] suggested the implementation of a privacy compliant framework, where informed consent is enhanced in order to give patients more control over how their images are used, while Indu et al. [52] proposed the use of only custom apps built exclusively for medical data sharing.

3.5. Digital Dentistry Might Solve Ethical Issues

Finally, almost one-third of the papers discussed not only ethical issues, but also mentioned how some of these technologies could be of assistance to solve ethical issues in dentistry and oral health. For instance, the application of digital technologies could result in empowerment of patients and democratization of oral health knowledge owing to increased and widespread information that could be easily retrieved on the Internet [32]. mHealth and teledentistry were argued to be powerful tools to (a) fight known inequalities in healthcare and provide better treatment and patient care in vulnerable populations thanks to the increased saturation of mobile phones and communication technologies that will allow them easier access to health information and remote treatment [41]; (b) overcome cultural and geographic barriers in oral health [40]; and (c) help eliminate the disparities in oral health care between rural and urban communities [42]. Provision of information about health care prevention and oral health issues through social media could positively influence and promote oral healthcare [46,49]. The implementation of research through correlation and data linkage between birth cohorts in the United Kingdom and oral health habits could ameliorate public oral health issues such as caries prevention for children and adolescents [34]. Finally, digital forensics, that is, the digital analysis of images, could help with the recognition of scientific misconduct in dental research [55].

4. Discussion

The analyzed literature raised a plethora of intertwined ethical issues across different technologies and practices in dentistry. Numerous issues are in line with the commonly mentioned ethical challenges that digital technologies are introducing in healthcare—privacy anonymity, security, and so on. On the other hand, additional aspects emerged for dental medicine—such as commercialization and image forgery—that are usually less associated with digitalization of healthcare and Big Data [28].

The most frequently mentioned ethical issues related to the increased digitalization of dentistry are those related to patient privacy, which is often associated with anonymization and confidentiality. This is in line with a study by Mittelstadt and Floridi [28] that highlighted how this cluster of issues related to patient privacy is the one that is most correlated by scholarly research with Big Data technologies such as data analytics, IOT, and social media use. In the era of digitalization, with increased implementation of EHRs and digital data management, issues of privacy become among the most paramount, notably also in dentistry, on account of the opportunities for patient treatment development and research offered by data linkage. Important ethical issues could be overlooked if it is assumed that dental health data are less sensitive than, for example, mental health or stigmatizing infectious disease data. On the contrary, dental health data are sensitive for a number of specific reasons. For example, economic or marketing discrimination, that is, inequality in pricing and offers that are given to costumers based on profiling, such as insurance or housing [59], or discrimination based on health data and health prediction [60], are practices that are creeping out of the exploitation of digital records and might be exacerbated by the analysis of dental records and the use of mHealth in dentistry.

Informed consent was another issue that was often mentioned by the selected papers, although surprisingly not in relationship to the reuse of EHR data. From an ethical and legal point of view, consent needs to be specific concerning three different activities: use for clinical care; clinical trials, where new Big Data technologies are used in dental patients; and secondary use of data for research or other purposes (such as marketing). For use in the clinical setting, issues of informed consent are not so prominent as the EHR would function as a substitute for a paper patient chart, leaving more concerns in the area of data security and patient privacy. However, as Big Data applications for secondary use of EHR data are becoming an increasingly implemented research practice and issues of consent for EHR and Big Data are quite often discussed for the biomedical context [28], more research should be spent in this area for the dental field. In fact, only three retrieved papers focused on EHR—they mostly targeted clinical care, and two of them were from before 2010, which may explain why they did not consider the implications of Big Data and secondary use of data from health records that are currently causing dilemmas of consent from both an ethical and a regulatory point of view [17,61]. Consent was also briefly mentioned by the retrieved papers in relation to data linkage and personalized medicine, but overall, the literature has not sufficiently analyzed the issue data linkage and secondary use of data for dentistry. In fact, electronic dental records increasingly include sensitive and complementary data about the patient, such as automatic tooth charting, general patient health information, development of treatment plans, radiographic captures of the mouth, and intraoral photography [43], which could be linked and analyzed for research and app development purposes without obtaining the appropriate patient's approval. Cvrkel [41], in the context of mHealth, suggested deflecting the discussion from privacy concerns to the development of high-quality consent practices for both clinical as well as secondary research use. On the basis of a recent study by Valenza et al. [62], which assessed the benefits of "Smart consent" strategies that take into account patients' preferences and desires regarding both treatment and the use of their dental data, we argue that the implementation of better consent policies and strategies could also be beneficial to electronic dental records in order to face not only privacy issues related to clinical care, but also issues of consent related to secondary use of data.

As might be expected, considerable space was given to digital photography and radiology in dentistry. Ethical issues were raised in two directions. First, concerns of patient privacy and anonymity and of data security were highlighted in relation to the storage and sharing of digital images [52,57,58]. These issues are of a comparable nature to those enumerated for EHR, mHealth, and teledentistry, which principally have to do with possible access to sensitive patient information by unwarranted parties and interception of digital communications. Interestingly, substantial weight was given to the topic of image forgery. According to the literature, image modification for fraudulent purposes such as insurance fraud and scientific misconduct is described as an expanding practice within dentistry [55,56]. The main problem is that the introduction of digital imagery in our society has exponentially increased the ease with which digital photographs can be manipulated and changed, both in the early and late stages of image production, to a point where essential information about the subject of the image might be falsified [63]. As a consequence, numerous scholars who focused on the epistemic status of photographs and digital imaging have tried to analyze the challenges that digital imaging poses to the epistemic consistency of images [63–65]. The question is, in our opinion, whether in the case of image modification in dentistry, a well-defined line can be settled on acceptable modifications that prevent misinterpretation or misreading by the observer, and modifications that would let the image fall in the category of image forgery. Following clear guidelines on the ethics of image modification [66] could assist practitioners in making the right choices, but might not be enough. Well-intentioned image modification, such as changing the background, modifying light sources, over and under exposure, cropping, color modification, and so on might unintentionally alter the epistemic consistency of an image, as the limit of acceptable alterations that digital images can endure, while maintaining their epistemic value is vague and undetermined [63].

Another interesting finding of this study is that numerous articles—almost one-third of the total and all theoretical papers—rather than expanding on the ethical issues that derive from the application of a medical/dental digital technology, focused on how digital communication could have an impact on the practice of dental care itself and on the doctor–dentist relationship. Some of the retrieved papers [44–49], in fact, highlighted how the inappropriate use of social media by dentists could compromise trust between dental practitioners and patients either owing to leakage of confidential information about patients, such as treatment outcomes or identifiable pictures, or displays of inappropriate behavior on their private social media pages. As the use of social media is permeating our everyday life, blurring the line between private and public, social media and online professionalism are topics that have been increasingly addressed in other areas of healthcare as well [67,68]. The ethical challenge here seems to be twofold. First, education regarding the professional use of social media for dental practitioners could be enhanced by the implementation of rules and social media policies that clearly state the "dos-and-don'ts" of managing a social media page, such as the following: do not post identifiable pictures of patients without their consent; do not discuss patient treatment on the page, and so on [48]. However, if a breach of confidentiality should occur through inattentiveness, the reach of the leaked information would be greater than in face to face exchanges, expanding exponentially the scale of the mistake [67]. Second, it becomes more challenging to implement strategies to appropriately educate dental practitioners about their private social media behavior. It has been argued by Greysen et al. [67] that some online content that might be flagged as unprofessional—such as posts concerning off-duty drinking and intoxication or the advertisement of radical political ideals that might question their professionalism—do not clearly violate any existing principle of medical professionalism, as they are done in the private sphere. In addition, even the interactions that a health practitioner might have with the private social media page of a patient become an intricate matter that might raise ethical dilemmas. By only accessing the page of their patient, the doctor could access private information such as their marital status, sexual orientation, or political orientation that might have an impact, either conscious or unconscious, on the practitioner's personal perception of the patient [69]. Things become even more complicated if the healthcare professional retrieves posts or photos on social media sites that depict patients participating in risk-taking or health-averse behaviors [67]. All of this information might create a fracture in the patient–doctor relationship, as implicit bias and conflict of interests might prevent medical practitioners from providing the patient with the best care [69,70].

In addition, another interesting challenge raised by almost all of the papers that discussed digital communication in dentistry was the issues of commercialization and conflict of interest that interfere with patient care. A strong focus of some of the papers was on the possible exertion of undue influence on the patient by producing misleading advertisement for private practices and state-of-the-art dental procedures. As Chambers et al. [44] argue, the dentist–patient relationship should never shift to one of customer–provider, and commercial interests should always be in a subordinate position to that of oral health, as the well-being of the patient should always come first. In addition, according to the American Dentist Associations' (ADA) Code of Conduct: "dentists who, in the regular conduct of their practices, engage in or employ auxiliaries in the marketing or sale of products or procedures to their patients must take care not to exploit the trust inherent in the dentist–patient relationship for their own financial gain [. . .] and no dentist shall advertise or solicit patients in any form of communication in a manner that is false or misleading in any material respect" [71].

Doing so would negate the patient's right to self-determination and accurate information [50]. As additional technological developments are being increasingly introduced in dental practices, it is of the utmost importance that strong measures are taken to limit commercial interests for dental practice.

In addition, while a substantial number of papers focused on digital photography and radiography, as well as the impact of digital communication for dental practice, this systematic review highlighted some gaps regarding some of the applications that data technologies have in dentistry and the possible ethical issues that might emerge as a consequence. For instance, the implementation of AI applications for diagnostic purposes in dentistry [12] or the sophistication of 3D imaging technologies for pre-operative clinical assessment [9] were not discussed in the retrieved literature. In addition, very few of the retrieved papers focused on the increased application of Big Data analytics and data linkage of health-related data. Shetty et al. [72] highlighted how the debate on digital dentistry is reflective of the traditional dental delivery model and usually focuses on micro trends in technology development such as technology-assisted services (e.g. computer-aided design/computer-aided manufacturing (CAD/CAM)), digital radiography, and electronic patient records. However, trends in the implementations of Big Data technologies such as mHealth, social media, AI, and the like are transforming oral healthcare through social and technical influences from outside the dental profession, as has been seen in relation to the social media use by dental providers. In addition, it has recently been argued that current literature on the topic of digital dentistry has a tendency to focus on its beneficial potentials or on the technical challenges of the discussed technology without appropriately addressing the ethical issues that these technologies might raise [32]. Also, our review indicates that, while a theoretical discussion on this topic is emerging, empirical studies on the ethical issues of digital implementations in dentistry are largely lacking. As a consequence, owing to the sensitive nature of data included in electronic dental records, the specific digital implementations in dental practice and research, and the gaps in the literature regarding the ethical analysis of some dental applications, it is of the outmost importance to conduct additional research, and especially more evidence-based studies, on the possible specific ethical issues related to the field of digital dentistry in order to appropriately understand and confront these issues.

Finally, only a few papers mentioned ethical issues that could be solved by digital dentistry. In addition to those mentioned in Section 3.5, there are two other contenders for useful applications of Big Data research. It has historically been very difficult to conduct epidemiological research on the relationship (if any) between the public health measure of adding fluoride to water supplies and the incidence of dental fluorosis in children owing to the very high number of variables and confounders involved in such research. Big Data analytics could make sense of this difficult area of research, helping to address the public health ethics of water fluoridation [73]. Similarly, antibiotic prophylaxis before dental treatment in patients who have undergone heart surgery remains a contentious area, with dentists tending to recommend against it despite heart surgeons supporting the prescription of antibiotics [74]. Big Data research could help to shed some light on this difficult ethical dilemma.

5. Conclusions

Our study highlighted how most of the issues presented for digital dental technologies such as electronic dental records, mHealth, and teledentistry, as well as developments in personalized medicine, are in line with those mostly discussed in the debate regarding the application of ICT in healthcare, namely, patient privacy, confidentiality and anonymity, data security, and informed consent. In addition to those issues, image forgery aimed at scientific misconduct and insurance fraud was frequently reported in the literature. Moreover, the present review identified how major concerns in the field of dentistry are related to the impact that an improper use of ICT could have on the dental practice and the doctor–patient relationship. In this context, issues of online professionalism were raised together with issues of aggressive or misleading social media or web. Finally, additional research should be conducted to properly assess the ethical issues that might emerge from the routine applications of increasingly novel technologies.

Author Contributions: Conceptualization, M.F., E.D.C., and D.S.; methodology, M.F. and E.D.C.; data analysis, M.F. and E.D.C.; writing—original draft preparation, M.F.; writing—review and editing, D.S., E.D.C., T.J., and B.S.E.; supervision, B.S.E.; funding acquisition, B.S.E. All authors have read and agreed to the published version of the manuscript.

Acknowledgments: The first author would like to thank Christophe Schneble for his support during data collection and analysis.

References

1. Lynch, C. How do your data grow? *Nature* **2008**, *455*, 28–29. [CrossRef]
2. Boyd, D.; Crawford, K. CRITICAL QUESTIONS FOR BIG DATA. *Info. Commun. Soc.* **2012**, *15*, 662–679. [CrossRef]
3. Mertz, L. Saving Lives and Money with Smarter Hospitals: Streaming analytics, other new tech help to balance costs and benefits. *IEEE Pulse* **2014**, *5*, 33–36. [CrossRef] [PubMed]
4. Cohen, I.G.; Amarasingham, R.; Shah, A.; Xie, B.; Lo, B. The Legal And Ethical Concerns That Arise From Using Complex Predictive Analytics In Health Care. *Heal. Aff.* **2014**, *33*, 1139–1147. [CrossRef] [PubMed]
5. Lee, C.H.; Yoon, H.-J. Medical big data: promise and challenges. *Kidney Res. Clin. Pr.* **2017**, *36*, 3–11. [CrossRef]
6. Liu, X.; Faes, L.; Kale, A.U.; Wagner, S.K.; Fu, D.J.; Bruynseels, A.; Mahendiran, T.; Moraes, G.; Shamdas, M.; Kern, C.; et al. A comparison of deep learning performance against health-care professionals in detecting diseases from medical imaging: a systematic review and meta-analysis. *Lancet Digit. Heal.* **2019**, *1*, e271–e297. [CrossRef]
7. Nilsen, W.J.; Kumar, S.; Shar, A.; Varoquiers, C.; Wiley, T.; Riley, W.T.; Pavel, M.; Atienza, A.A. Advancing the Science of mHealth. *J. Heal. Commun.* **2012**, *17*, 5–10. [CrossRef]
8. Fasbinder, D.J. Digital dentistry: innovation for restorative treatment. *Compend. Contin. Educ. Dent.* **2010**, *31*, 2–11.
9. Joda, T.; Wolfart, S.; Reich, S.; Zitzmann, N.U. Virtual Dental Patient: How Long Until It's Here? *Curr. Oral Heal. Rep.* **2018**, *5*, 116–120. [CrossRef]
10. Finkelstein, J.; Ba, F.Z.; Bs, S.A.L.; Cappelli, D. Using big data to promote precision oral health in the context of a learning healthcare system. *J. Public Heal. Dent.* **2020**, *80*, S43–S58. [CrossRef]
11. Joda, T.; Waltimo, T.; Pauli-Magnus, C.; Probst-Hensch, N.; Zitzmann, N.U. Population-Based Linkage of Big Data in Dental Research. *Int. J. Environ. Res. Public Heal.* **2018**, *15*, 2357. [CrossRef] [PubMed]
12. Joda, T.; Waltimo, T.; Probst-Hensch, N.; Pauli-Magnus, C.; Zitzmann, N.U. Health Data in Dentistry: An Attempt to Master the Digital Challenge. *Public Heal. Genom.* **2019** *22*, 1–7. [CrossRef] [PubMed]

13. Hogan, R.; Goodwin, M.; Boothman, N.; Iafolla, T.; Pretty, I.A. Further opportunities for digital imaging in dental epidemiology. *J. Dent.* **2018**, *74*, S2–S9. [CrossRef] [PubMed]

14. Vandenberghe, B. The digital patient – Imaging science in dentistry. *J. Dent.* **2018**, *74*, S21–S26. [CrossRef]

15. Brodt, E.D.; Skelly, A.C.; Dettori, J.R.; Hashimoto, R.E. Administrative Database Studies: Goldmine or Goose Chase? *Evid Based Spine Care J.* **2014**, *5*, 74–76. [CrossRef]

16. Liang, H.; Tsui, B.Y.; Ni, H.; Valentim, C.C.S.; Baxter, S.L.; Liu, G.; Cai, W.; Kermany, D.S.; Sun, X.; Chen, J.; et al. Evaluation and accurate diagnoses of pediatric diseases using artificial intelligence. *Nat. Med.* **2019**, *25*, 433–438. [CrossRef]

17. Ioannidis, J.P. Informed consent, big data, and the oxymoron of research that is not research. *Am. J. Bioeth.* **2013**, *13*, 40–42. [CrossRef]

18. Martani, A.; Geneviève, L.D.; Pauli-Magnus, C.; McLennan, S.; Elger, B.S. Regulating the Secondary Use of Data for Research: Arguments Against Genetic Exceptionalism. *Front. Genet.* **2019**, *10*, 1254. [CrossRef]

19. Francis, J.G.; Francis, L.P. Privacy, Confidentiality, and Justice. *J. Soc. Philos.* **2014**, *45*, 408–431. [CrossRef]

20. Schneble, C.O.; Elger, B.S.; Shaw, D. The Cambridge Analytica affair and Internet-mediated research. *EMBO Rep.* **2018**, *19*, e46579. [CrossRef]

21. Schneble, C.O.; Elger, B.S.; Shaw, D. Google's Project Nightingale highlights the necessity of data science ethics review. *EMBO Mol. Med.* **2020**, *12*(3), e12053. [CrossRef] [PubMed]

22. McMahon, A.; Buyx, A.; Prainsack, B. Big Data Governance Needs More Collective Responsibility: The Role of Harm Mitigation in the Governance of Data Use in Medicine and Beyond. *Med Law Rev.* **2019**, *28*, 155–182. [CrossRef] [PubMed]

23. Choudhury, S.; Fishman, J.R.; McGowan, M.L.; Juengst, E. Big data, open science and the brain: lessons learned from genomics. *Front. Hum. Neurosci.* **2014**, *8*, 239. [CrossRef] [PubMed]

24. Favaretto, M.; De Clercq, E.; Elger, B.S. Big Data and discrimination: perils, promises and solutions. A systematic review. *J. Big Data* **2019**, *6*, 12. [CrossRef]

25. Geneviève, L.D.; Martani, A.; Shaw, D.M.; Elger, B.S.; Wangmo, T. Structural racism in precision medicine: leaving no one behind. *BMC Med Ethic* **2020**, *21*, 1–13. [CrossRef]

26. Martani, A.; Shaw, D.; Elger, B.S. Stay fit or get bit - ethical issues in sharing health data with insurers' apps. *Swiss Med Wkly.* **2019**, *149*, w20089. [CrossRef]

27. Martin, K.E.M. Ethical Implications and Accountability of Algorithms. *SSRN Electron. J.* **2018**, *160*, 835–850. [CrossRef]

28. Mittelstadt, B.D.; Floridi, L. The ethics of big data: current and foreseeable issues in biomedical contexts. *Sci. Eng. Ethics* **2016**, *22*, 303–341. [CrossRef]

29. Esfandiari, S.; Feine, J. Health technology assessment in oral health. *Int. J. Oral Maxillofac. Implant.* **2011**, *26*, 93–100.

30. Moher, D.; Shamseer, L.; Clarke, M.; Ghersi, D.; Liberati, A.; Petticrew, M.; Shekelle, P.G.; Stewart, L.A. Preferred reporting items for systematic review and meta-analysis protocols (PRISMA-P) 2015 statement. *Syst. Rev.* **2015**, *4*, 1. [CrossRef]

31. Rodgers, M.; Sowden, A.; Petticrew, M.; Arai, L.; Roberts, H.M.; Britten, N.; Popay, J. Testing Methodological Guidance on the Conduct of Narrative Synthesis in Systematic Reviews. *Evaluation* **2009**, *15*, 49–73. [CrossRef]

32. Gross, D.; Gross, K.; Wilhelmy, S. Digitalization in dentistry: ethical challenges and implications. *Quintessence Int.* **2019**, *50*, 830–838. [PubMed]

33. Knott, N.J. The use of information and communication technology (ICT) in dentistry. *Br. Dent. J.* **2013**, *214*, 151–153. [CrossRef] [PubMed]

34. Day, P.F.; Petherick, E.; Godson, J.; Owen, J.; Douglas, G. A feasibility study to explore the governance processes required for linkage between dental epidemiological, and birth cohort, data in the UK. *Community Dent. Health* **2018**, *35*, 228–234.

35. Zijlstra-Shaw, S.; Stokes, C.W. Learning analytics and dental education; choices and challenges. *Eur. J. Dent. Educ.* **2018**, *22*, e658–e660. [CrossRef]

36. Eng, G.; Chen, A.; Vess, T.; Ginsburg, G.S. Genome technologies and personalized dental medicine. *Oral Dis.* **2011**, *18*, 223–235. [CrossRef]

37. Boden, D.F. What Guidance Is There for Ethical Records Transfer and Fee Charges? *J. Am. Dent. Assoc.* **2008**, *139*, 197–198. [CrossRef]

38. A Cederberg, R.; A Valenza, J. Ethics and the electronic health record in dental school clinics. *J. Dent. Educ.* **2012** *76*, 584–589.

39. Szekely, D.G.; Milam, S.; A Khademi, J. Legal issues of the electronic dental record: Security and confidentiality. *J. Dent. Educ.* **1996**, *60*, 19–23.

40. Da Costa, A.L.P.; Silva, A.A.; Pereira, C.B. Tele-orthodontics: Tool aid to clinical practice and continuing education. *Dental Press J. Orthod. Rev.* **2012**, *16*, 15–21.

41. Cvrkel, T. The ethics of mHealth: Moving forward. *J. Dent.* **2018**, *74*, S15–S20. [CrossRef] [PubMed]

42. Nutalapati, R.; Boyapati, R.; Jampani, N.D.; Dontula, B.S.K. Applications of teledentistry: A literature review and update. *J. Int. Soc. Prev. Community Dent.* **2011**, *1*, 37–44. [CrossRef]

43. Cederberg, R.; Walji, M.; Valenza, J. *Electronic Health Records in Dentistry: Clinical Challenges and Ethical Issues*; Springer Science and Business Media LLC: Cham, Switzerland, 2014; pp. 1–12.

44. Chambers, D.W. Position paper on digital communication in dentistry. *J. Am. Coll. Dent.* **2012**, *79*, 19–30. [PubMed]

45. Neville, P.; Waylen, A.E. Social media and dentistry: some reflections on e-professionalism. *Br. Dent. J.* **2015**, *218*, 475–478. [CrossRef] [PubMed]

46. Oakley, M.; Spallek, H. Social media in dental education: a call for research and action. *J. Dent. Educ.* **2012**, *76*, 279–287. [PubMed]

47. Peltier, B.; Curley, A. The ethics of social media in dental practice: Ethical tools and professional responses. *J. Calif. Dent. Assoc.* **2013**, *41*, 507–513. [PubMed]

48. Spallek, H.; Turner, S.P.; Donate-Bartfield, E.; Chambers, D.; McAndrew, M.; Zarkowski, P.; Karimbux, N. Social Media in the Dental School Environment, Part A: Benefits, Challenges, and Recommendations for Use. *J. Dent. Educ.* **2015**, *79*, 1140–1152.

49. Sykes, L.M.; Harryparsad, A.; Evans, W.G.; Gani, F. Social Media and Dentistry: Part 8: Ethical, legal, and professional concerns with the use of internet sites by health care professionals. *SADJ* **2017**, *72*, 132–136.

50. Swirsky, E.S.; Michaels, C.; Stuefen, S.; Halasz, M. Hanging the digital shingle. *J. Am. Dent. Assoc.* **2018**, *149*, 81–85. [CrossRef]

51. Calberson, F.L.; Hommez, G.M.; De Moor, R.J. Fraudulent Use of Digital Radiography: Methods to Detect and Protect Digital Radiographs. *J. Endod.* **2008**, *34*, 530–536. [CrossRef]

52. Indu, M.; Sunil, S.; Rathy, R.; Binu, M. Imaging and image management: A survey on current outlook and awareness in pathology practice. *J. Oral Maxillofac. Pathol.* **2015**, *19*, 153–157. [CrossRef] [PubMed]

53. Kapoor, P. Photo-editing in Orthodontics: How Much is Too Much? *Int. J. Orthod.* **2015**, *26*, 17–23.

54. Khelemsky, R. The ethics of routine use of advanced diagnostic technology. *J. Am. Coll. Dent.* **2011**, *78*, 35–39. [PubMed]

55. Luther, F. Scientific Misconduct. *J. Dent. Res.* **2010**, *89*, 1364–1367. [CrossRef]

56. Rao, S.; Singh, N.; Kumar, R.; Thomas, A. More than meets the eye: Digital fraud in dentistry. *J. Indian Soc. Pedod. Prev. Dent.* **2010**, *28*, 241. [CrossRef]

57. Stieber, J.C.; Nelson, T.M.; E Huebner, C. Considerations for use of dental photography and electronic media in dental education and clinical practice. *J. Dent. Educ.* **2015**, *79*, 432–438.

58. Wentworth, R.B. What ethical responsibilities do I have with regard to radiographs for my patients? *J. Am. Dent. Assoc.* **2010**, *141*, 718–720. [CrossRef]

59. Peppet, S.R. Regulating the internet of things: first steps toward managing discrimination, privacy, security and consent. *Tex. L. Rev.* **2014**, *93*, 85.

60. Hoffman, S. Employing e-health: the impact of electronic health records on the workplace. *Kan. JL Pub. Pol'y* **2009**, *19*, 409.

61. Starkbaum, J.; Felt, U. Negotiating the reuse of health-data: Research, Big Data, and the European General Data Protection Regulation. *Big Data Soc.* **2019**, *6*, 2053951719862594. [CrossRef]

62. Valenza, J.A.; Taylor, D.; Walji, M.F.; Johnson, C.W. Assessing the benefit of a personalized EHR-generated informed consent in a dental school setting. *J. Dent. Educ.* **2014**, *78*, 1182–1193. [PubMed]

63. Benovsky, J. The Limits of Photography. *Int. J. Philos. Stud.* **2014**, *22*, 716–733. [CrossRef]

64. Hopkins, R. Factive Pictorial Experience: What's Special about Photographs? *Nous* **2010**, *46*, 709–731. [CrossRef]

65. Alcarez, A.L. Epistemic function and ontology of analog and digital images. *CA* **2015**, *13*, 11.

66. Cromey, D. Avoiding twisted pixels: ethical guidelines for the appropriate use and manipulation of scientific digital images. *Sci. Eng. Ethic* **2010**, *16*, 639–667. [CrossRef]

67. Greysen, R.; Kind, T.; Chretien, K.C. Online Professionalism and the Mirror of Social Media. *J. Gen. Intern. Med.* **2010**, *25*, 1227–1229. [CrossRef]

68. Ventola, C.L. Social Media and Health Care Professionals: Benefits, Risks, and Best Practices. *J. Formul. Manag.* **2014**, *39*, 491–520.

69. Fitzgerald, C.; Hurst, S. Implicit bias in healthcare professionals: A systematic review. *BMC Med. Ethics* **2017**, *18*, 19. [CrossRef]

70. Garrison, N.O.; Ibañez, G.E. Attitudes of Health Care Providers toward LGBT Patients: The Need for Cultural Sensitivity Training. *Am. J. Public Heal.* **2016**, *106*, 570. [CrossRef]

71. McCarley, D.H. ADA Principles of Ethics and Code of Professional Conduct. *Tex. Dent. J.* **2011**, *128*, 728–732.

72. Shetty, V.; Yamamoto, J.; Yale, K. Re-architecting oral healthcare for the 21st century. *J. Dent.* **2018**, *74*, S10–S14. [CrossRef] [PubMed]

73. Shaw, D.M. Weeping and wailing and gnashing of teeth: The legal fiction of water fluoridation. *Med Law Int.* **2012**, *12*, 11–27. [CrossRef]

74. Shaw, D.; Conway, D. Pascal's Wager, infective endocarditis and the "no-lose" philosophy in medicine. *Heart* **2009**, *96*, 15–18. [CrossRef] [PubMed]

12

Marginal and Internal Fit of Ceramic Restorations Fabricated Using Digital Scanning and Conventional Impressions

Jeong-Hyeon Lee [1,2,†], Keunbada Son [2,3,†]⬤ and Kyu-Bok Lee [1,2,*]

[1] Department of Prosthodontics, School of Dentistry, Kyungpook National University, 2177 Dalgubeol-daero, Jung-gu, Daegu 41940, Korea; prossn@naver.com
[2] Advanced Dental Device Development Institute (A3DI), Kyungpook National University, 2177 Dalgubeol-daero, Jung-gu, Daegu 41940, Korea; sonkeunbada@gmail.com
[3] Department of Dental Science, Graduate School, Kyungpook National University, 2177 Dalgubeol-daero, Jung-gu, Daegu 41940, Korea
* Correspondence: kblee@knu.ac.kr
† These authors contributed equally to this work (co-first author).

Abstract: This clinical study was designed with the aim of fabricating four ceramic crowns using the conventional method and digital methods with three different intraoral scanners and evaluate the marginal and internal fit as well as clinician satisfaction. We enrolled 20 subjects who required ceramic crowns in the upper or lower molar or the premolar. Impressions were obtained using digital scans, with conventional impressions (polyvinyl siloxane and desktop scanner) and three different intraoral scanners (EZIS PO, i500, and CS3600). Four lithium disilicate glass-ceramic crowns were fabricated for each patient. In the oral cavity, the proximal and occlusal adjustments were performed, and the marginal fit and internal fit were evaluated using the silicone replica technique. The clinician satisfaction score of the four crowns was evaluated as per the evaluations of the proximal and occlusal contacts made during the adjustment process and the marginal and internal fit. For statistical analysis, the differences among the groups were analyzed with one-way analysis of variance and Tukey HSD test as a post-test; Pearson correlation analysis was used for analyzing the correlations ($\alpha = 0.05$). There was a significant difference in the marginal and internal fit of the ceramic crowns fabricated using three intraoral scanner types and one desktop scanner type ($p < 0.001$); there was a significant difference in the clinician satisfaction scores ($p = 0.04$). The clinician satisfaction score and marginal fit were significantly correlated (absolute marginal discrepancy and marginal gap) ($p < 0.05$). An impression technique should be considered for fabricating a ceramic crown with excellent goodness-of-fit. Further, higher clinician satisfaction could be obtained by reproducing the excellent goodness-of-fit using the intraoral scanning method as compared to the conventional method.

Keywords: marginal and internal fit; intraoral scanner; conventional method; ceramic crown; digital workflow

1. Introduction

In the processes of fabricating and restoring prostheses, it is crucial to take impressions accurately [1–3]. The use of conventional impression material for taking impressions causes the patient discomfort, such as gagging; further, there may be various problems, such as the possibility of deformation of the impression material and contamination by the saliva and blood in the oral cavity [3,4]. In contrast, the use of an intraoral canner for taking a digital impression is a method that obtains impressions via direct scanning [5,6]. Moreover, it is possible to correct it and check the bite, looking at the three-dimensional (3D) virtual cast displayed in real time on the monitor [7]. In the conventional method that uses impression material, dental stone, investing material, and alloy, etc., there are differences in the expansion and contraction rate of each material; therefore, the goodness-of-fit of the prostheses may differ, depending on the proficiency of the dental technician [8]. However, prosthesis fabrication using an intraoral scanner offers the advantage in that the work process can be standardized [9]. Furthermore, digital impression taking is unlikely to cause the deformation of the impression material, and the additional scan and work are easy [9]. In addition, compared to conventional impression taking, this method involves a lower cost and less time; thus, this method tends to be used increasingly [10].

An intraoral scanner is an essential tool in chairside computer-aided design and computer-aided manufacturing (CAD/CAM) system because it allows the acquisition of a virtual cast directly from the patient's oral cavity without the need for any additional work process [11–15]. In the dental clinic, where quick fabrication is necessary, lithium disilicate ceramic material is preferred because it takes less milling time and less crystallization time [16]. The lithium disilicate ceramic crown is superior to a zirconia crown in terms of better aesthetics, faster fabrication, and easier post-processing process [17,18].

The accuracy of the impression obtained from the patient's oral cavity is important for the fabrication of a well-fitting prosthesis [13–16]. The deformation of the impression may lead to poor marginal and internal fit of the prostheses along with inaccurate working cast fabrication [13,14]. This may cause issues, such as plaque deposits in the oral cavity, secondary caries, cement dissolution, and periodontal disease [13]. Furthermore, the poor internal fit may cause loss of the retention force of the prostheses and lower fracture resistance [14,16]. In general, it is judged that the clinically allowable marginal fit of the fixed prostheses is 100–120 μm [17–20]. Previous studies fabricated zirconia coping, using an intraoral scanner, and reported about 100 μm as the marginal fit [21,22]. Many earlier trials have shown various results of the marginal fit [23–26]; however, few studies have studied the marginal and internal fit of the crowns fabricated using various intraoral scanners.

Several studies have compared the conventional method to the digital method [27–31]. However, the results were different and inconsistent [29–31]. Some studies have demonstrated superior accuracy of the conventional method [23–25], and some have shown better results using the digital method [27,28]. However, most previous studies were in vitro trials that performed extraoral evaluations, and various conditions that might be reflected in the oral cavity (obstacles, such as saliva, limited scan space, tongue, and cheek) have not been reflected [23–25]. Thus, in vivo studies conducted directly in the oral cavity with the conventional method of impression taking and intraoral scanning are continuously needed. In addition, most previous studies have compared the marginal and internal fit of the crowns fabricated using the conventional and digital method. There is insufficient research on the comparison of the ceramic crowns fabricated with different intraoral scanners [23–25].

In the present clinical study, we fabricated four ceramic crowns for each patient using the conventional method and the digital method using three different intraoral scanners and compare the marginal and internal fit of the ceramic crowns with respect to clinician satisfaction. The first null hypothesis is that there would be no differences in the marginal and internal fit of the prostheses fabricated using the conventional and digital methods. The second null hypothesis is that the marginal and internal fit of the ceramic crowns and clinician satisfaction were not correlated.

2. Materials and Methods

The present clinical test was conducted after obtaining approval from the IRB of the Kyungpook National University Dental Hospital (Approval Number: KNUDH-2019-02-02-02). The present clinical study was conducted from April 2019 to April 2020. Twenty subjects (10 women and 10 men) who required a ceramic crown on the upper or lower molar or premolar were enrolled. Of the participants, those with poor oral hygiene or more than one crown; those with parafunctional activities, such as bruxism, clenching, and grinding; those with acute or chronic temporomandibular joint dysfunction sensation or mental abnormalities; and those with serious medical conditions; as well as those who were a pregnant or breastfeeding were excluded. Based on the pilot experiment, training was provided for all the processes involved in the fabrication of ceramic crowns; using power software (G*Power version 3.1.9.2; Heinrich-Heine-Universität Düsseldorf, Düsseldorf, Germany), 20 participants were selected for the analyses (actual power = 96.1%; power = 95%; $\alpha = 0.05$).

All the subjects were trained for intraoral scanning, crown design using CAD software, and all digital workflows, including the CAM process in advance. All the intraoral processes were prepared by one skilled dentist. The dentist was blinded to the information about the type of crown. Abutment teeth were ground as per the standard crown treatment guidelines [32]. All the abutment teeth were ground, using diamond rotary cutting instruments (852.FG.010; Jota AG, Rüthi, SG, Switzerland) to have 0.5-mm supragingival finish line, 2-mm occlusal reduction, and 6-degree convergence angle; the line range was rounded.

Impressions were obtained, using a conventional impression (desktop scanner) and three intraoral scanner types for each patient (Figure 1). All the scanners used in the present clinical study were calibrated immediately before performing scanning, and scanning was done under uniform conditions of ambient light and surface condition of the dried tooth by a single skilled operator. The same skilled dentist (J.-H.L.) conducted all the clinical tests, and four ceramic crowns were fabricated for each patient.

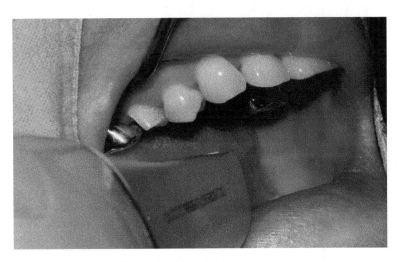

Figure 1. Intraoral scanning.

Group 1: Conventional impression (polyvinyl siloxane (PVS) (Aquasil Ultra; Dentsply Sirona, Bensheim, Germany) (PVS group)
Group 2: Intraoral scanner (EZIS PO; DDS, Seoul, South Korea) (EZIS PO group)
Group 3: Intraoral scanner (i500; MEDIT, Seoul, South Korea) (i500 group)
Group 4: Intraoral scanner (CS3600; Carestream Dental, Atlanta USA) (CS3600 group)

For the PVS Group, an impression was taken, using PVS impression and a double-arch tray (Dual Arch Impression Tray; 3M, MN, USA) in the oral cavity. For the material of the obtained impression, a working cast was fabricated, using Type IV dental stone (FUGIROCK; GC, Leuven, Belgium). The fabricated working cast was scanned with a desktop scanner (E1; 3Shape, Copenhagen, Denmark) and converted to an STL file. All the processes of the working cast fabrication, desktop scanning, and ceramic crown fabrication were performed by a skilled dental technician. For Intraoral Scan Groups, three intraoral scanner types were used, including EZIS PO, i500, and CS3600. All the digital scans were performed as per the manufacturers' instructions. All the intraoral scanning processes were performed by a skilled dentist (J.-H.L.).

In the scan file obtained from each group, the cement space was set at 80 μm in the dental CAD software (EZIS VR; DDS, Seoul, Korea), and the crown was designed for the anatomical shape (Figure 2). After the design preparation was complete, crowns were fabricated, using four-axis milling equipment (EZIS HM; DDS, Seoul, Korea). For the crown material, lithium disilicate glass-ceramic block (IPS e.max CAD; Ivoclar Vivadent AG, Schaan, Liechtenstein) was used. The milled ceramic crown was cleaned using the method recommended by the manufacturer, and it was crystallized and finished. Four ceramic crowns were fabricated for each patient, and 80 ceramic crowns were fabricated for 20 patients.

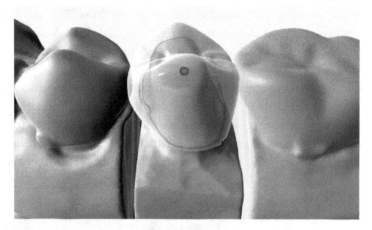

Figure 2. Computer-aided design of a crown.

Four crowns were tried for each patient intraorally and adjusted to enable optimum proximal and occlusal contacts. The marginal and internal fit for the adjustment and cementation in the oral cavity was subjected to clinical evaluation. The marginal fit was checked for appropriateness by probing with a dental explorer (5 XTS™ EXPLORER; Hu-Friedy, Chicago, IL, USA), and the internal fit was checked with silicone paste (Fit Checker; GC, Tokyo, Japan). After trying that in by putting the silicone paste, it was hardened under the patient's bite force (Figure 3), and the transparent region of the silicon was marked on the intaglio surface of the crown, using graphite and adjusted with a diamond rotary cutting instrument. Finally, the occlusal contacts of the ceramic crown were adjusted. Using articulating paper (AccuFilm II; Parkell, Inc., Farmingdale, NY, USA), the regions of earlier contacts or interference were checked during the centric occlusion and eccentric occlusion and carefully removed, using diamond rotary cutting instruments. Using shim stock foil, proximal, and occlusal contacts were checked, and the final grinding was performed as per the recommendation of the manufacturer of the lithium disilicate glass-ceramic.

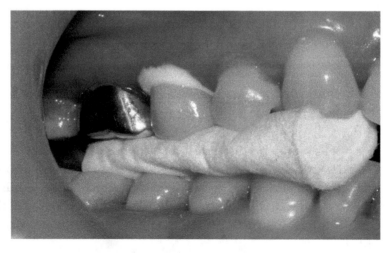

Figure 3. Taking silicone film for checking the fit.

For each patient, the marginal and internal fit of four ceramic crowns was evaluated, using the silicone replica technique. After all the adjustments were made, silicone indicator paste (Fit Checker; GC, Tokyo, Japan) was injected into the intaglio surface of each crown, and the position of the crown was maintained at the patient's bite force till the end of the silicon polymerization process. After the hardening of the silicone indicator paste, the ceramic crown was removed, and a light-body PVS impression was (Aquasil Ultra; Dentsply Sirona, Bensheim, Germany) was injected in the intaglio surface of the crown and hardened for five minutes to support the thin silicon layer. The silicon in which the space between the ceramic crown and the abutment tooth was duplicated was cut from the crown in the medial-mesiodistal and buccolingual directions, and the gap was evaluated at 60× magnification with an industrial video microscope system (IMS 1080P; SOMETECH, Seoul, Korea). With respect to the position of measurement, marginal fit (absolute marginal discrepancy and marginal gap) and internal fit (chamfer, axial, angle, and occlusal gap) were measured (Figure 4). In the internal fit, the chamfer gap was evaluated at the central point of the chamfer region, and the angle gap was assessed at the central point of the angle region. The axial gap was evaluated at the central point between the chamfer gap and the angle gap, and the occlusal gap was measured at the center of the occlusal region and the central point of the axial gap.

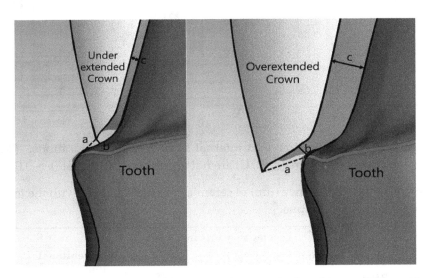

Figure 4. Schematic showing measurement positions for marginal and internal fit. a, Absolute marginal discrepancy. b, Marginal gap. c, Internal gap.

One prosthetic dentist evaluated the quality of the four crowns for each patient based on the clinician satisfaction score. The order of the four crowns was set based on the evaluations of the proximal and occlusal contacts performed in the adjustment process and the marginal and internal fit. The crown showing the best quality was assigned four points and that with the lowest quality was scored one point. The best ceramic crown was chosen and cemented as per the standard prosthetic protocol.

All the data were analyzed using SPSS statistical software (IBM, Armonk, NY, USA). First, the normality of the data was investigated using Shapiro–Wilk test. The data were normal, and the equality of dispersion was evaluated using the Levene test. As per the result, the differences among the groups were analyzed using One-way ANOVA and Tukey HSD test as a post-test ($\alpha = 0.05$).

Moreover, in order to analyze the correlations between the marginal and internal fit and the clinician satisfaction score, Pearson correlation analysis was used. The correlations were divided as per the size of the Pearson correlation coefficient (PCC), as reported previously [33]. The results of the correlation analysis among the variables were explained through the following criteria by the previous studies [14,16,33]: perfect (PCC = +1 or −1), strong (PCC = +0.7–+0.9 or −0.7––0.9), moderate (PCC = +0.4–+0.6 or −0.4––0.6), and weak (PCC = +0.1–+0.3 or −0.1––0.3) ($\alpha = 0.05$).

3. Results

There were significant differences in the marginal and internal fit of the ceramic crowns fabricated using three intraoral scanner types and one desktop scanner type ($p < 0.001$; Figure 5; Table 1). There was no significant difference in the marginal gap as per the three intraoral scanner types ($p > 0.05$; Figure 5; Table 1). There was a higher value for the gap of the marginal fit (absolute marginal discrepancy and marginal gap) in the desktop scanner as compared to that in the three intraoral scanner types ($p < 0.001$; Figure 5; Table 1). There was a significant difference in the internal fit based on the three intraoral scanner types and the desktop scanner ($p < 0.001$); however, no special tendency was observed among the groups (Figure 5; Table 1).

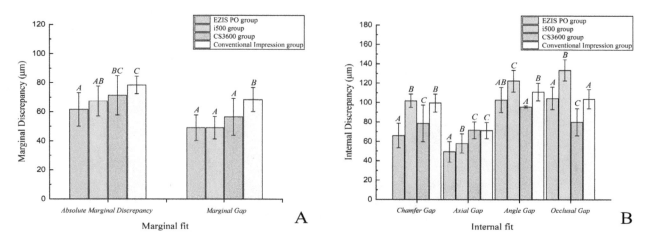

Figure 5. Comparison of the marginal and internal fit of ceramic restorations. (**A**) Marginal fit. (**B**) Internal fit. Same uppercase letters (A, B, C) are not significantly different ($p > 0.05$).

Table 1. Comparison of the discrepancy (μm) of ceramic crowns fabricated with the intraoral scanners and conventional impression technique.

Measurement Position	Discrepancy (Mean ± SD)				F	p
	Intraoral Scanner Group			Conventional Impression Technique		
	EZIS PO	i500	CS3600			
Absolute Marginal Discrepancy	61.6 ± 11.5 A	67.4 ± 10.2 A,B	71.3 ± 13.5 B,C	78.4 ± 6 C	8.758	<0.001 *
Marginal Gap	49.1 ± 8.8 A	49.1 ± 7.7 A	56.5 ± 12.7 A	68.4 ± 8.3 B	17.771	<0.001 *
Chamfer Gap	65.9 ± 12.7 A	101.9 ± 6.9 B	78.5 ± 18.8 C	99.5 ± 9.3 B	36.483	<0.001 *
Axial Gap	49.2 ± 10.6 A	58 ± 10 B	71.6 ± 8.6 C	71.3 ± 8.3 C	26.547	<0.001 *
Angle Gap	102.8 ± 12.9 A,B	122.4 ± 11.2 C	95.7 ± 12.8 A	111.2 ± 9 B	19.505	<0.001 *
Occlusal Gap	104.5 ± 11.6 A	133.5 ± 11 B	80 ± 13.9 C	103.7 ± 9.9 A	69.547	<0.001 *

* $p < 0.05$; significance was determined using one-way ANOVA. Different letters (A, B, C) indicate that the difference between the groups was significant, as determined using Tukey's HSD post hoc test ($p < 0.05$).

There were significant differences in the clinician satisfaction score of the ceramic crowns fabricated with three intraoral scanner types and one desktop scanner type ($p = 0.04$; Figure 6; Table 2). The value of the clinician satisfaction score was lower in the desktop scanner as compared to that in the three intraoral scanner types ($p < 0.001$; Figure 6; Table 2), while there were no significant differences as per the three intraoral scanner types ($p > 0.05$; Figure 6; Table 2).

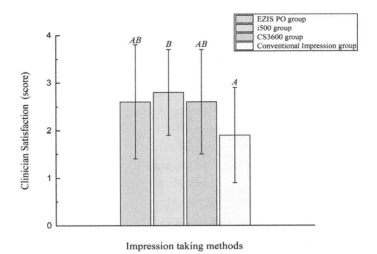

Figure 6. Comparison of clinician satisfaction score of ceramic restorations. Same uppercase letters denote that the difference was not significant ($p > 0.05$).

Table 2. Comparison of the marginal and internal fit of ceramic crowns fabricated with the intraoral scanners and conventional impression technique.

	Intraoral Scanner Group			Conventional Impression Technique	F	p
	EZIS PO	**i500**	**CS3600**			
Clinician satisfaction (Mean ± SD, Score)	2.6 ± 1.2 A,B	2.8 ± 0.9 B	2.6 ± 1.1 A,B	1.9 ± 1 A	2.909	0.04 *

* $p < 0.05$; significance was determined using one-way ANOVA. Different letters (A, B, C) indicate that the difference between the groups was significant, as determined by Tukey's HSD post hoc test ($p < 0.05$).

Clinician satisfaction score and marginal fit (absolute marginal discrepancy and marginal gap) had a significant correlation ($p < 0.05$; Table 3). The clinician satisfaction score and absolute marginal discrepancy showed a weak negative correlation ($p = 0.015$; PCC = −0.271; Table 3); the clinician satisfaction score and marginal gap showed a general negative correlation ($p < 0.001$; PCC = −0.403; Table 3).

Table 3. Correlation coefficient between the clinical satisfaction score and the marginal and internal fit.

	Absolute Marginal Discrepancy		Marginal Gap		Chamfer Gap	
	p	PCC	p	PCC	p	PCC
Clinician Satisfaction	0.015	−0.271	<0.001	−0.403	0.207	-
	Axial Gap		**Angle Gap**		**Occlusal Gap**	
	p	PCC	p	PCC	p	PCC
	0.166	-	0.526	-	0.457	-

4. Discussion

The present clinical study aimed to fabricate ceramic crowns using the conventional method and the digital method with three different intraoral scanners and compare the marginal and internal fit of the ceramic crowns with clinician satisfaction. Thus, the first null hypothesis stated that there would be no differences between the marginal and internal fit of the ceramic crowns fabricated using the four methods and clinician satisfaction; however, this hypothesis was false for all the ceramic crowns ($p < 0.001$). The second null hypothesis stated that there would be no correlation between the marginal and internal fit of the ceramic crowns and clinician satisfaction; this hypothesis was partially dismissed only with respect to the correlation between the marginal fit and clinician satisfaction ($p < 0.001$).

In Chairside CAD/CAM workflow, the use of an intraoral scanner is essential [11,12]. However, previous studies did not investigate the impact of the type of intraoral scanner in the clinical environment on the marginal and internal fit of the ceramic crown. The present results suggest that conventional impression and intraoral scanner type may affect the marginal and internal fit of the ceramic prostheses and the clinician's satisfaction score; thus, clinicians should consider the method for acquiring a virtual cast for the fabrication of an excellent ceramic crown.

Most previous studies report the goodness-of-fit of the prostheses based on the type of the restoring material [13,14]. Moreover, these studies mostly evaluated if the marginal fit could be applied in the clinical setting [15,16]. In many previous studies, the clinically allowable range of the marginal fit is assumed to be a value from 100 μm to 120 μm [17–19], and a range of 50–100 μm is recommended for the internal fit [20–22]. In the present trial, all the ceramic crowns that were fabricated using the conventional method and the digital method with three different intraoral scanners were in the clinically allowable range of marginal fit. However, the internal fit (angle and occlusal gap) had a value exceeding the gap of 100 μm except for CS3600 Group.

Many previous studies have compared the marginal fit and internal fit of the prostheses that was fabricated as per various dental CAD/CAM workflows. Ortorp A. et al. reported poorer marginal fit in the digital workflow (222.5 ± 124.6 μm) as compared to that in the conventional workflow (118 ± 49.7 μm) [23]. Varol S. et al. reported poorer marginal fit in the digital workflow (86.17 ± 27.61 μm) as compared to that in the conventional workflow (77.26 ± 29.23 μm) [24]. In a similar manner, Bayramoglu E. et al. reported poorer marginal fit in the digital workflow (120.4 ± 54.5 μm) as compared to that in the conventional workflow (75.4 ± 16.6 μm) [25]. However, Massignan Berejuk H. et al. reported poorer marginal fit in the conventional workflow (11.56 ± 8.74 μm) as compared to that in the digital workflow (1.85 ± 1.50 μm) [26]. Previous studies have shown different results. Several earlier researches have reported superior marginal fit of prostheses fabricated using the conventional method in a working cast with a physical impression material than that with an intraoral scanner [23–25]. However, recently, the use of chairside CAD/CAM workflow has increased, and many intraoral scanners have recently been developed [27,28]. Thus, most recent studies have reported better marginal fit of prostheses fabricated using an intraoral scanner than that of those fabricated using the conventional method [27,28]. In keeping with these results, in the present study, the method for fabrication with three kinds of intraoral scanner showed better marginal and internal fit of the prostheses than the conventional method. As per a systematic review of the multi-unit fixed dental prosthesis fabricated using the digital workflow, Russo LL et al. reported that studies of a single crown fabricated with the digital workflow are generally conducted; however, few studies of a multi-unit fixed dental prosthesis have been performed, and it is important to perform additional studies to confirm the clinical reliability of the findings [29]. Thus, in addition to the evaluation of the single ceramic crown conducted in the present study, it is necessary to perform a study on the multi-unit fixed dental prosthesis.

In the present clinical study, we found a significant correlation between the clinician satisfaction score and the marginal fit (absolute marginal discrepancy and marginal gap) ($p < 0.05$). However, there was no correlation between the clinician satisfaction score and the internal fit ($p > 0.05$) because the marginal fit was recognized as the most important factor in the process wherein clinicians check the prostheses in the oral cavity. Many previous studies have reported that marginal fit is an important element that influences the prognosis of the fixed dental prosthesis [13,20–26]. Based on the present results, clinicians can use the intraoral scanning method rather than the conventional method for the fabrication of ceramic crowns with excellent goodness-of-fit and realize high clinician satisfaction by reproducing the excellent goodness-of-fit obtained using the intraoral scanning method.

Previous studies have shown a difference in the scanning accuracy based on the intraoral scanner used [11,12]. In the present study, there were significant differences in the marginal fit and internal fit of the ceramic crowns that were fabricated, based on the three intraoral scanner types ($p < 0.001$); however, all values were within the clinically allowable range (within 120 μm), and there were no big differences. Moreover, there were no significant differences in the clinicians' satisfaction among the ceramic crowns fabricated with the three intraoral scanner types ($p > 0.05$). It is judged that there was no impact on the clinician satisfaction because all the ceramic crowns fabricated with the three intraoral scanner types were in the clinically allowable range (within 120 μm). Further, it is necessary to conduct additional studies to evaluate the three intraoral scanner types used in the present study and examine the impact of the scanning accuracy on the marginal fit and the internal fit.

The present clinical study has certain limitations. It is necessary to conduct additional studies on various intraoral scanners other than those used in the present study. Moreover, it is crucial to perform additional studies using materials other than the lithium disilicate glass-ceramic material that was used in the present clinical study, such as zirconia. We believe that it is important to conduct a study of the multi-unit fixed dental prosthesis. Finally, additional studies on the prognosis should be conducted as a continuation of the present clinical study.

5. Conclusions

Based on the findings of this clinical study, the following conclusions were drawn:

1. There was an impact on the marginal and internal fit of the ceramic crowns based on the type of intraoral scanner that was used; however, there was no difference in the clinicians' satisfaction with the prostheses.
2. The ceramic crowns fabricated using an intraoral scanner showed superior marginal fit and internal fit as well as higher clinician satisfaction than those fabricated using the conventional method with PVS impression.
3. The excellent marginal fit of the fabricated ceramic crowns can achieve high clinician satisfaction.
4. Thus, clinicians should consider the use of the impression method for fabricating a ceramic crown with excellent goodness-of-fit and can realize high clinician satisfaction by reproducing excellent goodness-of-fit using the intraoral scanning method rather than the conventional method.

Author Contributions: Conceptualization, J.-H.L. and K.S.; funding acquisition, K.-B.L.; methodology, J.-H.L. and K.S.; validation, J.-H.L. and K.S.; formal analysis, J.-H.L.; investigation, J.-H.L.; data curation, J.-H.L.; software, J.-H.L. and K.S.; writing—original draft, J.-H.L. and K.S.; visualization, K.S.; supervision, K.-B.L.; project administration, K.-B.L. All authors have read and agreed to the published version of the manuscript.

Acknowledgments: The authors thank the researchers from the Advanced Dental Device Development Institute, Kyungpook National University, for their time and contributions to the study.

References

1. Falahchai, M.; Hemmati, Y.B.; Asli, H.N.; Emadi, I. Marginal gap of monolithic zirconia endocrowns fabricated by using digital scanning and conventional impressions. *J. Prosthet. Dent.* **2020**. [CrossRef] [PubMed]
2. Porrelli, D.; Berton, F.; Piloni, A.C.; Kobau, I.; Stacchi, C.; Di Lenarda, R.; Rizzo, R. Evaluating the stability of extended-pour alginate impression materials by using an optical scanning and digital method. *J. Prosthet. Dent.* **2020**. [CrossRef] [PubMed]
3. Sahin, V.; Jodati, H.; Evis, Z. Effect of storage time on mechanical properties of extended-pour irreversible hydrocolloid impression materials. *J. Prosthet. Dent.* **2020**, *124*, 69–74. [CrossRef] [PubMed]
4. Bohner, L.O.L.; Canto, G.D.L.; Marció, B.S.; Laganá, D.C.; Sesma, N.; Neto, P.T. Computer-aided analysis of digital dental impressions obtained from intraoral and extraoral scanners. *J. Prosthet. Dent.* **2017**, *118*, 617–623. [CrossRef]
5. Michelinakis, G.; Apostolakis, D.; Tsagarakis, A.; Kourakis, G.; Pavlakis, E. A comparison of accuracy of 3 intraoral scanners: A single-blinded in vitro study. *J. Prosthet. Dent.* **2019**. [CrossRef]
6. Park, J.M.; Kim, R.J.Y.; Lee, K.W. Comparative reproducibility analysis of 6 intraoral scanners used on complex intracoronal preparations. *J. Prosthet. Dent.* **2020**, *123*, 113–120. [CrossRef]

7.   Braian, M.; Wennerberg, A. Trueness and precision of 5 intraoral scanners for scanning edentulous and dentate complete-arch mandibular casts: A comparative in vitro study. *J. Prosthet. Dent.* **2019**, *122*, 129–136. [CrossRef]

8.   Stimmelmayr, M.; Groesser, J.; Beuer, F.; Erdelt, K.; Krennmair, G.; Sachs, C.; Güth, J.F. Accuracy and mechanical performance of passivated and conventional fabricated 3-unit fixed dental prosthesis on multi-unit abutments. *J. Prosthodont. Res.* **2017**, *61*, 403–411. [CrossRef]

9.   Hayama, H.; Fueki, K.; Wadachi, J.; Wakabayashi, N. Trueness and precision of digital impressions obtained using an intraoral scanner with different head size in the partially edentulous mandible. *J. Prosthodont. Res.* **2018**, *62*, 347–352. [CrossRef]

10. Kihara, H.; Hatakeyama, W.; Komine, F.; Takafuji, K.; Takahashi, T.; Yokota, J.; Kondo, H. Accuracy and practicality of intraoral scanner in dentistry: A literature review. *J. Prosthodont. Res.* **2020**, *64*, 109–113. [CrossRef]

11. Park, G.H.; Son, K.; Lee, K.B. Feasibility of using an intraoral scanner for a complete-arch digital scan. *J. Prosthet. Dent.* **2019**, *121*, 803–810. [CrossRef] [PubMed]

12. Son, K.; Lee, K.B. Effect of Tooth Types on the Accuracy of Dental 3D Scanners: An In Vitro Study. *Materials* **2020**, *13*, 1744. [CrossRef] [PubMed]

13. Son, K.; Lee, S.; Kang, S.H.; Park, J.; Lee, K.B.; Jeon, M.; Yun, B.J. A comparison study of marginal and internal fit assessment methods for fixed dental prostheses. *J. Clin. Med.* **2019**, *8*, 785. [CrossRef] [PubMed]

14. Jang, D.; Son, K.; Lee, K.B. A Comparative study of the fitness and trueness of a three-unit fixed dental prosthesis fabricated using two digital workflows. *Appl. Sci.* **2019**, *9*, 2778. [CrossRef]

15. Kang, B.H.; Son, K.; Lee, K.B. Accuracy of five intraoral scanners and two laboratory scanners for a complete arch: A comparative in vitro study. *Appl. Sci.* **2020**, *10*, 74. [CrossRef]

16. Lee, K.; Son, K.; Lee, K.B. Effects of Trueness and Surface Microhardness on the Fitness of Ceramic Crowns. *Appl. Sci.* **2020**, *10*, 1858. [CrossRef]

17. Alajaji, N.K.; Bardwell, D.; Finkelman, M.; Ali, A. Micro-CT Evaluation of Ceramic Inlays: Comparison of the Marginal and Internal Fit of Five and Three-Axis CAM Systems with a Heat Press Technique. *J. Esthet. Restor. Dent.* **2017**, *29*, 49–58. [CrossRef]

18. Roperto, R.; Assaf, H.; Soares-Porto, T.; Lang, L.; Teich, S. Are different generations of CAD/CAM milling machines capable to fabricate restorations with similar quality? *J. Clin. Exp. Dent.* **2016**, *8*, e423.

19. Sachs, C.; Groesser, J.; Stadelmann, M.; Schweiger, J.; Erdelt, K.; Beuer, F. Full-arch prostheses from translucent zirconia: Accuracy of fit. *Dent. Mater.* **2014**, *30*, 817–823. [CrossRef]

20. Colpani, J.T.; Borba, M.; Della Bona, Á. Evaluation of marginal and internal fit of ceramic crown copings. *Dent. Mater.* **2013**, *29*, 174–180. [CrossRef]

21. Mously, H.A.; Finkelman, M.; Zandparsa, R.; Hirayama, H. Marginal and internal adaptation of ceramic crown restorations fabricated with CAD/CAM technology and the heat-press technique. *J. Prosthet. Dent.* **2014**, *112*, 249–256. [CrossRef] [PubMed]

22. Lins, L.; Bemfica, V.; Queiroz, C.; Canabarro, A. In vitro evaluation of the internal and marginal misfit of CAD/CAM zirconia copings. *J. Prosthet. Dent.* **2015**, *113*, 205–211. [CrossRef] [PubMed]

23. Örtorp, A.; Jönsson, D.; Mouhsen, A.; von Steyern, P.V. The fit of cobalt–chromium three-unit fixed dental prostheses fabricated with four different techniques: A comparative in vitro study. *Dent. Mater.* **2011**, *27*, 356–363. [CrossRef] [PubMed]

24. Varol, S.; Kulak-Özkan, Y. In Vitro Comparison of Marginal and Internal Fit of Press-on-Metal Ceramic (PoM) Restorations with Zirconium-Supported and Conventional Metal Ceramic Fixed Partial Dentures Before and After Veneering. *J. Prosthodont.* **2015**, *24*, 387–393. [CrossRef]

25. Bayramoğlu, E.; Özkan, Y.K.; Yildiz, C. Comparison of marginal and internal fit of press-on-metal and conventional ceramic systems for three-and four-unit implant-supported partial fixed dental prostheses: An in vitro study. *J. Prosthet. Dent.* **2015**, *114*, 52–58. [CrossRef]

26. Massignan Berejuk, H.; Hideo Shimizu, R.; Aparecida de Mattias Sartori, I.; Valgas, L.; Tiossi, R. Vertical microgap and passivity of fit of three-unit implant-supported frameworks fabricated using different techniques. *Int. J. Oral Maxillofac. Implants* **2014**, *29*, 1064–1070. [CrossRef]

27. Rapone, B.; Palmisano, C.; Ferrara, E.; Di Venere, D.; Albanese, G.; Corsalini, M. The Accuracy of Three Intraoral Scanners in the Oral Environment with and without Saliva: A Comparative Study. *Appl. Sci.* **2020**, *10*, 7762. [CrossRef]

28. Lee, S.J.; Kim, S.W.; Lee, J.J.; Cheong, C.W. Comparison of Intraoral and Extraoral Digital Scanners: Evaluation of Surface Topography and Precision. *Dent. J.* **2020**, *8*, 52. [CrossRef]

29. Russo, L.L.; Caradonna, G.; Biancardino, M.; De Lillo, A.; Troiano, G.; Guida, L. Digital versus conventional workflow for the fabrication of multiunit fixed prostheses: A systematic review and meta-analysis of vertical marginal fit in controlled in vitro studies. *J. Prosthet. Dent.* **2019**, *122*, 435–440. [CrossRef]

30. Hasanzade, M.; Shirani, M.; Afrashtehfar, K.I.; Naseri, P.; Alikhasi, M. In Vivo and In Vitro Comparison of Internal and Marginal Fit of Digital and Conventional Impressions for Full-Coverage Fixed Restorations: A Systematic Review and Meta-analysis. *J. Evid. Based Dent. Pract.* **2019**, *19*, 236–254. [CrossRef]

31. Hasanzade, M.; Aminikhah, M.; Afrashtehfar, K.I.; Alikhasi, M. Marginal and internal adaptation of single crowns and fixed dental prostheses by using digital and conventional workflows: A systematic review and meta-analysis. *J. Prosthet. Dent.* **2020**, in press. [CrossRef] [PubMed]

32. Goodacre, C.J.; Campagni, W.V.; Aquilino, S.A. Tooth preparations for complete crowns: An art form based on scientific principles. *J. Prosthet. Dent.* **2001**, *85*, 363–376. [CrossRef] [PubMed]

33. Dancey, C.; Reidy, J. *Statistics without Maths for Psychology: Pearson Higher*; Pearson: London, UK, 2014.

13

Digital Oral Medicine for the Elderly

Christian E. Besimo *, Nicola U. Zitzmann and Tim Joda

Department of Reconstructive Dentistry, University Center for Dental Medicine Basel, University of Basel, 4058 Basel, Switzerland; n.zitzmann@unibas.ch (N.U.Z.); tim.joda@unibas.ch (T.J.)
* Correspondence: christian.besimo@bluewin.ch

Abstract: Sustainable oral care of the elderly requires a holistic view of aging, which must extend far beyond the narrow field of dental expertise to help reduce the effects of sociobiological changes on oral health in good time. Digital technologies now extend into all aspects of daily life. This review summarizes the diverse digital opportunities that may help address the complex challenges in Gerodontology. Systemic patient management is at the center of these descriptions, while the application of digital tools for purely dental treatment protocols is deliberately avoided.

Keywords: oral medicine; oral healthcare; dentistry; gerodontology; elderly patient; digital transformation; big data; patient-centered outcomes

1. Introduction

The steady aging of human populations is a development that affects not only the industrialized world, but also emerging and developing countries. It is estimated that about half of all people who have ever lived to an age of 65 years old or older are alive today. We are living through an exponential population expansion and demographic transition. Therefore, it is necessary to understand the sociological and biological changes facing the elderly population and to master the current and future challenges in dental healthcare for aging patients [1].

This opinion letter, based on an ongoing evaluation of the sociodemographic changes due to aging, focuses on digital technologies, which could help deal with the complex challenges in oral medicine for the growing elderly.

2. A Silent Revolution

2.1. Social Change

Old age is changing fundamentally and to an extent that justifies the term 'social revolution', albeit one that is proceeding quietly. This change is characterized by the objective of being able to live in a self-determined manner and in a private environment for as long as possible, even when in need of healthcare. In this context, a transfer to a care institution is only foreseen in the case of an extreme emergency and to be delayed for as long as possible. This development will contribute to the progressive delaying of the fourth age, which is marked by the need for advanced assistance and care, and will further reduce the average length of stay in institutions. In Switzerland, individuals aged 65 years and older only stay in nursing homes for one year [2].

It is important to recognize the goal-oriented willingness and the high degree of creativity that senior citizens, either currently working or retired, display in their third age (traditionally 65–80 years old). However, these factors do not allow for any reliable prognoses regarding changes in lifestyles in old age and force the professional groups, institutions, and organizations concerned with aging to continually adapt their strategies and concepts [2]. This awareness has also reached the political arena in Switzerland, so that in future, there will be a growing reluctance to plan new inpatient care places and priority will be given to outpatient care in terms of cost-effectiveness [3,4].

2.2. Consequences for Health

The biological limit for life expectancy at birth and after reaching the age of 65 is still not predictable. Medical advances, healthy nutrition, good education, and improving working conditions continue to favor an increasingly longer third age and will reduce the risk and duration of the fourth age [2].

The preventive and restorative success of dentistry have led to people with an increasing number of teeth (including implant-supported reconstructions). However, despite their knowledge of the importance of regular dental check-ups for oral and general health, the elderly will inevitably gradually withdraw from this care, beginning between the ages of 60 and 65 [5]. The risk of psychosocial (loneliness, poverty) and medical problems (multimorbidity, polypharmacy), which increase with age, play a central role in withdrawing from care with major consequences for dental and oral health in the long term. Oral diseases do not only occur in old age when the need for help and care begins, but much earlier, because the social and biological factors mentioned above increasingly affect the resources needed to maintain oral hygiene and to receive regular care from the personal dental team. Even if the fourth age is delayed, the oral health issues still inevitably arise, and are then complicated further by the additional comorbidities of aging [6].

Facing these complex challenges, it is important for dentists to learn to perceive the human being holistically—in her or his entirety—and to establish a close network with other medical disciplines, institutions, organizations, authorities, and relatives who are concerned with the care of aging people. It is important to be aware that the range of stakeholders involved is growing and becoming more volatile, as the shift from inpatient to outpatient care increases [7,8].

3. Digital Opportunities

People participating in the digital community generate a rapidly growing amount of data every day. This is also increasingly true for senior citizens. Scientific use of this data offers the opportunity to gain a deeper and more dynamic insight into the lifestyle of aging people, for example, through analyzing digital shopping activities and payment transactions. This could allow a better and more up-to-date understanding of the changing lifestyles of the elderly. It is conceivable that algorithms could be developed that can identify sociobiological threats at an early stage by monitoring changes in behavior. Such algorithms would also be important for the dental care of aging people and thus for oral health. This would be one of several opportunities to achieve a paradigm shift in geriatric dentistry and to promote preventive rather than palliative care concepts that are still predominant [9,10].

3.1. In Frigo Veritas (The Truth Lies in the Fridge)

The "In Frigo Veritas" study conducted in Geneva in the 1990s demonstrated that the contents of the refrigerators of senior citizens was associated with the likelihood of hospitalization in the following month (11). Monitoring the nutritional provisions available to an elderly individual could therefore identify those at risk early. The use of shopping lists of food products, which are already electronically recorded today with the help of customer cards, could be considered here. This data alone would already allow individual conclusions to be drawn about the quantity, quality, and course of food. A link to intelligent refrigerator systems that can document the consumption and replenishment of food would also be conceivable. This would allow continuous conclusions to be drawn in real time on the nutritional situation and thus the morbidity risk in an out-of-home care setting [11]. This application could also be used in dentistry for therapeutic decision making or for the ongoing assessment of the care capacity of aging people threatened by sociobiological risks. In addition, nutritional counselling and guidance, supported by nutritional algorithms, could be carried out in a simplified, individualized and continuous manner, before, during, and/or after dental interventions such as tooth extractions or the insertion of fixed and removable dentures [12].

3.2. Intelligent, Individually Usable Systems

The personal health data generated in medicine, including dentistry, or by intelligent systems suitable for everyday use, such as smartphones, watches or other devices, open up a wide range of application options that will go far beyond the recording of acute emergency situations in in-home and out-of-home care settings. On the one hand, the cumulative use of medically relevant data does not only offer significantly expanded perspectives for research, but also for patient care. Today, it is already feasible to record vital data in real time using the aforementioned intelligent everyday systems. It can be assumed that the availability and variety of such systems will continuously increase in the near future and will also be usefully applied in dentistry [13,14].

3.3. Stop Walking When Talking

Nowadays, electronic pedometers are used to obtain discounts from health insurance companies. Similarly, we are already able to analyze gait regularity and thus the risk of falls among older people in specialized mobility centers, with or without multitasking, and to draw conclusions about diseases, side effects of medication, and cognitive performance [15]. The transfer of such systems to shoe insoles, for example, not only has the potential to obtain and link incomparably more empirical data on gait safety in elderly people living in a private household, but also to monitor their mobility in real time. In this context, the effects of therapeutic interventions on gait safety, such as those that aim to optimize occlusion, could be dynamically monitored [16].

4. Interdisciplinary Networking

As mentioned previously, the (dental) medical care of aging people living in private households is faced with growing interdisciplinary challenges. On the one hand, healthcare providers have to establish a network to harness the knowledge of the various disciplines by means of suitable digital systems to make it not only accessible for interdisciplinary research, but also clinically usable under growing organizational and legal requirements. On the other hand, everyday clinical practice requires dynamic, real-time networking among the growing number of stakeholders in the care of the elderly, which will increase significantly and become more volatile as outpatient care expands. Here, intelligent tools are needed that enable compatible, rapid, and secure interdisciplinary data exchange on a patient-by-patient basis to support individually tailored decision-making based on algorithms [17].

Finally, it is expected that routine sequencing of the genome in the case of disease will become established within the next five to ten years, as the costs of this procedure have been significantly reduced from $100,000 to $1000 over the last 20 years [18]. This should also contribute to the individualization of prevention, diagnostics, and therapy in dentistry, especially for older people with increasing psychosocial and medical risks. The latter could possibly be detected earlier and counteracted more effectively [19].

5. Ethical and Legal Responsibilities

We have learned from the hitherto short history of the digitalization of our world that this development is accelerating at a breathtaking rate. This calls for an urgent and internationally valid regulation for the protection of personal data of individuals, while enabling the exchange of personal information between stakeholders for the benefit of the individual. This has been pioneered by the basic data protection regulation of the European Union [20]. Such a set of rules must compensate for the existing socio-economic asymmetry of a data-driven economy, which ensures the right to a copy of personal data and thus digital self-determination. However, the right to a copy of personal data also requires the development of cooperatively managed databases that are able to manage the digital information in a fiduciary capacity and in a comparable way to financial institutions. In this way, it would be ensured that people could come into possession of all their health-related data to use these under regulated conditions for their own benefit or to make data available to research and thus to the community [21].

In addition, society must ensure that (dental) medicine, which is increasingly controlled by guidelines and algorithms, does not lose sight of the individual person. It is true that large amounts of data can increase the reliability of answers to individual questions. Nevertheless, it remains to be hoped that big data will not lead to further commercialization or industrialization of medicine, and thus, neglect the healing power of a systemic doctor-patient relationship, but rather that it will nurture this relationship [22,23].

6. Conclusions

The global demographic change is characterized by an exponential population expansion and sociobiological transition towards a growing number of older patients. Sustainable oral healthcare of the elderly must comprise a holistic view of aging, far beyond the narrow field of dental diagnostics and modernized treatment protocols. Digital health data generated in dental medicine, or by daily used systems, such as smartphones, tablets, and watches, open up a wide range of application options in (oral) healthcare to master the complex challenges in Gerodontology. Scientific use of this data offers broad insights into the lifestyle of aging patients for the early identification of social threats and changing behaviors.

Medical and dental healthcare providers have to establish an interdisciplinary network using these digital systems for routine clinical practice. Smart digital applications are needed, which enable compatible, rapid, and secure interdisciplinary data exchange on a patient-by-patient level to support individually tailored decision-making based on the knowledge of all stakeholders in the care of the elderly in in-home and out-of-home care settings. The digital transformation has the opportunity to achieve a paradigm shift in geriatric dentistry and to promote preventive rather than palliative healthcare concepts.

Author Contributions: Conceptualization, C.E.B. and T.J.; methodology, C.E.B. and T.J.; writing—original draft preparation, C.E.B.; writing—review and editing, T.J. and N.U.Z.; supervision, T.J.; project administration, T.J. All authors have read and agreed to the published version of the manuscript.

References

1. WHO. *World Report on Ageing and Health*; World Health Organization: Geneva, Switzerland, 2015.
2. Höpflinger, F.; Bayer-Oglesby, L.; Zumbrunn, A. *Pflegebedürftigkeit und Langzeitpflege im Alter. Aktualisierte Szenarien für die Schweiz*; Verlag Hans Huber: Bern, Switzerland, 2011; pp. 33–66.
3. Gesundheitsdirektion Kanton Zürich. *Bedarfsentwicklung und Steuerung der Stationären Pflegeplätze*; Kanton Zürich: Zürich, Switzerland, 2018.
4. Gesundheitsdepartement des Kantons Basel-Stadt. *Gesundheitsversorgungsbericht über die Spitäler, Pflegeheime, Tagespflegeheime und Spitex-Einrichtungen im Kanton Basel-Stadt*; Kanton Basel-Stadt: Basel, Switzerland, 2018.
5. Biffar, R.; Klinke-Wilberg, T. Gesundheit der Älterwerdenden und Inanspruchnahme ärztlicher Dienste—zahnmedizinische Konsequenzen und Aufgaben. *Senioren-Zahnmedizin* **2013**, *1*, 35–42.
6. Tavares, M.; Lindefjeld Calabi, K.A.; San Martin, L. Systemic diseases and oral health. *Dent. Clin. N. Am.* **2014**, *58*, 797–814. [CrossRef] [PubMed]
7. Plasschaert, A.J.M.; Holbrook, W.P.; Delap, E.; Martinez, C.; Walmsley, A.D. Profile and competences for the European dentist. *Eur. J. Dent. Educ.* **2005**, *9*, 98–107. [CrossRef] [PubMed]
8. Besimo, C. Paradigmenwechsel zugunsten einer besseren oralen Gesundheit im Alter. *Swiss Dent. J.* **2015**, *125*, 599–604. [PubMed]
9. March, S. Individual Data Linkage of Survey Data with Claims Data in Germany—An Overview Based on a Cohort Study. *Int. J. Environ. Res. Public Health* **2017**, *14*, 1543–1558. [CrossRef] [PubMed]

10. Joda, T.; Waltimo, T.; Pauli-Magnus, C.; Probst-Hensch, N.; Zitzmann, N.U. Population-Based Linkage of Big Data in Dental Research. *Int. J. Environ. Res. Public Health* **2018**, *15*, 2357–2361. [CrossRef] [PubMed]

11. Boumandjel, N.; Herrmann, F.; Girod, V.; Sieber, C.; Rapin, C.H. Refrigerator content and hospital admission in old people. *Lancet* **2000**, *356*, 563. [CrossRef]

12. Kiss, C.M.; Besimo, C.; Ulrich, A.; Kressig, R.W. Ernährung und Gesundheit im Alter. *Aktuel Ernahrungsmed* **2016**, *41*, 27–35.

13. Majumder, S.; Deen, M.J. Smartphone Sensors for Health Monitoring and Diagnosis. *Sensors* **2019**, *19*, 2164. [CrossRef] [PubMed]

14. Reeder, D.; David, A. Health at hand: A systematic review of smart watch uses for health and wellness. *J. Biomed. Inform.* **2016**, *63*, 269–276. [CrossRef] [PubMed]

15. Beauchet, O.; Blumen, H.M.; Callisaya, M.L.; De Cock, A.M.; Kressig, R.W.; Srikanth, V.; Steinmetz, J.P.; Verghese, J.; Allali, G. Spatiotemporal gait characteristics associated with cognitive impairment: A multicenter cross-sectional study, the intercontinental "Gait, cOgnitiOn & Decline" initiative. *Curr. Alzheimer Res.* **2018**, *23*, 273–282.

16. Brand, C.; Bridenbaugh, A.A.; Perkovac, M.; Glenz, F.; Besimo, C.; Marinello, C.P. The effect of tooth loss on gait stability of community-dwelling older adults. *Gerodontology* **2015**, *32*, 296–301. [CrossRef] [PubMed]

17. Lehne, M.; Sass, J.; Essenwanger, A.; Schepers, J.; Thun, S. Why digital medicine depends on interoperability. *NPJ Digit. Med.* **2019**, *20*, 79. [CrossRef] [PubMed]

18. The Cost of Sequencing a Human Genome. Available online: https://www.genome.gov/about-genomics/fact-sheets/Sequencing-Human-Genome-cost (accessed on 30 October 2019).

19. Payne, K.; Gavan, S.P.; Wright, S.J.; Thompson, A.J. Cost-effectiveness analyses of genetic and genomic diagnostic tests. *Nat. Rev. Genet.* **2018**, *19*, 235–246. [CrossRef] [PubMed]

20. Verordnung (EU) 2016/679 des europäischen Parlaments und des Rates. vom 27. April 2016. zum Schutz natürlicher Personen bei der Verarbeitung personenbezogener Daten, zum freien Datenverkehr und zur Aufhebung der Richtlinie 45/96/EG (Datenschutz-Grundverordnung). Available online: https://eur-lex.europa.eu/eli/reg/2016/679/oj (accessed on 27 April 2016).

21. Hafen, E. Why Citizens Should Have Control of Their Own Data. Available online: https://ethz.ch/en/news-and-events/eth-news/news/2018/04/ernst-hafen-midata.html (accessed on 24 April 2018).

22. Joda, T.; Waltimo, T.; Probst-Hensch, N.; Pauli-Magnus, C.; Zitzmann, N.U. Health data in dentistry: An attempt to master the digital challenge. *Public Health Genom.* **2019**, *22*, 1–7. [CrossRef] [PubMed]

23. Joda, T.; Bornstein, M.M.; Jung, R.E.; Ferrari, M.; Waltimo, T.; Zitzmann, N.U. Recent trends and future direction of dental research in the digital era. *Int. J. Environ. Res. Public Health* **2020**, *17*, 1987. [CrossRef] [PubMed]

14

Influence of Preparation Design, Marginal Gingiva Location and Tooth Morphology on the Accuracy of Digital Impressions for Full-Crown Restorations: An In Vitro Investigation

Selina A. Bernauer [1], Johannes Müller [2], Nicola U. Zitzmann [1]🆔 and Tim Joda [1,*]🆔

[1] Department of Reconstructive Dentistry, UZB University Center for Dental Medicine Basel, University of Basel, 4058 Basel, Switzerland; selina.bernauer@unibas.ch (S.A.B.); n.zitzmann@unibas.ch (N.U.Z.)

[2] Private Practice, 80634 Munich, Germany; dr.johannes.a.mueller@gmail.com

* Correspondence: tim.joda@unibas.ch

Abstract: (1) Background: Intraoral optical scanning (IOS) has gained increased importance in prosthodontics. The aim of this in vitro study was to analyze the IOS accuracy for treatment with full crowns, considering possible influencing factors. (2) Methods: Two tooth morphologies, each with four different finish-line designs for tooth preparation and epi- or supragingival locations, were digitally designed, 3D-printed, and post-processed for 16 sample abutment teeth. Specimens were digitized using a laboratory scanner to generate reference STLs (Standard Tessellation Language), and were secondary-scanned with two IOS systems five times each in a complete-arch model scenario (Trios 3 Pod, Primescan AC). For accuracy, a best-fit algorithm (Final Surface) was used to analyze deviations of the abutment teeth based on 160 IOS-STLs compared to the reference STLs (16 preparations × 2 IOS-systems × 5 scans per tooth). (3) Results: Analysis revealed homogenous findings with high accuracy for intra- and inter-group comparisons for both IOS systems, with mean values of 80% quantiles from 20 ± 2 μm to 50 ± 5 μm. Supragingival finishing lines demonstrated significantly higher accuracy than epigingival margins when comparing each preparation ($p < 0.05$), whereas tangential preparations exhibited similar results independent of the gingival location. Morphology of anterior versus posterior teeth showed slightly better results in favor of molars in combination with shoulder preparations only. (4) Conclusion: The clinical challenge for the treatment with full crowns following digital impressions is the location of the prospective restoration margin related to the distance to the gingiva. However, the overall accuracy for all abutment teeth was very high; thus, the factors tested are unlikely to have a strong clinical impact.

Keywords: fixed prosthodontics; full crown; tooth preparation; intraoral optical scanning (IOS); digital dentistry

1. Introduction

Continuous technical development has expanded opportunities in reconstructive dentistry and prosthodontics [1]. In particular, intraoral optical scanning (IOS), computer-aided design, and computer-aided manufacturing (CAD/CAM) have fostered complete digital workflows for the treatment of fixed dental prostheses (FDPs) [2]. IOS has become indispensable in everyday dental practice, in university education [3,4], and in dental laboratories [5–7].

Digital impressions have been proven to be more time-efficient compared to conventional impressions, and a majority of patients have preferred the digital impression technique rather than the conventional approach with plastic materials [8–10]. At the same time, IOS has simplified the process chain between dentist and dental technician. Complete digital workflows have rendered various work steps superfluous such as tray preparation, disinfecting, shipping of the conventional impression, and further preparations for the fabrication of gypsum dental casts [11]. IOS technology offers new possibilities for clinical routine in selected indications, especially in the field of fixed prosthodontics. By taking a digital impression, the intraoral situation is visually recorded with neither the mucosa nor the teeth needing to be physically touched. This prevents possible gingival displacement or tooth movement from the application of conventional elastomeric impression material [12–14]. IOS is also advantageous for the treatment of periodontally compromised dentitions with recessions, enlarged interdental spaces, and dental undercuts (such as pontics or cantilevers), which make an accurate impression difficult [15]. Additionally, IOS opens the door to chairside CAD/CAM systems that could offer treatment protocols with single-unit restorations in one clinical session [16]. In contrast to conventional impressions, technical factors must be taken into account when using a digital approach. IOS requires a direct line of sight on the object in order to create 3D surface files, which are known as standard tessellation language (STL) [17]. Additional studies have shown that a supragingival preparation margin in the impression is more accurate [17,18].

Besides the technical development related to digital impressions, the finish-line design for tooth preparation has remained a crucial aspect for the abutment tooth [19,20]. Are the same finish-line designs applicable for full-crown restorations, or are adjustments required to facilitate the application of IOS? The challenge is now to analyze the existing parameters of tooth preparation in order to identify the best design for an accurate IOS and further STL processing for clinically acceptable restorations, while considering minimal invasiveness combined with modern materials and adhesive luting technology [21].

The aim of this in vitro study was to analyze the influence of different finish lines for complete crown preparations, their locations related to the gingival margin, and tooth morphology on the accuracy of digital impressions. The null hypotheses tested were that the IOS accuracy does not depend on the finish-line design (tangential, narrow chamfer, wide chamfer, and shoulder), the gingival positioning of the finishing line (epi- and supragingival), or on tooth morphology (incisor and molar); secondly, there is no difference in performance between the IOS systems used (Trios 3 Pod, 3Shape, Copenhagen, Denmark and Cerec Primescan AC, Dentsply Sirona, Bensheim, Germany).

2. Materials and Methods

A maxillary dental training model was used as reference (Dental Model AG-3, Frasaco, Tettnang, Germany). A maxillary central incisor (FDI 11) was selected to represent the anterior tooth morphology, while a first maxillary molar (FDI 16) was chosen to represent posterior sites. Based on a standardized complete crown preparation, two typodonts were manually prepared with a supragingival finishing line, 0.4 mm chamfer, and a 4–6° convergence angle. Substance removal was incisal 2.0 mm, palatal 1.0 mm, and labial 1.0–1.5 mm for tooth 11, and occlusal 1.5 mm and labial 1.0 mm, palatal 1.0 mm, and interdental 1.0 mm for the molar. All practical work steps were performed by the same operator (S.B.), a postgraduate prosthodontic resident, and each step was supervised by a senior clinician and board-certified prosthodontist (J.M.).

Both prepared typodonts were digitized with a laboratory desktop scanner (Series 7, Institute Straumann AG, Basel, Switzerland), and these served as the basis for the digital designs of the virtual modifications to create the test specimens, involving four different finish-line designs for both morphologies. These designs were digitally computed with the software Geomatic Design X (3D Systems, Rock Hill, SC, USA) and saved as STL files. The following finish-line designs were applied: tangential, narrow chamfer (0.4 mm), wide chamfer (0.8 mm), and shoulder (0.8 mm). Each design was applied in an epigingival or a 1.0 mm supragingival position, resulting in a total of eight tooth preparations for the anterior and another eight for the posterior region. Figure 1 displays the study setup with 16 different specimens (Figure 1).

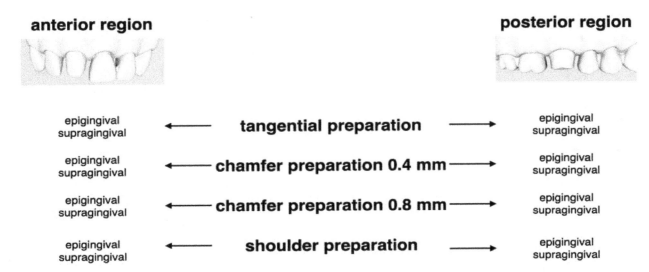

Figure 1. Trial setting: Four different preparation designs in anterior and posterior regions separated for epi- and supragingival finishing lines.

Finally, the 16 virtual tooth preparations were 3D-printed for the production of standardized replicas (3D-Printer Objet260 Connex2, Stratasys, Eden Prairie, MN, USA). The color of the rubber-like material used was a mixture of Vero White Plus RGD 835 and Tango Black Plus FLX 980. This mixture resulted in the color DM8515 (Stratasys, Eden Prairie, MN, USA). All 3D-printed teeth were mounted in the reference model and manually finalized with diamond burs (Intensive SA, Montagnola, Switzerland) and Sof-Lex discs (3M ESPE AG, Saint Paul, MN, USA) to achieve an exact finishing line and a smooth surface. In order to avoid potential deviations due to printing errors and to visualize the manual corrections, all teeth were removed from the reference model and digitized with the same laboratory desktop scanner that was used for the initial digitalization.

Successively, all 16 3D-printed teeth were remounted in the reference model and scanned by one experienced operator (S.B.) with two IOS systems (Trios 3 Pod and Cerec Primescan AC). Each preparation, including adjacent teeth, was captured five times in order to minimize potential scanning errors. The scans were carried out according to the manufacturer's recommendations.

For accuracy of analysis, a total of 160 IOS-STLs (16 specimens × 2 IOS-systems × 5 scans = 160 STLs) were then superimposed to the corresponding original reference STLs with the software Final Surface (GFaI e.V., Berlin, Germany). A best-fit algorithm was applied for deviation analysis in order to minimize the distances between the two surfaces being compared. Here, the distance to the surface of the IOS-STL to be examined was considered for all surfaces of the matching reference STL. Scanning data beyond 2 mm from the finishing lines were digitally cut to guarantee an accurate fine registration. Trimmed scan data obtained from five scans by each IOS were paired, and these pairs were inspected (STL-1 vs. STL-2, STL-1 vs. STL-3, STL-1 vs. STL-3, etc.). Deviations between polygons formed by the point cloud constituting the two superimposed scans were calculated, and the distance data of all superimposed pairs were summarized [22].

Numerical variables of interest were descriptively analyzed with sample means for 80% quantiles including standard deviation. Since the IOS-STLs under investigation appeared with a plus or minus of data points compared to the reference STLs, the use of 80% quantiles ensured error minimization regarding "too small" and "too large" areas for deviation analysis. Statistics were carried out using R 4.0.3 (The R Project for Statistical Computing, Vienna, Austria), and a significance level was set at 0.05.

3. Results

Trios 3 Pod and Primescan AC could successfully capture all selected preparations as tangential, narrow and wide chamfer, and shoulder, respectively (Figure 2). Intra- and intergroup analyses comparing both IOS systems revealed homogenous results with high accuracy representing mean values of 80% quantiles ranging from 20 ± 2 μm to 50 ± 5 μm throughout all tested abutment teeth (Tables 1 and 2). Supragingival finishing lines demonstrated significantly higher accuracy than epigingival margins when comparing preparation designs against each other ($p < 0.05$), whereas tangential preparations exhibited similar results independent of the gingival location of the finishing line. Morphology of anterior versus posterior teeth showed slightly better results in favor of molars in combination with shoulder preparations only.

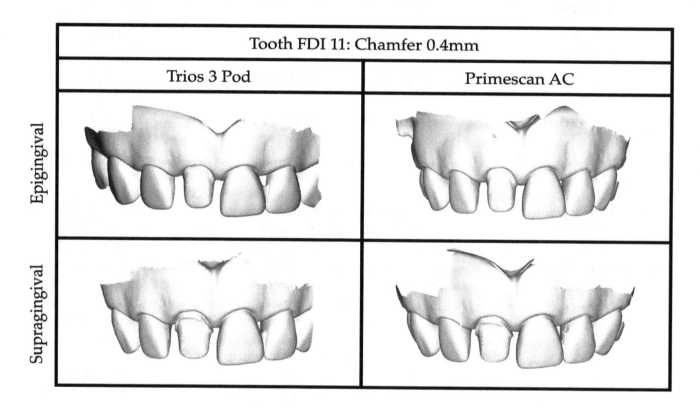

Figure 2. 3D color mapping depicting sample abutment teeth in position FDI 11 with epi-/supragingival 0.4 mm chamfer captured with Trios 3/Primescan AC and superimposition to the corresponding references (Final Surface, GFaI e.V., Berlin, Germany).

Table 1. Anterior tooth morphology: Deviation (in μm) of IOS-STLs compared to the reference STLs summarizing mean values of 80% quantiles, including standard deviations (SD) of the different preparation designs separated for epi- and supragingival finishing lines ([a–f] $p < 0.05$).

		Trios 3 Pod	Primescan AC
Epigingival	Tangential	34 ± 6	35 ± 5
	Chamfer 0.4 mm	[a] 38 ± 4	[b] 40 ± 6
	Chamfer 0.8 mm	[c] 42 ± 5	[d] 45 ± 6
	Shoulder	[e] 48 ± 5	[f] 50 ± 5
Supragingival	Tangential	30 ± 1	31 ± 2
	Chamfer 0.4 mm	[a] 28 ± 3	[b] 26 ± 2
	Chamfer 0.8 mm	[b] 29 ± 3	[d] 30 ± 3
	Shoulder	[e] 40 ± 6	[f] 39 ± 5

([a] $p = 0.0036$, [b] $p = 0.001$, [c] $p = 0.0013$, [d] $p = 0.0008$, [e] $p = 0.0008$, [f] $p = 0.0025$)

Table 2. Posterior tooth morphology: Deviation (in μm) of IOS-STLs compared to the reference STLs summarizing mean values of 80% quantiles, including standard deviations (SD) of the different preparation designs separated for epi- and supragingival finishing lines ([a–f] $p < 0.05$).

		Trios 3 Pod	Primescan AC
Epigingival	Tangential	30 ± 4	31 ± 4
	Chamfer 0.4 mm	[a] 40 ± 6	[b] 39 ± 4
	Chamfer 0.8 mm	[c] 39 ± 4	[d] 41 ± 5
	Shoulder	[e] 34 ± 4	[f] 36 ± 5
Supragingival	Tangential	29 ± 3	30 ± 3
	Chamfer 0.4 mm	[a] 28 ± 3	[b] 32 ± 3
	Chamfer 0.8 mm	[c] 27 ± 2	[d] 27 ± 1
	Shoulder	[e] 21 ± 2	[f] 20 ± 2

([a] $p = 0.0018$, [b] $p = 0.0128$, [c] $p = 0.0018$, [d] $p = 0.001$, [e] $p = 0.0013$, [f] $p = 0.0006$)

4. Discussion

The aim of this in vitro study was to analyze IOS accuracy for complete crown restorations, considering maxillary incisor and molar tooth morphologies with four different finish-line designs (tangential, narrow chamfer, wide chamfer, and shoulder) in epi- and supragingival margin positions. The results demonstrated that all specimens were successfully digitized with high accuracy independently of the IOS device used. However, the supragingival finishing lines were captured significantly better than the epigingivally located margins. Therefore, the hypothesis that IOS accuracy does not depend on any of the factors listed above was partially rejected.

IOS technology offers new possibilities for clinical routine in selected indications, especially in the field of fixed prosthodontics with all the advantages mentioned above. In the present study, the position of the finishing line with respect to the gingiva showed differences between epi- and supragingival margins. IOS recorded the supragingival preparations more precisely. Two further investigations have also demonstrated higher reproducibility for supragingival finishing lines [17,18]. Divergent literature states that the supra- and epigingival margins can be scanned without significant differences. In that mentioned in vitro study, supragingival finishing lines were made visible by gingival retraction [23]. The significant difference between the epi- and supragingival margins could be attributed to the absence of gingival retraction. Sufficient soft-tissue management is a crucial success factor and, therefore, should be ensured in clinical routine.

Based on the results of this in vitro investigation, it can be recommended that, to ensure a higher predictability of digital impression-taking in clinical routine, the finishing line must be clearly visible, with healthy gingiva surrounded a full 360°. Therefore, complete-crown finishing lines should be prepared supragingivally whenever possible using IOS [19,24], including proper soft-tissue management during impression taking, which remains a crucial success factor for any kind of impression technique [25] until future technology can provide novel IOS possibilities for scanning through tissue and liquids.

Today, IOS requires a direct line of sight on the object being scanned, and a minimal distance of 0.5 mm between adjacent teeth seems to be the critical threshold for the optical resolving power [17]. Otherwise, the IOS software takes over to calculate the preparation margins virtually, instead of capturing the intraoral situation with optical precision. Not all surfaces of a tooth seem to be recorded with the same accuracy; for example, distal and lingual surfaces have shown the lowest accuracy [26,27]. Finally, the complexity of the geometry to be scanned has an impact on the accuracy as well. Supragingival complete crown preparations have demonstrated significantly better results than intracoronal inlay preparations using different IOS systems [28]. For more complex preparations, e.g., for post copings or adhesive attachments, capturing with IOS is currently not feasible.

However, what are the limitations of digital impressions for treatment with complete crown restorations? Do any influencing factors affect the successful use of IOS in clinical routine?

Based on the results of the present trial, conventional crown preparation designs can be applied with a digital capturing by IOS while considering minimal invasiveness. It is possible to focus on the desired requirements for single-unit restorations in everyday clinical practice. The anatomical position and morphology of the area to be restored must be analyzed first. Moreover, the selected material has to be considered when selecting the preparation characteristics. Basically, the following parameters have been summarized for metal-based complete crowns: (i) convergence angle between two opposing prepared axial surfaces in the range of 10° to 22°; (ii) retentive vertical surfaces of at least 3 mm and a height-to-diameter ratio of at least 0.4 to provide adequate resistance form; (iii) teeth should be reduced uniformly to facilitate esthetic dental work, as well as anatomically to keep the teeth's characteristic geometric shape and to avoid pulp trauma [19].

The translation from in vitro to in vivo always involves difficulties. The presented trial setting reflects ideal and constant conditions. The clinical real-world scenario has to tackle multi-factor challenges such as irregular tooth preparations in terms of design and distance to the gingival margin, different dental surfaces, perfused soft tissue, saliva and sulcus fluids, limited access in the oral cavity, and patient movement. It was also not possible to work with gingival retraction in this in vitro setting. This study was carried out in a stable single-jaw setting using a typodont model with ideally prepared artificial abutment teeth. The absence of saliva, tongue, mouth opening, and individual patient anatomy simplified IOS scanability [29]. The impact of mouth opening, in particular, needs be further investigated for mandibular impressions in vivo. During IOS, patients must maintain an extensive mouth opening for a longer time compared to the conventional approach. This could lead to slight deformations of the mandible [30,31]. With the conventional method, the mouth must only initially be opened wide; however, during the setting time of the material, the patient can almost rest in a relaxing position. In vivo, this could lead to deviations in scanning accuracy between anterior and posterior areas, which could not be detected in this in vitro setting. Additionally, only two IOS devices were used, which reduces the power of generalization, and the operators could not be blinded for the intervention and the type of scanner used. For further studies, it would be useful to include a greater variety of IOS scanners and also to perform subgingival preparations in vivo, where appropriate soft-tissue management could be applied.

5. Conclusions

Within the limitations of this study, the following can be concluded:

(1) the overall accuracy for all abutment teeth was very high, without significant differences in the performance of 3Shape Trios 3 Pod versus Cerec Primescan AC;
(2) the supragingival finishing lines were captured significantly better than the epigingivally located margins using IOS. If the clinical situation allows, a supragingival margin should be chosen accordingly;
(3) the tooth morphology seems to be a negligible factor for IOS accuracy in terms of single-unit complete crown restorations.

Author Contributions: Conceptualization, S.A.B., J.M. and T.J.; methodology, S.A.B., J.M. and T.J.; software, S.A.B. and T.J.; validation, S.A.B. and T.J.; investigation, S.A.B. and J.M.; resources, J.M. and T.J.; data curation, S.A.B. and T.J.; writing—original draft preparation, S.A.B.; writing—review and editing, S.A.B., N.U.Z. and T.J.; visualization, S.A.B. and T.J.; supervision, J.M. and T.J. All authors have read and agreed to the published version of the manuscript.

Acknowledgments: The authors thank Institute Straumann AG, Basel, Switzerland, for their support of the study by donating the prepared teeth. Thanks also go to Dentsply Sirona for making the Cerec Primescan AC scanner available.

References

1. Joda, T.; Ferrari, M.; Gallucci, G.O.; Wittneben, J.; Brägger, U. Digital technology in fixed implant prosthodontics. *Periodontolgy 2000* **2016**, *73*, 178–192. [CrossRef] [PubMed]
2. Joda, T.; Zarone, F.; Ferrari, M. The complete digital workflow in fixed prosthodontics: A systematic review. *BMC Oral Health* **2017**, *17*, 1–9. [CrossRef] [PubMed]
3. Zitzmann, N.U.; Matthisson, L.; Ohla, H.; Joda, T. Digital Undergraduate Education in Dentistry: A Systematic Review. *Int. J. Environ. Res. Public Health* **2020**, *17*, 3269. [CrossRef] [PubMed]
4. Zitzmann, N.U.; Kovaltschuk, I.; Lenherr, P.; Dedem, P.; Joda, T. Dental Students' Perceptions of Digital and Conventional Impression Techniques: A Randomized Controlled Trial. *J. Dent. Educ.* **2017**, *81*, 1227–1232. [CrossRef]
5. Joda, T.; Gallucci, G.O. The virtual patient in dental medicine. *Clin. Oral Implant. Res.* **2014**, *26*, 725–726. [CrossRef]
6. Schoenbaum, T.R. Dentistry in the digital age: An update. *Dent. Today* **2012**, *31*, 12–13.
7. Eaton, K.A.; Reynolds, P.A.; Grayden, S.K.; Wilson, N.H.F. A vision of dental education in the third millennium. *Br. Dent. J.* **2008**, *205*, 261–271. [CrossRef]
8. Schepke, U.; Meijer, H.J.A.; Kerdijk, W.; Cune, M.S. Digital versus analog complete-arch impressions for single-unit premolar implant crowns: Operating time and patient preference. *J. Prosthet. Dent.* **2015**, *114*, 403–406. [CrossRef]
9. Joda, T.; Lenherr, P.; Dedem, P.; Kovaltschuk, I.; Bragger, U.; Zitzmann, N.U. Time efficiency, difficulty, and operator's preference comparing digital and conventional implant impressions: A randomized controlled trial. *Clin. Oral Implant. Res.* **2017**, *28*, 1318–1323. [CrossRef]
10. Yuzbasioglu, E.; Kurt, H.; Turunc, R.; Bilir, H. Comparison of digital and conventional impression techniques: Evaluation of patients' perception, treatment comfort, effectiveness and clinical outcomes. *BMC Oral Health* **2014**, *14*, 10. [CrossRef]
11. Christensen, G.J. Impressions are changing: Deciding on conventional, digital or digital plus in-office milling. *J. Am. Dent. Assoc. (1939)* **2009**, *140*, 1301–1304. [CrossRef] [PubMed]
12. Gintaute, A.; Straface, A.; Zitzmann, N.U.; Joda, T. Die Modellgussprothese 2.0: Digital von A bis Z? *Swiss. Dent. J.* **2020**, *130*, 229–235. [PubMed]
13. Masri, R.; Driscoll, C.F.; Burkhardt, J.; von Fraunhofer, A.; Romberg, E. Pressure generated on a simulated oral analog by impression materials in custom trays of different designs. *J. Prosthodont.* **2002**, *11*, 155–160. [CrossRef] [PubMed]
14. Al-Ahmad, A.; Masri, R.; Driscoll, C.F.; Von Fraunhofer, J.; Romberg, E. Pressure Generated on a Simulated Mandibular Oral Analog by Impression Materials in Custom Trays of Different Design. *J. Prosthodont.* **2006**, *15*, 95–101. [CrossRef]
15. Schlenz, M.A.; Schubert, V.; Schmidt, A.; Wöstmann, B.; Ruf, S.; Klaus, K. Digital versus Conventional Impression Taking Focusing on Interdental Areas: A Clinical Trial. *Int. J. Environ. Res. Public Health* **2020**, *17*, 4725. [CrossRef]
16. Baroudi, K.; Ibraheem, S.N. Assessment of Chair-side Computer-Aided Design and Computer-Aided Manufacturing Restorations: A Review of the Literature. *J. Int. Oral Health* **2015**, *7*, 96–104.
17. Ferrari, M.; Keeling, A.; Mandelli, F.; Giudice, G.L.; Garcia-Godoy, F.; Joda, T. The ability of marginal detection using different intraoral scanning systems: A pilot randomized controlled trial. *Am. J. Dent.* **2018**, *31*, 272–276.
18. Keeling, A.; Wu, J.; Ferrari, M. Confounding factors affecting the marginal quality of an intra-oral scan. *J. Dent.* **2017**, *59*, 33–40. [CrossRef]
19. Goodacre, C.J. Designing tooth preparations for optimal success. *Dent. Clin. N. Am.* **2004**, *48*, 359–385. [CrossRef]
20. Ahmed, W.M.; Shariati, B.; Gazzaz, A.Z.; Sayed, M.E.; Carvalho, R.M. Fit of tooth-supported zirconia single crowns—A systematic review of the literature. *Clin. Exp. Dent. Res.* **2020**. [CrossRef]
21. Balevi, B. Limited evidence on the best position for prosthetic margins. *Evidence-Based Dent.* **2013**, *14*, 103–104. [CrossRef] [PubMed]

22. Mühlemann, S.; Greter, E.A.; Park, J.M.; Hämmerle, C.H.F.; Thoma, D.S. Precision of digital implant models compared to conventional implant models for posterior single implant crowns: A within-subject comparison. *Clin. Oral Implant. Res.* **2018**, *29*, 931–936. [CrossRef] [PubMed]

23. Koulivand, S.; Ghodsi, S.; Siadat, H.; Alikhasi, M. A clinical comparison of digital and conventional impression techniques regarding finish line locations and impression time. *J. Esthet. Restor. Dent.* **2020**, *32*, 236–243. [CrossRef] [PubMed]

24. Valderhaugw, J.; Birkeland, J. Periodontal conditions in patients 5 years following insertion of fixed prostheses: Pocket depth and loss of attachment. *J. Oral Rehabil.* **1976**, *3*, 237–243. [CrossRef]

25. Shetty, K. Gingival tissue management: A necessity or a liability. *Triv. Dent. J.* **2011**, *2*, 112–119.

26. Roperto, R.; Oliveira, M.; Porto, T.; Ferreira, L.; Melo, L.; Akkus, A. Can Tooth Preparation Design Affect the Fit of CAD/CAM Restorations? *Compend. Contin. Educ. Dent. (Jamesburg, NJ: 1995)* **2017**, *38*, e13–e17.

27. Chiu, A.; Chen, Y.W.; Hayashi, J.; Sadr, A. Accuracy of CAD/CAM Digital Impressions with Different Intraoral Scanner Parameters. *Sensors* **2020**, *20*, 1157. [CrossRef]

28. Ashraf, Y.; Sabet, A.; Hamdy, A.; Ebeid, K. Influence of Preparation Type and Tooth Geometry on the Accuracy of Different Intraoral Scanners. *J. Prosthodont.* **2020**. [CrossRef]

29. Fluegge, T.V.; Schlager, S.; Nelson, K.; Nahles, S.; Metzger, M.C. Precision of intraoral digital dental impressions with iTero and extraoral digitization with the iTero and a model scanner. *Am. J. Orthod. Dentofac. Orthop.* **2013**, *144*, 471–478. [CrossRef]

30. Chen, D.C.; Lai, Y.L.; Chi, L.Y.; Lee, S.Y. Contributing factors of mandibular deformation during mouth opening. *J. Dent.* **2000**, *28*, 583–588. [CrossRef]

31. Law, C.; Bennani, V.; Lyons, K.; Swain, M.V. Mandibular Flexure and Its Significance on Implant Fixed Prostheses: A Review. *J. Prosthodont.* **2012**, *21*, 219–224. [CrossRef] [PubMed]

15

Current Applications, Opportunities and Limitations of AI for 3D Imaging in Dental Research and Practice

Kuofeng Hung [1], Andy Wai Kan Yeung [1], Ray Tanaka [1] and Michael M. Bornstein [1,2,*]

[1]   Oral and Maxillofacial Radiology, Applied Oral Sciences and Community Dental Care, Faculty of Dentistry, The University of Hong Kong, Hong Kong 999077, China; hungkf@connect.hku.hk (K.H.); ndyeung@hku.hk (A.W.K.Y.); rayt3@hku.hk (R.T.)
[2]   Department of Oral Health & Medicine, University Center for Dental Medicine Basel UZB, University of Basel, 4058 Basel, Switzerland
*   Correspondence: michael.bornstein@unibas.ch

Abstract: The increasing use of three-dimensional (3D) imaging techniques in dental medicine has boosted the development and use of artificial intelligence (AI) systems for various clinical problems. Cone beam computed tomography (CBCT) and intraoral/facial scans are potential sources of image data to develop 3D image-based AI systems for automated diagnosis, treatment planning, and prediction of treatment outcome. This review focuses on current developments and performance of AI for 3D imaging in dentomaxillofacial radiology (DMFR) as well as intraoral and facial scanning. In DMFR, machine learning-based algorithms proposed in the literature focus on three main applications, including automated diagnosis of dental and maxillofacial diseases, localization of anatomical landmarks for orthodontic and orthognathic treatment planning, and general improvement of image quality. Automatic recognition of teeth and diagnosis of facial deformations using AI systems based on intraoral and facial scanning will very likely be a field of increased interest in the future. The review is aimed at providing dental practitioners and interested colleagues in healthcare with a comprehensive understanding of the current trend of AI developments in the field of 3D imaging in dental medicine.

Keywords: artificial intelligence; AI; machine learning; ML; cone beam computed tomography (CBCT); intraoral scanning; facial scanning

---

1. Introduction

Artificial intelligence (AI) is generally defined as intelligent computer programs capable of learning and applying knowledge to accomplish complex tasks such as to predict treatment outcomes, recognize objects, and answer questions [1]. Nowadays, AI technologies are widespread and penetrate many applications of our daily life, such as Amazon's online shopping recommendations, Facebook's image recognition, Netflix's streaming videos, and the smartphone's voice assistant [2]. For such daily life applications, it is characteristic that the initial use of an AI-driven system will give a more generalized outcome based on big data, and after repeated use by the individual, it will gradually present a more adapted and personalized outcome in accordance with the user's characteristics. The remarkable success of AI in various fields of our daily life has inspired and is stimulating the development of AI systems in the field of medicine and, also, more specifically, dental medicine [3,4].

Radiology is deemed to be the front door for AI into medicine as digitally coded diagnostic images are more easily translated into computer language [5]. Thus, diagnostic images are seen as one of the primary sources of data used to develop AI systems for the purpose of an automated prediction of disease risk (such as osteoporotic bone fractures [6]), detection of pathologies (such as coronary artery calcification as a predictor for atherosclerosis [7]), and diagnosis of disease (such as skin cancers in dermatology [8]). Machine learning is a key component of AI, and commonly applied to develop image-based AI systems. Through a synergism between radiologists and the medical AI system used, increased work efficiency and more precise outcomes regarding the final diagnosis of various diseases are expected to be achieved [9,10].

In the field of dental and maxillofacial radiology (DMFR), reports on AI models used for diagnostic purposes and treatment planning cover a wide range of clinical applications, including automated localization of craniofacial anatomical structures/pathological changes, classification of maxillofacial cysts and/or tumors, and diagnosis of caries and periodontal lesions [11]. According to the literature related to clinical applications of AI in DMFR, most of the proposed machine learning algorithms were developed using two-dimensional (2D) diagnostic images, such as periapical, panoramic, and cephalometric radiographs [11]. However, 2D images have several limitations, including image magnification and distortion, superimposition of anatomical structures, and the lack of three-dimensional information for relevant landmarks/pathological changes. These may lower the diagnostic accuracy of the AI models trained using only 2D images [12]. For example, a 2D image-based AI model built for the detection of periodontal bone defects might not be able to detect three-walled bony defects, loss of buccal/oral cortical bone plates, or bone defects around overlapping teeth. Three-dimensional (3D) imaging techniques, including cone beam computed tomography (CBCT), as well as intraoral and facial scanning systems, are increasingly used in dental practice. CBCT imaging allows for the visualization and assessment of bony anatomic structures and/or pathological changes in 3D with high diagnostic accuracy and precision. The use of CBCT is of great help when conventional 2D imaging techniques do not provide sufficient information for diagnosis and treatment planning purposes [13]. Intraoral and facial scanning systems are reported to be reproducible and reliable to capture 3D soft-tissue images that can be used for digital treatment planning systems [14,15]. CBCT and intraoral/facial scans are considered as an ideal data source for developing AI models to overcome the limitations of 2D image-based algorithms [12,15]. Thus, the aim of this review is to describe current developments and to assess the performance of AI models for 3D imaging in DMFR, as well as intraoral and facial scanning.

2. Current Use of AI for 3D Imaging in DMFR

A literature search was conducted using PubMed to identify all existing studies of AI applications for 3D imaging in DMFR and intraoral/facial scanning. The search was conducted without restriction on the publication period but was limited to studies in English. The keywords used for the search were combinations of terms including "artificial intelligence", "AI", "machine learning", "deep learning", "convolutional neural networks", "automatic", "automated", "three-dimensional imaging", "3D imaging", "cone beam computed tomography", "CBCT", "three-dimensional scan", "3D scan", "intraoral scan", "intraoral scanning", "facial scan", "facial scanning", and/or "dentistry". Reviews, conference papers, and studies using clinical/nonclinical image data were eligible for the initial screening process. Initially, titles of the identified studies were manually screened, and subsequently, abstracts of the relevant studies were read to identify studies for further full-text reading. Furthermore, references of included articles were examined to identify further relevant articles. As a result, approximately 650 publications were initially screened, and 23 publications were eventually included in the present review for data extraction (details provided in Tables 1 and 2).

The methodological quality of the included studies was evaluated using the assessment criteria proposed by Hung et al. [11]. For proposed AI models for diagnosis/classification of a certain condition, four studies [16–19] were rated as having a "high" or an "unclear" risk of concern in the domain of subject selection because the testing dataset only consisted of images from subjects with the condition of interest. With regard to the selection of reference standards, all studies were considered as "low" risk of concern as expert judgment and clinical or pathological examination was applied as the reference standard. Concerns regarding the risk of bias were relatively high in the domain of index test, as ten [16,17,20–27] of the included studies did not test their AI models on independent images unused for developing the algorithms.

Table 1 exhibits the included studies regarding the use of AI for 3D imaging in DMFR. These studies focused on three main applications, including automated diagnosis of dental and maxillofacial diseases [16–20,28–32], localization of anatomical landmarks for orthodontic and orthognathic treatment planning [21,22,33–35], and improvement of image quality [23,36].

2.1. Automated Diagnosis of Dental and Maxillofacial Diseases

The basic principle of the learning algorithms for diagnostic purposes is to explore associations between the input image and output diagnosis. Theoretically, a machine learning algorithm is initially built using hand-crafted detectors of image features in a predefined framework, subsequently trained with the training data, iteratively adapted to minimize the error at the output, and eventually tested with the unseen testing data to verify its validity [37]. Deep learning, a subset of machine learning, is able to automatically learn to extract relevant image features without the requirement of the manual design of image feature detectors, which is currently considered as the most suitable method to develop image-based diagnostic AI models [12].

The workflow of the proposed machine learning algorithms for diagnostic purpose can be mainly categorized as (see Figure 1).

1. Input image data;
2. Image preprocessing;
3. Selection of the region of interest (ROI);
4. Segmentation of lesions;
5. Extraction of selected texture features in the segmented lesions;
6. Analysis of the extracted features;
7. Output of the diagnosis or classification.

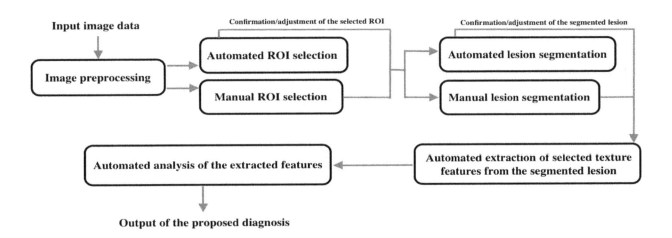

Figure 1. The workflow of the proposed machine learning algorithms for diagnostic purposes.

Table 1. Characteristics of studies describing machine learning-based artificial intelligence (AI) models applied in dentomaxillofacial radiology (DMFR).

Author (Year)	Application	Imaging Modality	AI Technique	Image Data Set Used to Develop the AI Model	Independent Testing Image Data Set / Validation Technique	Performance
				Diagnosis of Dental and Maxillofacial Diseases		
Okada [16] (2015)	Diagnosis of periapical cysts and granuloma	CBCT	LDA	28 scans from patients with periapical cysts or granuloma	7-fold CV	94.1% (accuracy)
Abdolali [17] (2017)	Diagnosis of radicular cysts, dentigerous cysts, and keratocysts	CBCT	SVM; SDA	96 scans from patients with radicular cysts, dentigerous cysts, or keratocysts	3-fold CV	94.29–96.48% (accuracy)
Yilmaz [18] (2017)	Diagnosis of periapical cysts and keratocysts	CBCT	k-NN; Naïve Bayes; Decision tree; Random forest; NN; SVM	50 scans from patients with cysts or tumors / 25 scans from patients with cysts or tumors	10-fold CV/LOOCV / 25 scans from patients with cysts or tumors	94–100% (accuracy)
Lee [19] (2020)	Diagnosis of periapical cysts, dentigerous cysts, and keratocysts	Panoramic radiography and CBCT	CNN	912 panoramic images and 789 CBCT scans	228 panoramic images and 197 CBCT scans	Panoramic radiography 0.847 (AUC); 88.2% (sensitivity); 77.0% (specificity) CBCT 0.914 (AUC); 96.1% (sensitivity); 77.1% (specificity)
Orhan [28] (2020)	Diagnosis of periapical pathology	CBCT	CNN	3900 scans acquired using multiple FOVs from 2800 patients with periapical lesions and 1100 subjects without periapical lesions	109 scans acquired using multiple FOVs from 153 patients with periapical lesions	92.8% (accuracy)
Abdolali [29] (2019)	Diagnosis of radiolucent lesion, maxillary sinus perforation, unerupted tooth, and root fracture	CBCT	Symmetry-based analysis model	686 scans acquired using a large FOV ($12 \times 15 \times 15$ cm³), collected from several dental imaging centers in Iran	459 scans acquired using a large FOV ($12 \times 15 \times 15$ cm³), collected from several dental imaging centers in Iran	0.85–0.92 (DSC)

Table 1. *Cont.*

Author (Year)	Application	Imaging Modality	AI Technique	Image Data Set Used to Develop the AI Model	Independent Testing Image Data Set / Validation Technique	Performance
Johari [30] (2017)	Detection of vertical root fractures	Periapical radiography and CBCT	CNN	180 periapical radiographs and 180 CBCT scans of the extracted teeth	60 periapical radiographs and 60 CBCT scans of the extracted teeth	Periapical radiography 70.0% (accuracy); 97.8% (sensitivity); 67.6% (specificity); CBCT 96.6% (accuracy); 93.3% (sensitivity); 100% (specificity)
Kise [32] (2019)	Diagnosis of Sjögren's syndrome	CT	CNN	400 scans (200 from 20 SjS patients and 200 from 20 control subjects) acquired using a large FOV	100 scans (50 from 5 SjS patients and 50 from 5 control subjects) acquired using a large FOV	96.0% (accuracy); 100% (sensitivity); 92.0% (specificity)
Kann [31] (2018)	Detection of lymph node metastasis and extranodal extension in patients with head and neck cancer	Contrast-enhanced CT	CNN	Images of 2875 CT-segmented lymph node samples with correlating pathology labels	Images of 131 lymph nodes (76 negative and 55 positive)	0.91 (AUC)
Ariji [20] (2019)	Detection of lymph node metastasis in patients with oral cancer	Contrast-enhanced CT	CNN	Images of 441 lymph nodes (314 negative and 127 positive) from 45 patients	5-fold CV	78.2% (accuracy); 75.4% (sensitivity); 81.0% (specificity), 0.80 (AUC)
Localization of Anatomical Landmarks for Orthodontic and Orthognathic Treatment Planning						
Cheng [33] (2011)	Localization of the odontoid process of the second vertebra	CBCT	Random forest	50 scans	23 scans	3.15 mm (mean deviation)
Shahidi [34] (2014)	Localization of 14 anatomical landmarks	CBCT	Feature-based and voxel similarity-based algorithms	8 scans acquired using a large FOV from subjects aged 10–45 years	20 scans acquired using a large FOV from subjects aged 10–45 years	3.40 mm (mean deviation)

Table 1. *Cont.*

Author (Year)	Application	Imaging Modality	AI Technique	Image Data Set Used to Develop the AI Model	Independent Testing Image Data Set / Validation Technique	Performance
Montufar [21] (2018)	Localization of 18 anatomical landmarks	CBCT	Active shape model	24 scans acquired using a large FOV	LOOCV	3.64 mm (mean deviation)
Montufar [22] (2018)	Localization of 18 anatomical landmarks	CBCT	Active shape model	24 scans acquired using a large FOV	LOOCV	2.51 mm (mean deviation)
Torosdagli [35] (2019)	Localization of 9 anatomical landmarks	CBCT	CNN	50 scans	48 scans	0.9382 (DSC); 93.42% (sensitivity); 99.97% (specificity),
Improvement of Image Quality						
Park [36] (2018)	Improvement of image resolution	CT	CNN	52 scans	13 scans	The CNN network can yield high-resolution images based on low-resolution images
Minnema [23] (2019)	Segmentation of CBCT scans affected by metal artifacts	CBCT	CNN	20 scans	Leave-2-out CV	The CNN network can accurately segment bony structures in CBCT scans affected by metal artifacts
Other						
Miki [38] (2017)	Tooth classification	CBCT	CNN	42 scans with the diameter of the FOV ranged from 5.1 to 20 cm	10 scans with the diameter of the FOV ranged from 5.1 to 20 cm	88.8% (accuracy)

AI, artificial intelligence; AUC, area under the receiver operating characteristic curve; CBCT, cone beam computed tomography; CNN, convolutional neural network; CT, computed tomography; CV, cross validation; DSC, dice similarity coefficient; FOV, field of view; k-NN, k-nearest neighbors; LDA, linear discriminant analysis; LOOCV, leave-one-out cross-validation; NN, neural network; SDA, sparse discriminant analysis; SjS, Sjögren's syndrome; SVM, support vector machine.

Some of the proposed machine learning algorithms were not fully automated and required manual operation/adjustment for the ROI selection or lesion segmentation. Okada et al. proposed a semiautomatic machine learning algorithm, using CBCT images to classify periapical cysts and granulomas [16]. This algorithm requires users to segment the target lesion before it proceeds to the next step (feature extraction). Yilmaz et al. proposed a semiautomatic algorithm, using CBCT images to classify periapical cysts and keratocysts [18]. In this algorithm, detection and segmentation of lesions are required to be performed manually. The users need to mark the lesion on different cross-sectional planes to predefine the volume of interest containing the lesion. Manual segmentation of cystic lesions on multiple CBCT slices is time-consuming, which limits the efficiency of the algorithms and also their implementation for routine clinical use. Lee et al. proposed deep learning algorithms, respectively, using panoramic radiographs and CBCT images for the detection and diagnosis of periapical cysts, dentigerous cysts, and keratocysts [19]. It was reported that automatic edge detection techniques can segment cystic lesions more efficiently and accurately than manual segmentation. This can shorten the execution time for the segmentation step and improve the usability of the proposed algorithms for clinical practice. Moreover, higher diagnostic accuracy was reported for CBCT image-based algorithms in comparison with panoramic image-based ones. This may result from a higher accuracy in detecting the lesion boundary in 3D and more quantitative features extracted from the voxel units. Abdolali et al. proposed an algorithm based on asymmetry analysis using CBCT images to automatically segment cystic lesions, including dentigerous cysts, radicular cysts, and keratocysts [39]. The algorithm exhibited promising performance with high true-positives and low false-positives. However, its limitations include a relatively low detection rate for small cysts, imperfect segmentation of keratocysts without well-defined boundaries, and the incapability of dealing with symmetric cysts crossing the midsagittal plane. Based on the proposed segmentation algorithm, Abdolali et al. developed another AI model using CBCT images to automatically classify dentigerous cysts, radicular cysts, and keratocysts [17]. This model exhibited high classification accuracies ranging from 94.29% to 96.48%. Subsequently, Abdolali et al. further proposed a fully automated medical-content-based image retrieval system for the diagnosis of four maxillofacial lesions/conditions, including radiolucent lesions, maxillary sinus perforation, unerupted teeth, and root fractures [29]. In this novel system, an improved version of a previously proposed segmentation algorithm [39] was incorporated. The diagnostic accuracy of the proposed system was 90%, with a significantly reduced segmentation time of three minutes per case. It was stated that this system is more effective than previous models proposed in the literature, and is promising for introduction into clinical practice in the near future.

Orhan et al. verified the performance of a deep learning algorithm using CBCT images to detect and volumetrically measure periapical lesions [28]. A detection rate of 92.8% and a significant positive correlation between the automated and manual measurements were reported. The differences between manual and automated measurements are mainly due to inaccurate lesion segmentation. Because of low soft-tissue contrast in CBCT images, the deep learning algorithm exhibits difficulties in perfectly distinguishing the lesion area from neighboring soft tissue when buccal/oral cortical perforations or endo-perio lesions occur. Johari et al. proposed deep learning algorithms using periapical and CBCT images to detect vertical root fractures [30]. The results showed that the proposed model resulted in higher diagnostic performance for CBCT images than periapicals. Furthermore, some studies have reported on the application of deep learning algorithms for the diagnosis of Sjögren's syndrome or lymph node metastasis. Kise et al. proposed a deep learning algorithm using CT images to assist inexperienced radiologists to semiautomatically diagnose Sjögren's syndrome [32]. The results exhibited that the diagnostic performance of the deep learning algorithm is comparable to experienced radiologists and is significantly higher than for inexperienced radiologists. The main limitation of the proposed algorithm is its semiautomatic nature, requiring manual image segmentation prior to performing automated diagnosis. For further ease and implementation in daily routine, a completely automated segmentation of the region of the parotid gland should be developed and incorporated into a fully automated diagnostic system. Kann et al. and Ariji et al., respectively, proposed deep learning algorithms using contrast-enhanced CT images to semiautomatically identify nodal metastasis in patients with oral/head and neck cancer [20,31]. The user of the respective programs is required to manually segment the contour of lymph nodes on multiple CT slices. Excellent performance was reported for both algorithms proposed, which was close to or even surpassed the diagnostic accuracy of experienced radiologists. Therefore, these deep learning algorithms have the potential to help guide oral/head and neck cancer patient management. Future investigations should focus on the development of a fully automated identification system to avoid manual segmentation of lymph nodes. This can significantly improve the efficiency of the AI system used and could enable wider use of this system in community clinics.

2.2. Automated Localization of Anatomical Landmarks for Orthodontic and Orthognathic Treatment Planning

The correct analysis of craniofacial anatomy and facial proportions is the basis of successful orthodontic and orthognathic treatment. Traditional orthodontic analysis is generally conducted on 2D cephalometric radiographs, which can be less accurate due to image magnification, superimposition of structures, inappropriate X-ray projection angle, and patient position. Since CBCT was introduced in dental medicine, 3D diagnosis and virtual treatment planning have been assessed as a more accurate option for orthodontic and orthognathic treatment [40]. Although 3D orthodontic analysis can be performed by a computer-aided digital tracing approach, it still requires orthodontists to manually locate anatomical landmarks on multiple CBCT slices. The manual localization process is tedious and time-consuming, which may currently discourage orthodontists from switching to a fully digital workflow. Cheng et al. proposed the first machine learning algorithm to automatically localize one key landmark on CBCT images and reported promising results [33]. Subsequently, a series of machine learning algorithms were developed for automated localization of several anatomical landmarks and analysis of dentofacial deformity. Shahidi et al. proposed a machine-learning algorithm to automatically locate 14 craniofacial landmarks on CBCT images, whereas the mean deviation (3.40 mm) for all of the automatically identified landmarks was higher than the mean deviation (1.41 mm) for the manually detected ones [34]. Montufar et al. proposed two different automatic landmark localization systems, respectively, based on active shape models and a hybrid approach using active shape models followed by a 3D knowledge-based searching algorithm [21,22]. The mean deviation (2.51 mm) for all of the automatically identified landmarks in the hybrid system was lower than that of the system only using active shape models (3.64 mm). Despite less localization deviation, the performance of automated localization in the proposed systems is still not accurate enough to meet clinical requirements. Therefore, the existing AI systems can only be recommended for the use of preliminary localization of the orthodontic landmarks, but manual correction is still necessary prior to further orthodontic analyses. This may be the main limitation of these AI systems and this needs to be improved for future clinical dissemination and use.

Orthodontic and orthognathic treatments in patients with craniofacial deformities are challenging. The aforementioned AI systems may not be able to effectively deal with such patients. Torosdagli et al. proposed a novel deep learning algorithm applied for fully automated mandible segmentation and landmarking in craniofacial anomalies on CBCT images [35]. The proposed algorithm allows for orthodontic analysis in patients with craniofacial deformities and showed excellent performance with a sensitivity of 93.42% and specificity of 99.97%. Future studies should consider widening the field of applications for AI systems, especially for different patient populations.

2.3. Automated Improvement of Image Quality

Radiation dose protection is of paramount importance in medicine and also for DMFR. It is reported that medical radiation exposure is the largest artificial radiation source and represents approximately 14% of the total annual dose of ionizing radiation for individuals [41]. Computed tomography (CT) imaging is widely used to assist clinical diagnosis in various fields of medicine. Reducing the scanning slice thickness is the general option to enhance the resolution of CT images. However, this will increase the noise level as well as radiation dose exposure to the patient. High-resolution CT images are recommended only when low-resolution CT images do not provide sufficient information for diagnosis and treatment planning purposes in individual cases [42]. The balance between the radiation dose and CT image resolution is the biggest concern for radiologists. To address this issue, Park et al. proposed a deep learning algorithm to enhance the thick-slice CT image resolution similar to that of a thin slice [36]. It is reported that the noise level of the enhanced CT images is even lower than the original images. Therefore, this algorithm has the potential to be a useful tool for enhancing the image resolution for CT scans as well as reducing the radiation dose and noise level. It is expected that such an algorithm can further be developed for CBCT scans.

The presence of metal artifacts in CT/CBCT images is another critical issue that can obscure neighboring anatomical structures and interfere with disease diagnosis. In dental medicine, metal artifacts are not uncommon in CBCT images due to materials used for dental restorations or orthodontic purposes. These metal artifacts not only interfere with disease diagnosis but, in some cases, impede the image segmentation of the teeth and bony structures in the maxilla and mandible for computer-guided treatment. Minnema et al. proposed a deep learning algorithm based on a mixed-scale dense convolutional neural network for the segmentation of teeth and bone on CBCT images affected by metal artifacts [23]. It is reported that the proposed algorithm can accurately classify metal artifacts as background and segment teeth and bony structures. The promising results prove that a convolutional neural network is capable of extracting the characteristic features in CBCT voxel units that cannot be distinguished by human eyes.

2.4. Other Applications

In addition to the above AI applications, automated tooth detection, classification, and numbering are also fields of great interest, and they have the potential to simplify the process of filling out digital dental charts [43]. Miki et al. developed a deep learning algorithm based on a convolutional neural network to automatically classify tooth types based on CBCT images [38]. Although this algorithm was designed for automated filling of dental charts for forensic identification purposes, it may also be valuable to incorporate it into the digital treatment planning system, especially for use in implantology and prosthetics. For example, such an application may contribute to the automated identification of missing teeth for the diagnosis and planning of implants or other prosthetic treatments.

3. Current Use of AI for Intraoral 3D Imaging and Facial Scanning

In recent years, computer-aided design and manufacturing (CAD/CAM) technology have been widely used in various fields of dentistry, especially in implantology, prosthetics, orthodontics, and maxillofacial surgery. For example, CAD/CAM technology can be used for the fabrication of surgical implant guides, provisional/definitive restorations, orthodontic appliances, and maxillofacial surgical templates. Most of these applications are based on 3D hard and soft tissue images generated by CBCT and optical scanning (such as intraoral/facial scanning and scanning of dental casts/impressions). Intraoral scanning is the most accurate method of digitalizing the 3D contour of teeth and gingiva [44]. As a result, the intraoral scanning technique is now gradually replacing the scanning of dental casts or impressions and is also frequently used in CAD/CAM systems. Tooth segmentation is a critical step, which is usually performed manually by trained dental practitioners in a digital workflow to design and fabricate restorations and orthodontic appliances. However, manual segmentation is time-consuming, poorly reproducible, and limited due to human error, which may eventually have a negative influence on treatment outcome. Ghazvinian Zanjani et al. and Kim et al., respectively, developed deep learning algorithms for automated tooth segmentation on digitalized 3D dental surface models resulting in high segmentation precision (Table 2) [24,45]. These algorithms can speed up the digital workflow and reduce human error. Furthermore, Lian et al. proposed an automated tooth labeling algorithm based on intraoral scanning [25]. This algorithm can simplify the process of tooth position rearrangements in orthodontic treatment planning.

Table 2 Characteristics of the machine learning-based AI models based on intraoral and facial scanning.

Author (Year)	Application	Imaging Modality	AI Technique	Image Data Set Used to Develop the AI Model	Independent Testing Image Data Set/Validation Technique	Performance
Ghazvinian Zanjani [24] (2019)	Tooth segmentation	Intraoral scanning	CNN	120 scans, comprising 60 upper jaws and 60 lower jaws.	5-fold CV	0.94 (intersection over union score)
Kim [45] (2020)	Tooth segmentation	Intraoral scanning	Generative adversarial network	10,000 cropped images	Approximate 350 cropped images	An average improvement of 0.004 mm in the tooth segmentation
Lian [25] (2020)	Tooth labelling	Intraoral scanning	CNN	30 scans of upper jaws	5-fold CV	0.894 to 0.970 (DSC)
Liu [27] (2016)	Identification of Autism Spectrum Disorder	Facial scanning	SVM	87 scans from children with and without Autism Spectrum Disorder	LOOCV	88.51% (accuracy)
Knoops [26] (2019)	Diagnosis and planning in plastic and reconstructive surgery	Facial scanning	Machine-learning-based 3D morphable model	4261 scans from healthy subjects and orthognathic patients	LOOCV	Diagnosis 95.5% (sensitivity); 95.2% (specificity) Surgical simulation 1.1 ± 0.3 mm (accuracy)

3D, three-dimensional; AI, artificial intelligence; CV, cross-validation; DSC, dice similarity coefficient; LOOCV, leave-one-out cross-validation; SVM, support vector machine.

Currently, only a few studies have reported on the use of machine learning techniques based on facial scanning (Table 2). Knoops et al. proposed an AI 3D-morphable model based on facial scanning to automatically analyze facial shape features for diagnosis and planning in plastic and reconstructive surgery [26]. In addition, this model is also able to predict patient-specific postoperative outcomes. The proposed model may improve the efficiency and accuracy in diagnosis and treatment planning, and help preoperative communication with the patient. However, this model can only perform an analysis based on 3D facial scanning alone. As facial scanning is unable to acquire volumetric bone data, the information about the underlying skeletal structures cannot be analyzed by this model. An updated model that can perform the analysis simultaneously on facial soft tissue and skeletal structures will be more realistic and probably more effective for clinical use.

Interestingly, facial scanning techniques in combination with AI can also be used for the diagnosis of neurodevelopmental disorders, such as autism spectrum disorder (ASD). Liu et al. explored the possibility of using a machine learning algorithm based on facial scanning to identify ASD and showed promising results with an accuracy of 88.51% (Table 2) [27]. This algorithm could be a supportive tool for the screening and diagnosis of ASD in clinical practice.

4. Limitations of the Included Studies

While the AI models proposed in the included studies have shown promising performance, several limitations are worth noting, which may affect the reliability of the proposed models. First, most of the proposed AI models were developed using a small number of images collected from the same institution over one defined time period (see details in Tables 1–3). Additionally, some classification models were only trained and tested using images from subjects with confirmed diseases (Table 3). These limitations might result in a risk of overfitting and a too optimistic appraisal of the proposed models. In addition, the images used to develop the algorithms might very likely be captured using the same device and imaging protocols, resulting in a lack of data heterogeneity (Table 3). This might cause a lack of generalizability and reliability of the proposed models and can result in inferior performance in clinical practice settings due to differences in variables, including devices, imaging protocols, and patient populations [46]. Thus, these models may still need to be verified by using adequate heterogeneous data collected from different dental institutions prior to being transferred and implemented into clinical practice.

Table 3. Conclusions and limitations of the included studies.

Author (Year)	Conclusion	Limitations (Risk of Bias *)
Okada [16] (2015)	The proposed model may assist clinicians to accurately differentiate periapical lesions.	• A small training dataset *; Lacking data heterogeneity *; Dataset only consisted of scans from subjects with the condition of interest *; Lacking independent unseen testing data *; Manual ROI selection; Long execution time.
Abdolali [17] (2017)	The proposed model can improve the accuracy of the diagnosis of dentigerous cysts, radicular cysts, and keratocysts, and may have a significant impact on future AI diagnostic systems.	• A small training dataset *; Lacking data heterogeneity *; Dataset only consisted of scans from subjects with the condition of interest *; Lacking independent unseen testing data *.
Yilmaz [18] (2017)	Periapical cysts and keratocysts can be classified with high accuracy with the proposed model. It can also contribute to the field of automated diagnosis of periapical lesions.	• A small training dataset *; Lacking data heterogeneity *; Dataset only consisted of scans from subjects with the condition of interest *; Manual detection and segmentation of lesions.
Lee [19] (2020)	Periapical cysts, dentigerous cysts, and keratocysts can be effectively detected and diagnosed with the proposed deep CNN algorithm, but the diagnosis of these lesions using radiological data alone, without histological examination, is still challenging.	• A relatively small training dataset *; Dataset only consisted of scans from subjects with the condition of interest *; Manual ROI selection; Potential overfitting problem in the training procedure *.
Orhan [28] (2020)	The proposed deep learning systems can be useful for detection and volumetric measurement of periapical lesions. The diagnostic performance was comparable to that of an oral and maxillofacial radiologist.	• Relatively inaccurate segmentation of lesions in close contact with neighboring soft tissue
Abdolali [29] (2019)	The proposed system is effective and can automatically diagnose various maxillofacial lesions/conditions. It can facilitate the introduction of content-based image retrieval in clinical CBCT applications.	• Relatively inaccurate detection of symmetric lesions
Johari [30] (2017)	The proposed deep learning model can be used for the diagnosis of vertical root fractures on CBCT images of endodontically treated and also vital teeth. With the aid of the model, the use of CBCT images is more effective than periapical radiographs.	• A small training dataset *; Ex-vivo data only containing sound extracted premolars *; Lacking data heterogeneity *; Unknown diagnostic performance on multirooted teeth and teeth with caries or filling materials *.

Table 3. *Cont.*

Author (Year)	Conclusion	Limitations (Risk of Bias *)
Kise [32] (2019)	The deep learning model showed high diagnostic accuracy for SjS, which is comparable to that of experienced radiologists. It is suggested that the model could be used to assist the diagnosis of SjS, especially for inexperienced radiologists.	• A small training dataset *; Lacking data heterogeneity *; Lacking subjects with other pathological changes of the parotid gland in the control subjects *; Manual ROI segmentation.
Kann [31] (2018)	The proposed deep learning model has the potential for use as a clinical decision-making tool to help guide head and neck cancer patient management.	• The process of individual lymph node CT labeling in correlation with pathology reports is subject to some degree of uncertainty and subjectivity *; Only lymph nodes for which a definitive correlation could be made were included in the labeled dataset, potentially biasing the dataset to those nodes that could be definitively correlated with pathologic report *.
Ariji [20] (2019)	The proposed deep learning model yielded diagnostic results comparable to that of radiologists, which suggests that the model may be valuable for diagnostic support.	• A small training dataset *; Lacking data heterogeneity *; Lacking independent unseen testing data *; Manual ROI segmentation;
Cheng [33] (2011)	The proposed model can efficiently assist clinicians in locating the odontoid process of the second vertebra.	• A small training dataset *; Lacking data heterogeneity *; Inaccurate localization performance.
Shahidi [34] (2014)	The localization performance of the proposed model was acceptable with a mean deviation of 3.40 mm for all automatically identified landmarks.	• A small training dataset *; Lacking data heterogeneity *; Inaccurate localization performance.
Montufar [21] (2018)	The proposed algorithm for automatically locating landmarks on CBCT volumes seems to be useful for 3D cephalometric analysis.	• A small training dataset *; Lacking data heterogeneity *; Lacking independent unseen testing data *; Inaccurate localization performance.
Montufar [22] (2018)	The proposed hybrid algorithm for automatic landmarking on CBCT volumes seems to be potentially useful for 3D cephalometric analysis.	• A small training dataset *; Lacking data heterogeneity *; Lacking independent unseen testing data *; Relatively inaccurate localization performance.
Torosdagli [35] (2019)	The proposed deep learning algorithm allows for orthodontic analysis in patients with craniofacial deformities exhibiting excellent performance.	• A small training dataset *; Lacking data heterogeneity *; Analysis of pseudo-3D images instead of fully 3D images *;

Table 3. *Cont.*

Author (Year)	Conclusion	Limitations (Risk of Bias *)
Park [36] (2018)	The proposed deep learning algorithm is useful for super-resolution and de-noising.	• A small training dataset *; Small anatomical structures may be easily buried and invisible in low-resolution images.
Minnema [23] (2019)	The proposed deep learning algorithm allows us to accurately classify metal artifacts as background noise, and to segment teeth and bony structures.	• A small training dataset *; Lacking independent unseen testing data *; Potential bias in the overall accuracy of the gold standard segmentations *.
Miki [38] (2017)	The proposed deep learning algorithm to classify tooth types on CBCTs yielded a high performance. This can be effectively used for automated preparation of dental charts and might be useful in forensic identification.	• A small training dataset *; Unstable classification performance due to the analyzed levels of the cross-sectional tooth images and metal artifacts;
Ghazvinian Zanjani [24] (2019)	The proposed end-to-end deep learning framework for the segmentation of individual teeth and the gingiva from intraoral scans outperforms state-of-the-art networks.	• A small training dataset *; Ex-vivo data *; Lacking independent unseen testing data *;
Kim [45] (2020)	The proposed automated segmentation method for full arch intraoral scan data is as accurate as a manual segmentation method. This tool could efficiently facilitate the digital setup process in orthodontic treatment.	• Ex-vivo data *; Unable to automatically detect the occlusion area.
Lian [25] (2020)	The proposed end-to-end deep neural network to automatically label individual teeth on raw dental surfaces acquired by 3D intraoral scanners outperforms the state-of-the-art methods for 3D shape segmentation.	• A small training dataset *; Scans only containing the maxillary dental surfaces with the complete 14 teeth *; Failed to properly handle missing teeth and additional braces in challenging cases; Lacking independent unseen testing data *;
Liu [27] (2016)	The proposed machine learning algorithm based on face scanning patterns could support current clinical practice of the screening and diagnosis of ASD	• A small training dataset *; Lacking independent unseen testing data *; Several influencing factors, such as age-/culture-adapted face scanning patterns and the characteristics of the ASD patients should be considered when applying the model to classify children with ASD *.
Knoops [26] (2019)	The proposed model can automatically analyze facial shape features and provide patient-specific treatment plans from a 3D facial scan. This may benefit the clinical decision-making process and improve clinical understanding of face shape as a marker for plastic and reconstructive surgery.	• Lacking independent unseen testing data *

3D, three-dimensional; AI, artificial intelligence; ASD, autism spectrum disorder; CBCT, cone beam computed tomography; CT, computed tomography; CNN, convolutional neural network; ROI, region of interest; SjS, Sjögren's syndrome; * risk of bias.

5. Conclusions

The AI models described in the included studies exhibited various potential applications for 3D imaging in dental medicine, such as automated diagnosis of cystic lesions, localization of anatomical landmarks, and classification/segmentation of teeth (see details in Table 3). The performance of most of the proposed machine learning algorithms was considered satisfactory for clinical use, but with room for improvement. Currently, none of the algorithms described are commercially available. It is expected that the developed AI systems will be available as open-source for others to verify their findings and this will eventually lead to true impact in different dental settings. By such an approach, they will also be more easily accessible and potentially user-friendly for dental practitioners.

Up to date, most of the proposed machine learning algorithms were designed to address specific clinical issues in various fields of dental medicine. In the future, it is expected that various relevant algorithms would be integrated into one intelligent workflow system specifically designed for dental clinic use [47]. After input of the patient's demographic data, medical history, clinical findings, 2D/3D diagnostic images, and/or intraoral/facial scans, the system could automatically conduct an overall analysis of the patient. The gathered data might contribute to a better understanding of the health condition of the respective patient and the development of personalized dental medicine, and subsequently, an individualized diagnosis, recommendations for comprehensive interdisciplinary treatment plans, and prediction of the treatment outcome and follow-up. This information will be provided to assist dental practitioners in making evidence-based decisions for each individual based on a real-time up-to-date big database. Furthermore, the capability of deep learning to analyze the information in each pixel/voxel unit may help to detect early lesions or unhealthy conditions that cannot be readily seen by human eyes. The future goals of AI development in dental medicine can be expected to not only improve patient care and radiologist's work but also surpass human experts in achieving more timely diagnoses. Long working hours and uncomfortable work environments may affect the performance of radiologists, whereas a more consistent performance of AI systems can be achieved regardless of working hours and conditions.

It is worth noting that although the development of AI in healthcare is vigorously supported by world-leading medical and technological institutions, the current evidence of AI applications for 3D imaging in dental medicine is very limited. The lack of adequate studies on this topic has resulted in the present methodological approach to provide findings from the literature rather than a pure systematic review. Thus, a selection bias could very likely not be eliminated due to the design of the study, which is certainly a relevant limitation of the present article. Nevertheless, the results presented might have a positive and stimulating impact on future studies and research in this field and hopefully will result in academic debate.

Author Contributions: Conceptualization, M.M.B.; Methodology, A.W.K.Y. and K.H.; Writing—Original Draft Preparation, K.H. and M.M.B.; Writing—Review and Editing, A.W.K.Y. and R.T.; Supervision, M.M.B.; Project Administration, M.M.B. All authors have read and agreed to the published version of the manuscript.

References

1. Stone, P.; Brooks, R.; Brynjolfsson, E.; Calo, R.; Etzioni, O.; Hager, G.; Hirschberg, J.; Kalyanakrishnan, S.; Kamar, E.; Kraus, S.; et al. Artificial Intelligence and Life in 2030. One Hundred Year Study on Artificial Intelligence: Report of the 2015–2016 Study Panel, Stanford University, Stanford, CA. Available online: https://ai100.stanford.edu/2016-report (accessed on 12 March 2020).
2. Gandomi, A.; Haider, M. Beyond the hype: Big data concepts, methods, and analytics. *Int. J. Inf. Manag.* **2015**, *35*, 137–144. [CrossRef]
3. Jiang, F.; Jiang, Y.; Zhi, H.; Dong, Y.; Li, H.; Ma, S.; Wang, Y.; Dong, Q.; Shen, H.; Wang, Y. Artificial intelligence in healthcare: Past, present and future. *Stroke Vasc. Neurol.* **2017**, *2*, 230–243. [CrossRef] [PubMed]

4.   Hamet, P.; Tremblay, J. Artificial intelligence in medicine. *Metabolism* **2017**, *69*, S36–S40. [CrossRef] [PubMed]

5.   Fazal, M.I.; Patel, M.E.; Tye, J.; Gupta, Y. The past, present and future role of artificial intelligence in imaging. *Eur. J. Radiol.* **2018**, *105*, 246–250. [CrossRef] [PubMed]

6.   Ferizi, U.; Besser, H.; Hysi, P.; Jacobs, J.; Rajapakse, C.S.; Chen, C.; Saha, P.K.; Honig, S.; Chang, G. Artificial intelligence applied to osteoporosis: A performance comparison of machine learning algorithms in predicting fragility fractures from MRI data. *J. Magn. Reson. Imaging* **2019**, *49*, 1029–1038. [CrossRef] [PubMed]

7.   Schuhbaeck, A.; Otaki, Y.; Achenbach, S.; Schneider, C.; Slomka, P.; Berman, D.S.; Dey, D. Coronary calcium scoring from contrast coronary CT angiography using a semiautomated standardized method. *J. Cardiovasc. Comput. Tomogr.* **2015**, *9*, 446–453. [CrossRef]

8.   Esteva, A.; Kuprel, B.; Novoa, R.A.; Ko, J.; Swetter, S.M.; Blau, H.M.; Thrun, S. Dermatologist-level classification of skin cancer with deep neural networks. *Nature* **2017**, *542*, 115–118. [CrossRef]

9.   Litjens, G.; Kooi, T.; Bejnordi, B.E.; Setio, A.A.A.; Ciompi, F.; Ghafoorian, M.; van der Laak, J.; van Ginneken, B.; Sánchez, C.I. A survey on deep learning in medical image analysis. *Med. Image Anal.* **2017**, *42*, 60–88. [CrossRef]

10.   Hosny, A.; Parmar, C.; Quackenbush, J.; Schwartz, L.H.; Aerts, H.J.W.L. Artificial intelligence in radiology. *Nat. Rev. Cancer* **2018**, *18*, 500–510. [CrossRef]

11.   Hung, K.; Montalvao, C.; Tanaka, R.; Kawai, T.; Bornstein, M.M. The use and performance of artificial intelligence applications in dental and maxillofacial radiology: A systematic review. *Dentomaxillofac. Radiol.* **2020**, *49*, 20190107. [CrossRef]

12.   Leite, A.F.; Vasconcelos, K.F.; Willems, H.; Jacobs, R. Radiomics and machine learning in oral healthcare. *Proteom. Clin. Appl.* **2020**, *14*, e1900040. [CrossRef] [PubMed]

13.   Pauwels, R.; Araki, K.; Siewerdsen, J.H.; Thongvigitmanee, S.S. Technical aspects of dental CBCT: State of the art. *Dentomaxillofac. Radiol.* **2015**, *44*, 20140224. [CrossRef] [PubMed]

14.   Baysal, A.; Sahan, A.O.; Ozturk, M.A.; Uysal, T. Reproducibility and reliability of three-dimensional soft tissue landmark identification using three-dimensional stereophotogrammetry. *Angle Orthod.* **2016**, *86*, 1004–1009. [CrossRef] [PubMed]

15.   Hwang, J.J.; Jung, Y.H.; Cho, B.H.; Heo, M.S. An overview of deep learning in the field of dentistry. *Imaging Sci. Dent.* **2019**, *49*, 1–7. [CrossRef]

16.   Okada, K.; Rysavy, S.; Flores, A.; Linguraru, M.G. Noninvasive differential diagnosis of dental periapical lesions in cone-beam CT scans. *Med. Phys.* **2015**, *42*, 1653–1665. [CrossRef]

17.   Abdolali, F.; Zoroofi, R.A.; Otake, Y.; Sato, Y. Automated classification of maxillofacial cysts in cone beam CT images using contourlet transformation and Spherical Harmonics. *Comput. Methods Programs Biomed.* **2017**, *139*, 197–207. [CrossRef]

18.   Yilmaz, E.; Kayikcioglu, T.; Kayipmaz, S. Computer-aided diagnosis of periapical cyst and keratocystic odontogenic tumor on cone beam computed tomography. *Comput. Methods Programs Biomed.* **2017**, *146*, 91–100. [CrossRef]

19.   Lee, J.H.; Kim, D.H.; Jeong, S.N. Diagnosis of cystic lesions using panoramic and cone beam computed tomographic images based on deep learning neural network. *Oral Dis.* **2020**, *26*, 152–158. [CrossRef]

20.   Ariji, Y.; Fukuda, M.; Kise, Y.; Nozawa, M.; Yanashita, Y.; Fujita, H.; Katsumata, A.; Ariji, E. Contrast-enhanced computed tomography image assessment of cervical lymph node metastasis in patients with oral cancer by using a deep learning system of artificial intelligence. *Oral Surg. Oral Med. Oral Pathol. Oral Radiol.* **2019**, *127*, 458–463. [CrossRef]

21.   Montufar, J.; Romero, M.; Scougall-Vilchis, R.J. Automatic 3-dimensional cephalometric landmarking based on active shape models in related projections. *Am. J. Orthod. Dentofac. Orthop.* **2018**, *153*, 449–458. [CrossRef]

22.   Montufar, J.; Romero, M.; Scougall-Vilchis, R.J. Hybrid approach for automatic cephalometric landmark annotation on cone-beam computed tomography volumes. *Am. J. Orthod. Dentofac. Orthop.* **2018**, *154*, 140–150. [CrossRef] [PubMed]

23.   Minnema, J.; van Eijnatten, M.; Hendriksen, A.A.; Liberton, N.; Pelt, D.M.; Batenburg, K.J.; Forouzanfar, T.; Wolff, J. Segmentation of dental cone-beam CT scans affected by metal artifacts using a mixed-scale dense convolutional neural network. *Med. Phys.* **2019**, *46*, 5027–5035. [CrossRef] [PubMed]

24.   Ghazvinian Zanjani, F.; Anssari Moin, D.; Verheij, B.; Claessen, F.; Cherici, T.; Tan, T.; de With, P.H.N. Deep learning approach to semantic segmentation in 3D point cloud intra-oral scans of teeth. *MIDL* **2019**, *102*, 557–571.

25. Lian, C.; Wang, L.; Wu, T.H.; Wang, F.; Yap, P.T.; Ko, C.C.; Shen, D. Deep multi-scale mesh feature learning for automated labeling of raw dental surfaces from 3D intraoral scanners. *IEEE Trans. Med. Imaging* **2020**, in press. [CrossRef]

26. Knoops, P.G.M.; Papaioannou, A.; Borghi, A.; Breakey, R.W.F.; Wilson, A.T.; Jeelani, O.; Zafeiriou, S.; Steinbacher, D.; Padwa, B.L.; Dunaway, D.J.; et al. A machine learning framework for automated diagnosis and computer-assisted planning in plastic and reconstructive surgery. *Sci. Rep.* **2019**, *9*, 13597. [CrossRef]

27. Liu, W.; Li, M.; Yi, L. Identifying children with autism spectrum disorder based on their face processing abnormality: A machine learning framework. *Autism Res.* **2016**, *9*, 888–998. [CrossRef]

28. Orhan, K.; Bayrakdar, I.S.; Ezhov, M.; Kravtsov, A.; Ozyurek, T. Evaluation of artificial intelligence for detecting periapical pathosis on cone-beam computed tomography scans. *Int. Endod. J.* **2020**, *53*, 680–689. [CrossRef]

29. Abdolali, F.; Zoroofi, R.A.; Otake, Y.; Sato, Y. A novel image-based retrieval system for characterization of maxillofacial lesions in cone beam CT images. *Int. J. Comput. Assist. Radiol. Surg.* **2019**, *14*, 785–796. [CrossRef]

30. Johari, M.; Esmaeili, F.; Andalib, A.; Garjani, S.; Saberkari, H. Detection of vertical root fractures in intact and endodontically treated premolar teeth by designing a probabilistic neural network: An ex vivo study. *Dentomaxillofac. Radiol.* **2017**, *46*, 20160107. [CrossRef]

31. Kann, B.H.; Aneja, S.; Loganadane, G.V.; Kelly, J.R.; Smith, S.M.; Decker, R.H.; Yu, J.B.; Park, H.S.; Yarbrough, W.G.; Malhotra, A.; et al. Pretreatment identification of head and neck cancer nodal metastasis and extranodal extension using deep learning neural networks. *Sci. Rep.* **2018**, *8*, 14036. [CrossRef]

32. Kise, Y.; Ikeda, H.; Fujii, T.; Fukuda, M.; Ariji, Y.; Fujita, H.; Katsumata, A.; Ariji, E. Preliminary study on the application of deep learning system to diagnosis of Sjögren's syndrome on CT images. *Dentomaxillofac. Radiol.* **2019**, *48*, 20190019. [CrossRef] [PubMed]

33. Cheng, E.; Chen, J.; Yang, J.; Deng, H.; Wu, Y.; Megalooikonomou, V.; Gable, B.; Ling, H. Automatic Dent-landmark detection in 3-D CBCT dental volumes. *Conf. Proc. IEEE Eng. Med. Biol. Soc.* **2011**, *2011*, 6204–6207. [PubMed]

34. Shahidi, S.; Bahrampour, E.; Soltanimehr, E.; Zamani, A.; Oshagh, M.; Moattari, M.; Mehdizadeh, A. The accuracy of a designed software for automated localization of craniofacial landmarks on CBCT images. *BMC Med. Imaging* **2014**, *14*, 32. [CrossRef] [PubMed]

35. Torosdagli, N.; Liberton, D.K.; Verma, P.; Sincan, M.; Lee, J.S.; Bagci, U. Deep geodesic learning for segmentation and anatomical landmarking. *IEEE Trans. Med. Imaging* **2019**, *38*, 919–931. [CrossRef] [PubMed]

36. Park, J.; Hwang, D.; Kim, K.Y.; Kang, S.K.; Kim, Y.K.; Lee, J.S. Computed tomography super-resolution using deep convolutional neural network. *Phys. Med. Biol.* **2018**, *63*, 145011. [CrossRef]

37. ter Haar Romeny, B.M. A deeper understanding of deep learning. In *Artificial Intelligence in Medical Imaging: Opportunities, Applications and Risks*, 1st ed.; Ranschaert, E.R., Morozov, S., Algra, P.R., Eds.; Springer: Berlin, Germany, 2019; pp. 25–38.

38. Miki, Y.; Muramatsu, C.; Hayashi, T.; Zhou, X.; Hara, T.; Katsumata, A.; Fujita, H. Classification of teeth in cone-beam CT using deep convolutional neural network. *Comput. Biol. Med.* **2017**, *80*, 24–29. [CrossRef]

39. Abdolali, F.; Zoroofi, R.A.; Otake, Y.; Sato, Y. Automatic segmentation of maxillofacial cysts in cone beam CT images. *Comput. Biol. Med.* **2016**, *72*, 108–119. [CrossRef]

40. Scarfe, W.C.; Azevedo, B.; Toghyani, S.; Farman, A.G. Cone beam computed tomographic imaging in orthodontics. *Aust. Dent. J.* **2017**, *62*, 33–50. [CrossRef]

41. Bornstein, M.M.; Yeung, W.K.A.; Montalvao, C.; Colsoul, N.; Parker, Q.A.; Jacobs, R. Facts and Fallacies of Radiation Risk in Dental Radiology. Available online: http://facdent.hku.hk/docs/ke/2019_Radiology_KE_booklet_en.pdf (accessed on 12 March 2020).

42. Yeung, A.W.K.; Jacobs, R.; Bornstein, M.M. Novel low-dose protocols using cone beam computed tomography in dental medicine: A review focusing on indications, limitations, and future possibilities. *Clin. Oral Investig.* **2019**, *23*, 2573–2581. [CrossRef]

43. Tuzoff, D.V.; Tuzova, L.N.; Bornstein, M.M.; Krasnov, A.S.; Kharchenko, M.A.; Nikolenko, S.I.; Sveshnikov, M.M.; Bednenko, G.B. Tooth detection and numbering in panoramic radiographs using convolutional neural networks. *Dentomaxillofac. Radiol.* **2019**, *48*, 20180051. [CrossRef]

44. Tomita, Y.; Uechi, J.; Konno, M.; Sasamoto, S.; Iijima, M.; Mizoguchi, I. Accuracy of digital models generated by conventional impression/plaster-model methods and intraoral scanning. *Dent. Mater. J.* **2018**, *37*, 628–633. [CrossRef] [PubMed]
45. Kim, T.; Cho, Y.; Kim, D.; Chang, M.; Kim, Y.J. Tooth segmentation of 3D scan data using generative adversarial networks. *Appl. Sci.* **2020**, *10*, 490. [CrossRef]
46. Morey, J.M.; Haney, N.M.; Kim, W. Applications of AI beyond image interpretation. In *Artificial Intelligence in Medical Imaging: Opportunities, Applications and Risks*, 1st ed.; Ranschaert, E.R., Morozov, S., Algra, P.R., Eds.; Springer: Berlin, Germany, 2019; pp. 129–144.
47. Chen, Y.W.; Stanley, K.; Att, W. Artificial intelligence in dentistry: Current applications and future perspectives. *Quintessence Int.* **2020**, *51*, 248–257. [PubMed]

Dental Caries Diagnosis and Detection Using Neural Networks

María Prados-Privado [1,2,3,*], **Javier García Villalón** [1], **Carlos Hugo Martínez-Martínez** [4], **Carlos Ivorra** [1] **and Juan Carlos Prados-Frutos** [3,5]

[1]   Asisa Dental, Research Department, C/José Abascal, 32, 28003 Madrid, Spain;
     javier.villalon@asisadental.com (J.G.V.); carlos.ivorra@asisadental.com (C.I.)

[2]   Department of Signal Theory and Communications, Higher Polytechnic School, Universidad de Alcala de Henares, Ctra, Madrid-Barcelona, Km. 33,600, 28805 Alcala de Henares, Spain

[3]   IDIBO GROUP (Group of High-Performance Research, Development and Innovation in Dental Biomaterials of Rey Juan Carlos University), Avenida de Atenas s/n, 28922 Alcorcon, Spain; juancarlos.prados@urjc.es

[4]   Faculty of Medicine, Universidad Complutense de Madrid, Plaza de Ramón y Cajal, s/n, 28040 Madrid, Spain; carlos.martinez@asisa.es

[5]   Department of Medical Specialties and Public Health, Faculty of Health Sciences, Universidad Rey Juan Carlos, Avenida de Atenas, 28922 Alcorcon, Spain

*   Correspondence: maria.prados@uah.es

Abstract: Dental caries is the most prevalent dental disease worldwide, and neural networks and artificial intelligence are increasingly being used in the field of dentistry. This systematic review aims to identify the state of the art of neural networks in caries detection and diagnosis. A search was conducted in PubMed, Institute of Electrical and Electronics Engineers (IEEE) Xplore, and ScienceDirect. Data extraction was performed independently by two reviewers. The quality of the selected studies was assessed using the Cochrane Handbook tool. Thirteen studies were included. Most of the included studies employed periapical, near-infrared light transillumination, and bitewing radiography. The image databases ranged from 87 to 3000 images, with a mean of 669 images. Seven of the included studies labeled the dental caries in each image by experienced dentists. Not all of the studies detailed how caries was defined, and not all detailed the type of carious lesion detected. Each study included in this review used a different neural network and different outcome metrics. All this variability complicates the conclusions that can be made about the reliability or not of a neural network to detect and diagnose caries. A comparison between neural network and dentist results is also necessary.

Keywords: artificial intelligence; caries; images; detection

1. Introduction

Machine learning is an application of artificial intelligence (AI) that provides systems the ability to automatically learn and improve from experience without being explicitly programmed [1,2]. Machine learning needs input data, such as images or text, to obtain an output through a model.

Neural networks can be classified according to their typology or network structure or according to their learning algorithm. According to its topology, we can distinguish, as a characteristic of a network, the number of layers; the type of layers, which can be hidden or visible; input or output; and the directionality of the neuron connections. Depending on the typology, we can distinguish monolayer or multilayer networks.

According to its learning algorithm or how the network learns the patterns, we can distinguish as characteristics if it is supervised, unsupervised, competitive, or by reinforcement [3]. The model in supervised learning is trained, employing a labeled database. By contrast, the expected output is unknown in unsupervised learning [1,4]. Reinforcement learning is a model that falls between supervised and unsupervised learning.

The most common form of machine learning is supervised learning. To work with images, it is necessary, first, to collect a large data set of images, and second, to label each category in each image, in this case, with caries detected by a dentist. Then the training process begins. During the training process, the user/modeler feeds the data to network, it passes through the network, and an output is computed based on the current set of model weights. To obtain the best score of all categories, an objective function to measure the error is computed. Then the algorithm modifies its internal parameters to have the highest score of all categories. Finally, after training, the performance of the system is measured on a different set of images called a test dataset. The validation test serves to test the ability of the model to obtain good answers on new images (inputs) that it has never seen during the training process [5].

Convolutional neural network (CNN) is a type of deep and feedforward network. CNNs are designed to process data that come in the form of multiple arrays as images, and their architecture is composed of several stages.

Artificial intelligence is used in dentistry to identify and detect different variables from images, such as teeth, caries, and implants. Deep learning has been demonstrated to be a good collection of techniques to assist medical practitioners in medical fields such as radiology [6,7].

One of the most frequent activities in dental practice is to detect early caries lesions or to provide treatment preventing more invasive therapies [8]. The International Caries Detection and Assessment System (ICDAS) was developed by an international team of caries researchers to integrate several new criteria systems into one standard system for caries detection and assessment [9]. A workshop was organized to discuss and reach consensus about definitions of the most common terms in cariology [10]. Full agreement was obtained of the definition of dental caries:

"Dental caries is a biofilm-mediated, diet-modulated, multifactorial, non-communicable, dynamic disease resulting in net mineral loss of dental hard tissues. It is determined by biological, behavioral, psychosocial, and environmental factors. As a consequence of this process, a caries lesion develops". [10]

The definition of initial caries lesions was also obtained with full agreement and was defined as a frequently used term for noncavited caries lesions that refer to the stage of severity. Sound enamel/dentin was defined, with a 100% agreement, as a tooth structure without clinically detectable alterations of the natural translucency, color, or texture. However, other terms, such as secondary caries/recurrent caries, residual caries, or "hidden" caries, did not obtain full agreement [10]. During the first two sessions, ICDAS was formed and, afterwards, those criteria were revised, modified, and called ICDAS II [11].

The visual-tactile detection method is generally used in dental practice, followed by radiographic caries detection [8]. Bitewing radiography is the most frequent technique in carious lesion detection. Several studies have compared the performance of CBCT to conventional or digital intraoral radiography, histology, or micro CT for enamel and dentin caries detection [12,13]. The conclusion was that CBCT did not improve the accuracy of caries detection [14].

Dental caries is the most prevalent dental disease worldwide, and neural networks and artificial intelligence are increasingly being used in the field of dentistry. Many studies have contributed to the field of dental caries detection using neural networks with different dental images. This review aims to evaluate studies investigating caries detection with artificial intelligence and neural networks. This literature review analyzed in each study the type of image, the total image database and its characteristics, the neural network employed to detect caries, the exclusion criterion of images, and whether the database had been modified before the training process. Then, it was analyzed as to how caries were defined, what type of caries were detected, and the outcome metrics and values.

2. Materials and Methods

2.1. Review Questions

(1) What are the neural networks used to detect and diagnosis dental caries?
(2) How is the database used in the construction of these networks?
(3) How are caries lesions defined, and in which teeth are they detected?
(4) What are the outcome metrics and the values obtained by those neural networks?

2.2. Search Strategy

The research questions were elaborated considering each of the components of the PICO(S) [15] strategy research questions, which are explained as follows: (P) neural networks and caries detection; (I) caries definition and which teeth are detected; (C) studies with neural network are used to detect and diagnosis dental caries; (O) outcome metrics and values; (S) neural networks.

An electronic search was performed in the following databases up until 15 August 2020: MEDLINE/PubMed, Institute of Electrical and Electronics Engineers (IEEE) Xplore, and ScienceDirect.

The search strategy used is detailed in Table 1.

Table 1. Search strategy.

Database	Search Strategy	Search Data
MEDLINE/PubMed	(deep learning OR artificial intelligence OR neural network *) AND caries NOT review	15 August 2020
IEEE Xplore	(deep learning OR artificial intelligence OR neural network) AND caries AND (detect OR detection OR diagnosis)	15 August 2020
ScienceDirect	(deep learning OR artificial intelligence OR neural network) AND caries AND (detect OR detection OR diagnosis)	15 August 2020

2.3. Study Selection and Items Collected

M.P.-P. and J.G.-V. performed the bibliographic search and selected the articles that fulfilled the inclusion criteria. Both authors collected all the data from the selected articles in duplicate and independently of each other. Disagreements between the two authors were reviewed using full text by a third author (J.C.P.-F.) to make the final decision. The references of the articles included in this study were manually reviewed.

The following items were collected: study (journal and year), type of image, total image database, database characteristics (pixels and examiners), neural network, image exclusion criteria, database modification (resized pixel), caries definition, caries type detected, teeth in which caries lesions were detected, outcome metrics (accuracy, sensitivity, specificity), and outcome metrics values.

2.4. Inclusion and Exclusion Criteria

The inclusion criteria were full manuscripts, including conference proceedings, that reported the use of neural networks for the detection and diagnosis of caries. There were no restrictions on the language or date of publication. Exclusion criteria were reviews, no dental caries application, no images, and no neural network employed.

2.5. Study Quality Assessment

The risk of bias from neural networks studies was evaluated by two of the authors (C.M.-M. and C.I.). To this end, the guidelines presented in the Cochrane Handbook [7] were followed, which incorporates seven domains: random sequence generation (selection bias); allocation concealment (selection bias); masking of participants and personnel (performance bias); masking of outcome assessment (detection bias); incomplete outcome data (attrition bias); selective reporting (reporting bias); and other biases.

The studies were classified into the following categories: low risk of bias—low risk of bias for all key domains; unclear risk of bias—unclear risk of bias for one or more key domains; high risk of bias—high risk of bias for one or more key domains.

2.6. Statistical Analysis

The mean, standard deviation (SD), median, and percentage were calculated for several variables. Statistical calculations were performed with IBM SPSS Statistics (SAS Institute Inc., Cary, NC, USA).

3. Results

3.1. Study Selection

Figure 1 details a flowchart of the study selection. All of the electronic search strategies resulted in 187 potential manuscripts. A total of 178 studies were excluded because they did not meet the inclusion criteria. Additionally, a manual search was carried out to analyze the references cited in ten of the articles that were included in this work. Finally, three more articles were incorporated from the manual search. In the end, a total of thirteen studies were analyzed.

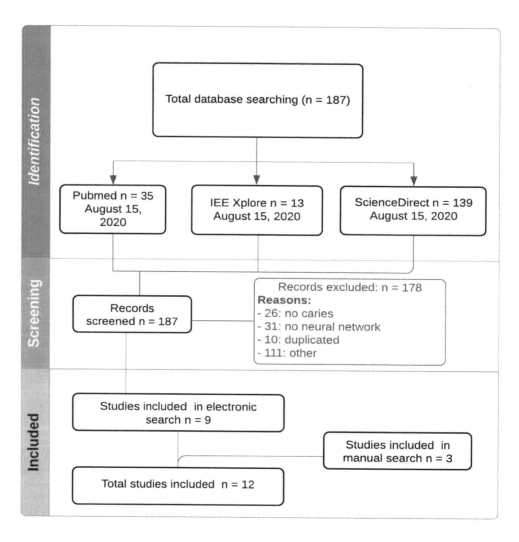

Figure 1. Flowchart.

3.2. Relevant Data about the Image Database and Neural Network of the Included Studies

Table 2 details the main characteristic of the studies included in the manuscript. Included studies were conducted between 2008 and 2020. All studies were published in English. Regarding the types of images, the most used were the periapical, the near-infrared light transilluminations, and the bitewings, each one appearing twice in each of the studies (16.66% in each study). The rest of the images used by a single study were panoramic radiographs, radiovisiography, intra-oral, in vivo with an intraoral camera and, and X-ray images (8.33%). Only two studies did not detail the type of image employed.

Image databases also varied from 87 to 3000 images, with a mean of 669.27 images, a standard deviation of 1153.76, and a median of 160 images. Seven (58.33%) of the included studies labeled the dental caries in each image by experienced dentists. Of those seven articles that used experts to indicate caries, five (71.42%) indicated that they use two experts ($n = 2$), one (14.28%) employed one expert, one employed four experts, and one employed 25 examiners. Three studies (25%) did not indicate the number of examiners.

Three studies detailed the exclusion criteria of the images. Six of the included studies detailed how images were standardized by resizing the number of pixels.

3.3. Relevant Data about Caries of the Included Studies

Table 3 details the main characteristic of carious lesion detection and outcome metrics of the included studies. Three studies (23.07%) detailed how caries are defined in their studies. One study explained that a caries lesion was considered where a radiolucent area appears on the structure. The other two considered the caries definition that follows the ICDAS II classification system. Seven (53.84%) of the included studies detailed the type of caries detected: three studies detected occlusal caries, while the other four studies detected proximal, enamel, and dentinal lesions; pre-cavitated lesions; and initial caries. Six of the included studies did not detail the type of caries detected by their neural network or define what they considered as caries.

Regarding the teeth where caries lesions are detected, seven studies (53.84%) did not detail in which teeth caries were detected, four studies (30.7%) employed molar and premolar teeth, and two (15.38%) of the included studies used posterior extracted teeth.

Eight of the included studies analyzed accuracy, obtaining the following outcomes: a range from 68.57 to 99% (mean ± SD of 90 ± 7%, median of 89%), a precision range from 0.615 to 0.987 (mean ± SD of 0.801 ± 0.263), and an AUC from 0.74 to 0.971 (mean ± SD of 0.815 ± 0.1).

Table 2. Main characteristics of image database and neural network.

Authors	Neural Network Task	Image	Total Image Database	Database Characteristics (Pixels and Examiners)	Neural Network	Image Exclusion Criterion	Database Modification (Resized and Other)	Journal	Year
Schwendicke et al. [16]	Classification	Near-infrared light transillumination	226	Pixel: 435 × 407 × 3. Examiners: two (clinical experience, 8–11 years)	Resnet18, Resnext50	-	Resized pixel: 224 × 224	Journal of Dentistry	2020
Geetha et al. [17]	Classification	Intra-oral digital radiography	105	Pixel: Examiners: a dentist	ANN with 10-fold cross validation	-	Resized pixel: 256 × 256	Health Information Science and Systems	2020
Casalengo et al. [18]	Segmentation	Near-infrared transillumination	217	Pixel: Examiners: by experts	CNN trained on a semantic segmentation task		Resized pixel: 256 × 320	Journal of Dental Research	2019
Moutselos et al. [19]	Segmentation and classification	In vivo with an intraoral camera	87	-	DNN Mask R-CNN, which extends Faster R-CNN by adding an FCN for predicting object masks.	1. Teeth with hypoplastic and/or hypomineralized. 2. Teeth with sealants on the occlusal surfaces.	-	Conf Proc IEEE Eng Med Biol Soc	2019
Lee et al. [20]	Classification	Periapical	3000	Pixel: Examiners: four calibrated board-certified dentists	CNN	1. Moderate-to-severe noise, haziness, distortion, and shadows. 2. Full crown or large partial inlay restoration. 3. Deciduous teeth.	Resized pixel: 299 × 299 Other: standardized contrast between gray/white matter and lesions.	Journal of Dentistry	2018
Sornam et al. [21]	Classification	Periapical	120	-	Feedforward Neural Network	-	-	IEEE International Conference on Power, Control, Signals, and Instrumentation Engineering (ICPCSI-2017)	2017

Table 2. *Cont.*

Authors	Neural Network Task	Image	Total Image Database	Database Characteristics (Pixels and Examiners)	Neural Network	Image Exclusion Criterion	Database Modification (Resized and Other)	Journal	Year
Singh et al. [22]	Detection	Panoramic radiographs	93	-	Radon Transformation (RT) and Discrete Cosine Transformation (DCT).	-	Resized pixel: 500 × 500	2017 8th International Conference on Computing, Communication and Networking Technologies (ICCCNT)	2017
Srivastava et al. [23]	Segmentation	Bitewing	3000	Pixel: Examiners: by certified dentists	FCNN (deep fully convolutional neural network)	-	-	NIPS 2017 workshop on Machine Learning for Health (NIPS 2017 ML4H)	2017
Prajapati et al. [24]	Classification	Radiovisiography	251	-	CNN	-	Resized pixel: 500 × 748	5th International Symposium on Computational and Business Intelligence	2017
Berdouses et al. [25]	Detection and classification	-	103	Pixel: Examiners: two	-	-	-	Computers in Biology and Medicine	2015
Devito et al. [26]	Detection	Bitewing	160	Pixel: Examiners: 25	Multilayer perceptron neural	-	-	Oral Med Oral Pathol Oral Radiol Endod	2008
Kuang et al. [27]	Segmentation	X-ray images	-	Pixel: 1000 × 800 Examiners: -	Back propagation Neural Network	-	-	Second International Symposium on Intelligent Information Technology Application	2008

CNN: Convolutional neural network.

Table 3. Main data about caries of the included studies.

Authors	Type of Study	Caries Definition	Caries Type Detected	Teeth	Outcome Metrics	Outcome Metrics Values
Schwendicke et al. [16]	in vitro	-	Occlusal and/or proximal caries	Premolar and molar	AUC, sensitivity, specificity, and positive/negative predictive values	0.74, 0.59, 0.76, 0.63, and 0.73
Geetha et al. [17]	in vitro	Loss of mineralization of these structures (radiolucent)	-	-	Accuracy, false positive rate, ROC, and precision	0.971, 0.028, 0.987
Casalengo et al. [18]	clinical	-	-	Upper and lower molars and premolars	IOU/AUC	72.7/83.6 and 85.6%
Moutselos et al. [19]		Classified from 1 to 6 using the ICDAS II classification system.	Caries on occlusal surfaces	-	Accuracy	0.889
Lee et al. [20]	in vitro	-	Dental caries, including enamel and dentinal carious lesions	Premolar, molar, and both premolar and molar	Accuracy, sensitivity, specificity, PPV, NPV, ROC curve, and AUC	82, 81, 83, 82.7, 81.4
Sornam et al. [21]	in vitro	-	-	-	Accuracy	99%
Singh et al. [22]	in vitro	-	-	-	Accuracy	86%
Srivastava et al. [23]	in vitro	-	-	-	Recall/Precision/F1-Score	0.805/0.615/0.7
Prajapati et al. [24]	in vitro	-	-	-	Accuracy	0.875
Berdouses et al. [25]	in vitro	ICDAS II	Pre-cavitated lesion and cavitated occlusal lesion	Posterior extracted human teeth	Accuracy	80%
Devito et al. [26]	in vitro	-	sound, enamel caries, enamel-dentine junction caries and, dentinal caries	Premolar and molar	ROC	0.717
Kuang et al. [27]	in vitro	-	Initial caries	-	Accuracy	68.57%

ICDAS: The International Caries Detection and Assessment System.

3.4. Study Quality Assessment

Evaluation of selection bias: All studies blinded image data.

Evaluation of performance bias: None of the studies indicated a blinding of staff or assessors.

Assessment of detection bias: All study results were blinded.

Evaluation of attrition bias: Not all of the studies reported complete results. Berdouses et al. [25] detailed all the results analyzed in the present review.

Evaluation of notification bias: Not all of the studies provided detailed information about the neural network parameters. Lee et al. [20] provided all the information.

Figure 2 shows a detailed description of the risk assessment of bias in the included studies.

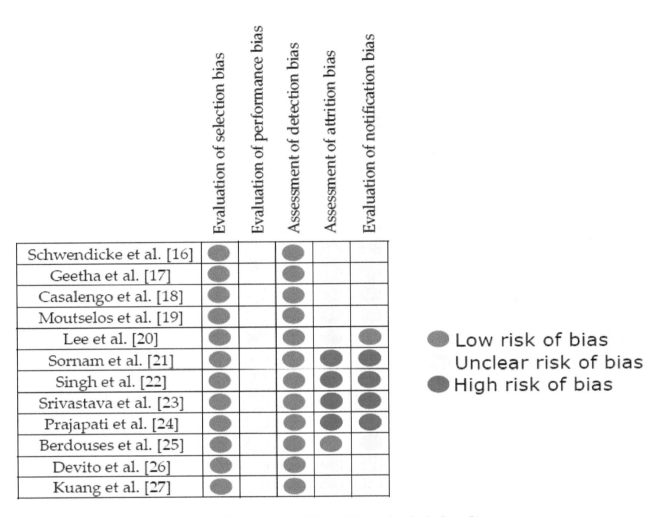

Figure 2. Assessment of risk of bias of included studies.

4. Discussion

The goal of this review is to visualize the state of the art of neural networks in detecting and diagnosing dental caries. The way in which each of the studies analyzes caries (definition, type, tooth), as well as the parameters of each neural network (type of network, characteristics of the database, and results), were studied.

A good definition of what is meant by caries and the type of caries lesions to be analyzed is essential to compare and analyze the results obtained in each study. Studies included in this review that detailed the use of ICDAS II obtained an accuracy between 80 and 88.9% (mean ± SD of 85.45 ± 6.29%), while the study that defined caries as a loss of mineralization of these structures (radiolucent) obtained an accuracy of 97.1%. However, 76% of the studies included in the present review did not detail how a caries lesion is defined.

Another bias factor is related to the training dataset. Images employed during the training process must be labeled by experts. Seven (58.33%) of the included studies indicated that examiners were used to label the images, although the experience and the number of those examiners varied from one study to another. Some studies analyzed the relation between caries detection and dentist experience. Bussaneli et al., concluded in their study that the experience of the examiner is not determinant to occlusal lesions in primary teeth but influenced the treatment decision of initial lesions [28]. However, when an artificial intelligence is trained with human observer's scores, the system can never exceed the trainer and, therefore, the performance depends on the quality of the input.

An important fact for artificial intelligence technology is the overfitting. Burnham and Anderson describes "the essence of overfitting is to have unknowingly extracted some of the residual variation as if that variation represented underlying model structure" [29]. A model is overfitted when it is so specific to the original data that trying to apply it to data collected in the future would result in problematic or erroneous outcomes and therefore less-than-optimal decisions [30].

The included studies in this review that detailed the use of examiners to obtain an accuracy ranged from 80 to 97% (mean ± SD of 88.7 ± 8.55%). The best result was obtained in the study that used only one examiner, and, therefore, the same criteria in caries detection was always used, followed by the study where four experts analyzed the images. Finally, the worst result in terms of accuracy was obtained by the study with two examiners. Regarding the experience of the examiners, only one study detailed the number of years of experience. However, these results were not completely related to the number of examiners; other factors such as neural network, dataset, and caries definition must be kept in mind. In this sense, the results detailed in Table 3 must be analyzed with caution, since each of the networks used in the studies has a different purpose, which means that the results are not comparable between them. The data analyzed in a general way helps us to get an idea about what percentages of accuracy, on average, are obtained in caries detection and diagnosis studies using neural networks.

One of the limitations of this review is that studies using artificial intelligence with different tasks have been taken into account. This means that, although the studies obtain the same metrics, they cannot be compared with each other. The reason is that each artificial intelligence is designed for one thing that makes comparison of results impossible. From each to future reviews, it is recommended to include studies whose artificial intelligence has the same purpose. The use of a large dataset is crucial for the performance of the deep learning model. It is possible to improve the technical capability employing a technique called data augmentation. This technique artificially inflates the training database by oversampling or data warping. Oversampling creates synthetic instances and adds them to the training dataset. However, data warping transforms the existing images [31].

The study from Geetha et al. [17] presents the highest accuracy of all the studies included in the present review. However, this study is a special case because the authors built their own feature extractor, which is rare nowadays, and used a very shallow neural network with only one hidden layer. Authors of that study used only 105 images and did 10-fold cross-validation, and, therefore, their model was not evaluated on a hold-out test set.

A great variety of architectures has been found in the studies included in this literature review. ResNets are residual networks that are CNNs designed to allow thousands of convolutional layers. Mask R-CNN is an extension of Faster R-CNN by adding a branch for predicting segmentation masks on each Region of Interest (ROI) [5]. Semantic image segmentation is the task of classifying each pixel in an image from a predefined set of classes, which has several applications in medical images. Six (50%) of the included studies detailed that, before starting the training process, they homogenized the size of the images (Table 2).

Shokri et al., analyzed the effect of filters on detecting proximal and occlusal caries employing intraoral images and concluded that the lowest accuracy in caries diagnosis was noted for the detection of enamel lesions on original radiographs (52%). However, this in vitro study induced caries by a demineralizing solution, and therefore induced carious lesions were more regular than those that developed naturally [32]. Belém et al. [33] analyzed the accuracy of detection of subsurface demineralization by different imaging modalities and concluded that original images had an accuracy of 73% and a sensitivity of 62%. Kositbowornchai et al. compared the accuracy of detecting occlusal caries lesions on original images and obtained a mean Receiver Operating Characteristic (ROC) curve of 0.75 [34]. Here, two of the studies analyzed enamel lesions with an accuracy of 82% and a ROC curve of 0.717. The studies that analyzed occlusal lesions in this review obtained an accuracy of 80 and 88.9%, and a precision of 45.3%.

Several studies analyzed the precision in the detection of caries depending on the type of image used. Schwendicke et al., concluded in their systematic review that fluorescence-based images showed a significantly higher accuracy, sensitivity, and specificity in detecting initial lesions than conventional radiographic images, and generally that radiographic caries detection is especially suitable for detecting dentine lesions and cavitated proximal lesions [8]. Here, two of the studies employed near-infrared transillumination images and obtained similar outcome metrics to the other studies with different image types.

Supervised learning is one where the learning process of the algorithm from the training dataset can be considered to be a process supervised by a teacher. The correct answer is previously known, and the algorithm iteratively makes its predictions at the same time as it is corrected by the teacher. Seven (58.33%) of the included studies labeled the dental caries in each image by experienced dentists. However, in addition to knowing the number of examiners and their experience, it is very important to know what the intra-examiner agreement is, that is, to know if the examiner's answers are the same if the categorization of the images is repeated a second time. It is also very important to know the inter-examiner agreement, that is, for the same image, how many examiners provide the same answer. None of the included studies mentioned the inter- and intra-examiner agreement. Intra- and inter-examiner agreement is evaluated by calculating Cohen's Kappa. According to Bulman and Osborn [35], values of Cohen's Kappa between 0.81 and 1.00 indicate almost perfect agreement.

Other graphical methods such as ROC (Receiver Operating Characteristic) curve or Bland-Altman plot can be employed to obtain information on those samples in which there is less agreement.

It is important to emphasize that manual labeling by experts provides a reference that is necessary for training and evaluating the model but does not necessarily represent ground truth [18]. The use of a histologic gold standard method is indispensable for the validation of a caries diagnostic method. None of the studies included in the present review mentioned the reference standard employed.

A quality analysis of the included studies was done using the Cochrane Handbook tool, which was employed to assess the risk of bias, concluding that in most domains, no data were given related to the transparency of the studies. This ensures that the data collected and analyzed have been managed in a controlled manner, avoiding all possible methodological errors. The criteria for allocation masking and randomization were not detailed in all of the studies, which is considered to be an unclear risk of bias. The present systematic review focused on the use of artificial intelligence in carious lesion diagnostic and detection; the bias is located in the lack of a reference standard and the inclusion of studies with different algorithms. However, the data presented above cannot be analyzed in isolation. Inter- and intra-examiner agreement must be taken into account in studies involving multiple examiners in order to obtain comparable and reliable results. This is a fundamental parameter to correctly define the variables that the neural network has to learn. That is, good agreement between examiners is essential to obtain good results once the image passes through the neural network. None of the studies using multiple examiners and included in this review detailed the concordance mentioned above in their respective studies. Neither was there a single parameter to compare the results obtained by the neural network, nor common parameters for the database. All these factors complicate the conclusions that can be made about the reliability or not of a neural network to detect and diagnose caries.

To be able to know if the neural networks give certain results, it is necessary to make a comparison with the results provided by the dentists, who should also have similar training and experience in order for comparisons to be made between them.

The diagnostic performance of artificial intelligence models varies between the different algorithms used and is still necessary to verify the generalizability and reliability of these models. For this, it would be necessary to use the ability to compare the results of the tasks of each algorithm before transferring and implement these models in clinical practice.

Author Contributions: Conceptualization, M.P.-P. and J.C.P.-F.; methodology, M.P.-P. and J.G.V.; data curation, M.P.-P. and J.G.V.; writing—original draft preparation, M.P.-P.; writing—review and editing, C.H.M.-M. and J.C.P.-F.; visualization, M.P.-P., J.G.V., C.H.M.-M., J.C.P.-F. and C.I.; supervision, C.I.; funding acquisition, C.H.M.-M. and C.I. All authors have read and agreed to the published version of the manuscript.

References

1. Pauwels, R. A brief introduction to concepts and applications of artificial intelligence in dental imaging. *Oral Radiol.* **2020**. [CrossRef]
2. Chen, Y.W.; Stanley, K.; Att, W. Artificial intelligence in dentistry: Current applications and future perspectives. *Quintessence Int.* **2020**, *51*, 248–257. [CrossRef]
3. Kohli, M.; Prevedello, L.M.; Filice, R.W.; Geis, J.R. Implementing Machine Learning in Radiology Practice and Research. *Am. J. Roentgenol.* **2017**, *208*, 754–760. [CrossRef]
4. Clarke, A.M.; Friedrich, J.; Tartaglia, E.M.; Marchesotti, S.; Senn, W.; Herzog, M.H. Human and Machine Learning in Non-Markovian Decision Making. *PLoS ONE* **2015**, *10*, e0123105. [CrossRef]
5. LeCun, Y.; Bengio, Y.; Hinton, G. Deep learning. *Nature* **2015**, *521*, 436–444. [CrossRef]
6. Schwendicke, F.; Golla, T.; Dreher, M.; Krois, J. Convolutional neural networks for dental image diagnostics: A scoping review. *J. Dent.* **2019**, *91*, 103226. [CrossRef]
7. Mazurowski, M.A.; Buda, M.; Saha, A.; Bashir, M.R. Deep learning in radiology: An overview of the concepts and a survey of the state of the art with focus on MRI. *J. Magn. Reson. Imaging* **2019**, *49*, 939–954. [CrossRef] [PubMed]
8. Schwendicke, F.; Tzschoppe, M.; Paris, S. Radiographic caries detection: A systematic review and meta-analysis. *J. Dent.* **2015**, *43*, 924–933. [CrossRef]
9. Gupta, M.; Srivastava, N.; Sharma, M.; Gugnani, N.; Pandit, I. International Caries Detection and Assessment System (ICDAS): A New Concept. *Int. J. Clin. Pediatr. Dent.* **2011**, *4*, 93–100. [CrossRef]
10. Machiulskiene, V.; Campus, G.; Carvalho, J.C.; Dige, I.; Ekstrand, K.R.; Jablonski-Momeni, A.; Maltz, M.; Manton, D.J.; Martignon, S.; Martinez-Mier, E.A.; et al. Terminology of Dental Caries and Dental Caries Management: Consensus Report of a Workshop Organized by ORCA and Cariology Research Group of IADR. *Caries Res.* **2020**, *54*, 7–14. [CrossRef]
11. Dikmen, B. Icdas II Criteria (International Caries Detection and Assessment System). *J. Istanb. Univ. Fac. Dent.* **2015**, *49*, 63. [CrossRef]
12. Valizadeh, S.; Tavakkoli, M.A.; Vasigh, H.K.; Azizi, Z.; Zarrabian, T. Evaluation of Cone Beam Computed Tomography (CBCT) System: Comparison with Intraoral Periapical Radiography in Proximal Caries Detection. *J. Dent. Res. Dent. Clin. Dent. Prospect.* **2012**, *6*, 1–5. [CrossRef]
13. Abogazalah, N.; Ando, M. Alternative methods to visual and radiographic examinations for approximal caries detection. *J. Oral Sci.* **2017**, *59*, 315–322. [CrossRef]
14. Zhang, Z.; Qu, X.; Li, G.; Zhang, Z.; Ma, X. The detection accuracies for proximal caries by cone-beam computerized tomography, film, and phosphor plates. *Oral Surg. Oral Med. Oral Pathol. Oral Radiol. Endodontol.* **2011**, *111*, 103–108. [CrossRef]
15. Centre for Reviews and Dissemination. *Systematic Reviews: CRD Guidance for Undertaking Reviews in Health Care*; University of York: York, UK, 2009; ISBN 978-1-900640-47-3.
16. Schwendicke, F.; Elhennawy, K.; Paris, S.; Friebertshäuser, P.; Krois, J. Deep Learning for Caries Lesion Detection in Near-Infrared Light Transillumination Images: A Pilot Study. *J. Dent.* **2019**, 103260. [CrossRef]
17. Geetha, V.; Aprameya, K.S.; Hinduja, D.M. Dental caries diagnosis in digital radiographs using back-propagation neural network. *Health Inf. Sci. Syst.* **2020**, *8*, 8–14. [CrossRef] [PubMed]
18. Casalegno, F.; Newton, T.; Daher, R.; Abdelaziz, M.; Lodi-Rizzini, A.; Schürmann, F.; Krejci, I.; Markram, H. Caries Detection with Near-Infrared Transillumination Using Deep Learning. *J. Dent. Res.* **2019**, *98*, 1227–1233. [CrossRef]
19. Moutselos, K.; Berdouses, E.; Oulis, C.; Maglogiannis, I. Recognizing Occlusal Caries in Dental Intraoral Images Using Deep Learning. In Proceedings of the 41st Annual International Conference of the IEEE Engineering in Medicine and Biology Society (EMBC), Berlin, Germany, 23–27 July 2019; pp. 1617–1620.
20. Lee, J.H.; Kim, D.H.; Jeong, S.N.; Choi, S.H. Detection and diagnosis of dental caries using a deep learning-based convolutional neural network algorithm. *J. Dent.* **2018**, *77*, 106–111. [CrossRef] [PubMed]
21. Sornam, M.; Prabhakaran, M. A new linear adaptive swarm intelligence approach using back propagation neural network for dental caries classification. In Proceedings of the IEEE International Conference on Power, Control, Signals and Instrumentation Engineering (ICPCSI), Chennai, India, 21–22 September 2017; pp. 2698–2703.

22. Singh, P.; Sehgal, P. Automated caries detection based on Radon transformation and DCT. In Proceedings of the 8th International Conference on Computing, Communication and Networking Technologies (ICCCNT), Delhi, India, 3–5 July 2017; pp. 1–6.

23. Srivastava, M.M.; Kumar, P.; Pradhan, L.; Varadarajan, S. Detection of Tooth caries in Bitewing Radiographs using Deep Learning. In Proceedings of the 31st Conference on Neural Information Processing Systems (NIPS), Long Beach, CA, USA, 4–9 December 2017; p. 4.

24. Prajapati, S.A.; Nagaraj, R.; Mitra, S. Classification of dental diseases using CNN and transfer learning. In Proceedings of the 5th International Symposium on Computational and Business Intelligence (ISCBI), Dubai, UAE, 11–14 August 2017; pp. 70–74.

25. Berdouses, E.D.; Koutsouri, G.D.; Tripoliti, E.E.; Matsopoulos, G.K.; Oulis, C.J.; Fotiadis, D.I. A computer-aided automated methodology for the detection and classification of occlusal caries from photographic color images. *Comput. Biol. Med.* **2015**, *62*, 119–135. [CrossRef]

26. Devito, K.L.; de Souza Barbosa, F.; Filho, W.N.F. An artificial multilayer perceptron neural network for diagnosis of proximal dental caries. *Oral Surg. Oral Med. Oral Pathol. Oral Radiol. Endodontol.* **2008**, *106*, 879–884. [CrossRef]

27. Kuang, W.; Ye, W. A Kernel-Modified SVM Based Computer-Aided Diagnosis System in Initial Caries. In Proceedings of the Second International Symposium on Intelligent Information Technology Application, Shanghai, China, 20–22 December 2008; pp. 207–211.

28. Bussaneli, D.G.; Boldieri, T.; Diniz, M.B.; Lima Rivera, L.M.; Santos-Pinto, L.; Cordeiro, R.D.C.L. Influence of professional experience on detection and treatment decision of occlusal caries lesions in primary teeth. *Int. J. Paediatr. Dent.* **2015**, *25*, 418–427. [CrossRef]

29. Burnham, K.P.; Anderson, D.R. *Model Selection and Multimodel Inference*; Burnham, K.P., Anderson, D.R., Eds.; Springer: New York, NY, USA, 2004; ISBN 978-0-387-95364-9.

30. Mutasa, S.; Sun, S.; Ha, R. Understanding artificial intelligence based radiology studies: What is overfitting? *Clin. Imaging* **2020**, *65*, 96–99. [CrossRef]

31. Shorten, C.; Khoshgoftaar, T.M. A survey on Image Data Augmentation for Deep Learning. *J. Big Data* **2019**, *6*, 60. [CrossRef]

32. Shokri, A.; Kasraei, S.; Lari, S.; Mahmoodzadeh, M.; Khaleghi, A.; Musavi, S.; Akheshteh, V. Efficacy of denoising and enhancement filters for detection of approximal and occlusal caries on digital intraoral radiographs. *J. Conserv. Dent.* **2018**, *21*, 162. [CrossRef]

33. Belém, M.D.F.; Ambrosano, G.M.B.; Tabchoury, C.P.M.; Ferreira-Santos, R.I.; Haiter-Neto, F. Performance of digital radiography with enhancement filters for the diagnosis of proximal caries. *Braz. Oral Res.* **2013**, *27*, 245–251. [CrossRef]

34. Kositbowornchai, S.; Basiw, M.; Promwang, Y.; Moragorn, H.; Sooksuntisakoonchai, N. Accuracy of diagnosing occlusal caries using enhanced digital images. *Dentomaxillofac. Radiol.* **2004**, *33*, 236–240. [CrossRef] [PubMed]

35. Bulman, J.S.; Osborn, J.F. Measuring diagnostic consistency. *Br. Dent. J.* **1989**, *166*, 377–381. [CrossRef]

Permissions

All chapters in this book were first published by MDPI; hereby published with permission under the Creative Commons Attribution License or equivalent. Every chapter published in this book has been scrutinized by our experts. Their significance has been extensively debated. The topics covered herein carry significant findings which will fuel the growth of the discipline. They may even be implemented as practical applications or may be referred to as a beginning point for another development.

The contributors of this book come from diverse backgrounds, making this book a truly international effort. This book will bring forth new frontiers with its revolutionizing research information and detailed analysis of the nascent developments around the world.

We would like to thank all the contributing authors for lending their expertise to make the book truly unique. They have played a crucial role in the development of this book. Without their invaluable contributions this book wouldn't have been possible. They have made vital efforts to compile up to date information on the varied aspects of this subject to make this book a valuable addition to the collection of many professionals and students.

This book was conceptualized with the vision of imparting up-to-date information and advanced data in this field. To ensure the same, a matchless editorial board was set up. Every individual on the board went through rigorous rounds of assessment to prove their worth. After which they invested a large part of their time researching and compiling the most relevant data for our readers.

The editorial board has been involved in producing this book since its inception. They have spent rigorous hours researching and exploring the diverse topics which have resulted in the successful publishing of this book. They have passed on their knowledge of decades through this book. To expedite this challenging task, the publisher supported the team at every step. A small team of assistant editors was also appointed to further simplify the editing procedure and attain best results for the readers.

Apart from the editorial board, the designing team has also invested a significant amount of their time in understanding the subject and creating the most relevant covers. They scrutinized every image to scout for the most suitable representation of the subject and create an appropriate cover for the book.

The publishing team has been an ardent support to the editorial, designing and production team. Their endless efforts to recruit the best for this project, has resulted in the accomplishment of this book. They are a veteran in the field of academics and their pool of knowledge is as vast as their experience in printing. Their expertise and guidance has proved useful at every step. Their uncompromising quality standards have made this book an exceptional effort. Their encouragement from time to time has been an inspiration for everyone.

The publisher and the editorial board hope that this book will prove to be a valuable piece of knowledge for researchers, students, practitioners and scholars across the globe.

List of Contributors

Dobrila Nesic, Yue Sun and Irena Sailer
Division of Fixed Prosthodontics and Biomaterials, University Clinic of Dental Medicine, University of Geneva, Rue Michel-Servet 1, CH-1211 Geneva 4, Switzerland

Birgit M. Schaefer
Geistlich Pharma AG, Bahnhofstrasse 40, CH-6110 Wolhusen, Switzerland

Nikola Saulacic
Department of Cranio-Maxillofacial Surgery, Inselspital, Bern University Hospital, University of Bern, Freiburgstrasse 10, CH-3010 Bern, Switzerland

Danilo Schneider and Constantinus Politis
OMFS IMPATH Research Group, Faculty of Medicine, Department of Imaging and Pathology, KU Leuven and Oral and Maxillofacial Surgery, University Hospitals Leuven, 3000 Leuven, Belgium

Ali Al-Rimawi
OMFS IMPATH Research Group, Faculty of Medicine, Department of Imaging and Pathology, KU Leuven and Oral and Maxillofacial Surgery, University Hospitals Leuven, 3000 Leuven, Belgium
Department of Dentistry, Royal Medical Services, Jordanian Armed Forces, 00962 Amman, Jordan

Mostafa EzEldeen
OMFS IMPATH Research Group, Faculty of Medicine, Department of Imaging and Pathology, KU Leuven and Oral and Maxillofacial Surgery, University Hospitals Leuven, 3000 Leuven, Belgium
Department of Oral Health Sciences, KU Leuven and Paediatric Dentistry and Special Dental Care, University Hospitals Leuven, 3000 Leuven, Belgium

Reinhilde Jacobs
OMFS IMPATH Research Group, Faculty of Medicine, Department of Imaging and Pathology, KU Leuven and Oral and Maxillofacial Surgery, University Hospitals Leuven, 3000 Leuven, Belgium
Department of Dental Medicine, Karolinska Institute, SE-171 77 Stockholm, Sweden

Yasaman Etemad-Shahidi, Omel Baneen Qallandar, Jessica Evenden, Frank Alifui-Segbaya and Khaled Elsayed Ahmed
School of Dentistry and Oral Health, Griffith University, Griffith Health Centre (G40), Office: 7.59, Brisbane, QLD 4215, Australia

Javier García Villalón and Carlos Ivorra
Asisa Dental, Research Department, C/José Abascal, 32, 28003 Madrid, Spain

María Prados-Privado
Asisa Dental, Research Department, C/José Abascal, 32, 28003 Madrid, Spain
Department of Signal Theory and Communications, Higher Polytechnic School, Universidad de Alcala de Henares, Ctra, Madrid-Barcelona, Km. 33,600, 28805 Alcala de Henares, Spain
IDIBO GROUP (Group of High-Performance Research, Development and Innovation in Dental Biomaterials of Rey Juan Carlos University), Avenida de Atenas s/n, 28922 Alcorcon, Spain

Carlos Hugo Martínez-Martínez
Faculty of Medicine, Universidad Complutense de Madrid, Plaza de Ramón y Cajal, s/n, 28040 Madrid, Spain

Juan Carlos Prados-Frutos
IDIBO GROUP (Group of High-Performance Research, Development and Innovation in Dental Biomaterials of Rey Juan Carlos University), Avenida de Atenas s/n, 28922 Alcorcon, Spain
Department of Medical Specialties and Public Health, Faculty of Health Sciences, Universidad Rey Juan Carlos, Avenida de Atenas, 28922 Alcorcon, Spain

Nadin Al-Haj Husain and Pedro Molinero-Mourelle
Department of Reconstructive Dentistry and Gerodontology, School of Dental Medicine, University of Bern, 3010 Bern, Switzerland

Mutlu Özcan
Division of Dental Biomaterials, Clinic for Reconstructive Dentistry, Center for Dental and Oral Medicine, University of Zurich, 8032 Zurich, Switzerland

Jens Fischer
Biomaterials and Technology, Department of Reconstructive Dentistry, University Center for Dental Medicine, University of Basel, 4058 Basel, Switzerland

Nadja Rohr
Biomaterials and Technology, Department of Reconstructive Dentistry, University Center for Dental Medicine, University of Basel, 4058 Basel, Switzerland
Department of Cell Biology, Rostock University Medical Center, 18057 Rostock, Germany

Claudia Bergemann and J Barbara Nebe
Department of Cell Biology, Rostock University Medical Center, 18057 Rostock, Germany

Katja Fricke
Leibniz Institute for Plasma Science and Technology e.V. (INP), 17489 Greifswald, Germany

Jeong-Hyeon Lee and Kyu-Bok Lee
Department of Prosthodontics, School of Dentistry, Kyungpook National University, 2177 Dalgubeol-daero, Jung-gu, Daegu 41940, Korea
Advanced Dental Device Development Institute (A3DI), Kyungpook National University, 2177 Dalgubeol-daero, Jung-gu, Daegu 41940, Korea

Keunbada Son
Advanced Dental Device Development Institute (A3DI), Kyungpook National University, 2177 Dalgubeol-daero, Jung-gu, Daegu 41940, Korea
Department of Dental Science, Graduate School, Kyungpook National University, 2177 Dalgubeol-daero, Jung-gu, Daegu 41940, Korea

Selina A. Bernauer, Nicola U. Zitzmann, Lea Matthisson and Tim Joda
Department of Reconstructive Dentistry, UZB University Center for Dental Medicine Basel, University of Basel, 4058 Basel, Switzerland

Johannes Müller
Private Practice, 80634 Munich, Germany

Maddalena Favaretto, David Shaw, Eva De Clercq and Bernice Simone Elger
Institute for Biomedical Ethics, University of Basel, 4056 Basel, Switzerland

Kuofeng Hung, Andy Wai Kan Yeung and Ray Tanaka
Oral and Maxillofacial Radiology, Applied Oral Sciences and Community Dental Care, Faculty of Dentistry, The University of Hong Kong, Hong Kong 999077, China

Sung Eun Choi
Department of Oral Health Policy and Epidemiology, Harvard School of Dental Medicine, Boston, MA 02115, USA

Michael M. Bornstein
Oral and Maxillofacial Radiology, Applied Oral Sciences and Community Dental Care, Faculty of Dentistry, The University of Hong Kong, Hong Kong 999077, China

Department of Oral Health & Medicine, University Center for Dental Medicine Basel UZB, University of Basel, 4058 Basel, Switzerland

Jane R. Barrow
Office of Global and Community Health, Harvard School of Dental Medicine, Boston, MA 02115, USA

Lisa Simon
Office of Global and Community Health, Harvard School of Dental Medicine, Boston, MA 02115, USA
Harvard Medical School, Boston, MA 02115, USA

Nathan Palmer
Department of Biomedical Informatics, Harvard Medical School, Boston, MA 02115, USA

Russell S. Phillips
Center for Primary Care, Harvard Medical School, Boston, MA 02115, USA

Sanjay Basu
Center for Primary Care, Harvard Medical School, Boston, MA 02115, USA
Research and Analytics, Collective Health, San Francisco, CA 94107, USA
School of Public Health, Imperial College London, London SW7 2BU, UK

Christian E. Besimo
Department of Reconstructive Dentistry, University Center for Dental Medicine Basel, University of Basel, 4058 Basel, Switzerland

Tuomas Waltimo
Department of Oral Health & Medicine, University Center for Dental Medicine Basel, University of Basel, 4058 Basel, Switzerland

Ronald E. Jung
Department of Reconstructive Dentistry, Center for Dental Medicine Basel, University of Zurich, 8032 Zurich, Switzerland

Marco Ferrari
Department of Prosthodontics & Dental Material, University School of Dental Medicine, University of Siena, 53100 Siena, Italy

Index

A
Acid Etching, 139, 143
Additive Manufacturing, 1-3, 6-7, 13-14, 22, 44, 46, 51, 58-60, 91, 132, 136
Artificial Intelligence, 131-133, 136-137, 150-151, 162, 189-190, 203-209, 215-219
Augmented Reality, 62-63, 136-137

B
Binder Jetting, 3, 45-46, 50
Biomaterials, 1-4, 7-8, 10-11, 13, 15-18, 105, 132, 136, 138-139, 148-149, 207
Biomedical Context, 150-151, 158
Bone Defects, 39, 190

C
Carious Lesions, 62, 80, 214, 216
Cell Spreading, 138-139, 141, 143, 146
Cell Viability, 138-139, 141, 143-144, 146
Cephalometric Radiographs, 190, 196
Ceramic Crown, 68, 70, 118, 124, 129, 165-169, 172-174
Computer Aided Manufacturing, 105
Computer-aided Design, 1-2, 4, 22, 32, 39, 58, 71, 105-107, 115, 132, 160, 166, 168, 181, 187, 197
Cone Beam Computed Tomography, 4, 16, 22-23, 29, 59, 157, 189-190, 204-205, 218
Continuous Liquid Interface Production, 45-46, 50
Conventional Method, 165-166, 171-173, 186

D
Dental Education, 62-65, 71-72, 74, 78-84, 102, 132-133, 136, 155, 162-163, 187
Dental Materials, 32, 40, 85
Dental Medicine, 1, 22, 62-63, 80, 85, 92, 105, 131-133, 135-136, 138, 150-151, 158, 162, 176, 179, 181, 187, 189, 196-197, 203, 205
Dental Models, 1, 29, 44-45, 53, 55, 57-60, 85-87, 89-91, 132, 136
Dental Practitioners, 95-97, 101, 157, 159, 189, 197, 203
Dental Research, 48, 79, 90, 92, 131-132, 134-136, 158, 161, 180, 189
Dentistry, 1-4, 6, 10, 12, 15-16, 20, 22-23, 29-30, 32-36, 38-42, 44, 55, 58-59, 62-66, 72, 103, 105, 125, 131-138, 147, 149-153, 155-163, 165, 174, 176-181, 187, 197, 204, 206-208, 212, 218
Diagnose Caries, 207, 217
Diagnostic Accuracy, 47, 58, 76, 190, 195-196, 201
Diagnostic Images, 189-190, 203
Digital Dentistry, 62, 78, 90, 131, 135, 150-151, 157, 160-161, 181
Digital Light Processing, 3, 14, 22-23, 44-46, 50, 53, 60

Digital Smile Design, 32-42
Digital Transformation, 79, 131-132, 135, 176, 179
Digital Workflow, 1, 4, 7, 10-11, 30, 32, 38-39, 42, 58, 60, 63, 80-81, 84-86, 90, 165, 172, 187, 196-197

E
Electronic Health Records, 93, 95, 134, 150, 153, 155, 163
Endosseous Surface, 138-139, 144
Ethical Issues, 150-153, 155, 157-163

F
Facial Scanning, 189-190, 197, 199
Feldspathic Ceramic, 110, 123, 126
Fixed Prosthodontics, 1, 30, 80, 90, 181-182, 185, 187
Full-arch, 44, 47, 53-54, 85-87, 89-90, 174, 237
Fused Filament Fabrication, 45-46, 50

G
Gene Expression, 138-139, 142, 145-147
Gingiva, 1, 7-8, 10-11, 19-21, 33, 75, 181, 185, 197

H
Human Osteoblasts, 138-139, 146-147
Hybrid Polymer, 105-106, 124-126

I
Implant Prosthodontics, 91, 136, 187
Implant Scanbodies, 220
Inclusion Criteria, 34, 37, 46-47, 51, 108, 209-210
Integrated Care, 92-93, 97, 100-101
Internet And Communication Technologies, 150
Internet Of Things, 131, 150, 163
Intraoral Optical Scanning, 62, 71, 181
Intraoral Scanner, 23, 50, 58-60, 85, 90, 165-167, 170-174, 188

L
Liquid Photopolymer, 45

M
Machine Learning, 131-133, 136-137, 189-191, 195-196, 199, 203-205, 207-208, 213, 218
Marginal And Internal Fit, 165-166, 168-174
Material Jetting, 3, 45-46, 50, 53
Medical-dental Integration, 92, 98-99, 101-102
Meshes, 18, 148
Meta-analysis, 18, 30, 54, 57, 78, 105-106, 108-111, 124-126, 128, 130, 147, 161-162, 175, 218
Microsimulation Model, 92-93

O

Oral Health, 11, 22, 29-30, 42, 44, 80, 90, 92-93, 101-103, 105, 128, 131, 136, 147, 150-152, 156-158, 160-162, 176-177, 179, 187, 189

Oral Healthcare, 131-132, 137, 151, 158, 160, 164, 176, 179, 204

Oral Rehabilitation, 39, 78

Oral Soft Tissues, 1

Orthodontic And Orthognathic Treatment Planning, 189, 191, 196

Orthodontics, 4, 10, 15, 23, 36-37, 39, 44, 50-51, 55, 64, 83, 163, 197, 205

P

Patient-centered Outcomes, 90, 131-132, 135, 176

Personalized Dental Medicine, 131, 162, 203

Plasma-polymerized Allylamine, 138-140, 142, 148

Prosthetic Rehabilitation, 32, 38-40

Prosthetic Treatment, 38

Prosthodontic Workflow, 44, 55

Prosthodontics, 1, 4, 12, 29-30, 37, 40, 42, 44, 55, 80, 85, 90-91, 131, 136, 150, 165, 181-182, 185, 187

R

Rapid Prototyping, 16, 29, 46, 59-60, 75, 83, 85-86, 91, 107, 131-132

Restorative Dentistry, 32, 34-36, 38-39, 41

S

Sandblasting, 138, 143, 146

Scientific Misconduct, 150, 158-159, 161, 163

Stereolithography, 2-3, 13, 23, 44-46, 50, 53, 58, 60

Systematic Review, 18, 20, 30, 44-45, 48, 55, 58, 61-63, 78, 80, 90, 105-106, 108-109, 124-125, 127-130, 136-137, 147, 150-151, 160-162, 164, 172, 175, 180, 187, 203-204, 207, 216-218

T

Tele-healthcare, 131, 134-135

Tissue Engineering, 1, 4, 10, 13-15, 17, 20, 149

Titanium Implants, 17, 138, 148

Tooth Autotransplantation, 22-23, 29

Tooth Preparation, 64, 66-67, 81, 86, 106, 112, 133, 181-182, 188

Treatment Outcomes, 10, 73, 83, 105, 159, 189

Treatment Planning, 5, 32, 38, 42, 44, 63, 65, 76, 100, 151, 189-191, 196-197, 199

V

Virtual Reality, 5, 15, 62-63, 66, 71-72, 80, 82-83, 131-133, 136

Z

Zirconia Implant, 14, 138, 144, 147, 149

Printed in the USA
CPSIA information can be obtained
at www.ICGtesting.com
JSHW051356091023
49903JS00006B/171

9 781639 276608